Practice-Based Nutrition Care

Editors

SCOTT KAHAN
ROBERT F. KUSHNER

MEDICAL CLINICS OF NORTH AMERICA

www.medical.theclinics.com

Consulting Editors
DOUGLAS S. PAAUW
EDWARD R. BOLLARD

November 2016 • Volume 100 • Number 6

ELSEVIER

1600 John F. Kennedy Boulevard • Suite 1800 • Philadelphia, Pennsylvania, 19103-2899

http://www.theclinics.com

MEDICAL CLINICS OF NORTH AMERICA Volume 100, Number 6
November 2016 ISSN 0025-7125, ISBN-13: 978-0-323-47688-1

Editor: Jessica McCool
Developmental Editor: Alison Swety

Medical Clinics of North America (ISSN 0025-7125) is published bimonthly by Elsevier Inc., 360 Park Avenue South, New York, NY 10010-1710. Months of publication are January, March, May, July, September, and November. Business and editorial offices: 1600 John F. Kennedy Boulevard, Suite 1800, Philadelphia, PA 19103-2899. Periodicals postage paid at New York, NY, and additional mailing offices. Subscription prices are USD $260.00 per year (US individuals), $531.00 per year (US institutions), $100.00 per year (US Students), $320.00 per year (Canadian individuals), $690.00 per year (Canadian institutions), $200.00 per year (Canadian and foreign students), $390.00 per year (foreign individuals), and $690.00 per year (foreign institutions). To receive student/resident rate, orders must be accompanied by name of affiliated institution, date of term, and the signature of program/residency coordinator on institution letterhead. Orders will be billed at individual rate until proof of status is received. Foreign air speed delivery is included in all Clinics' subscription prices. All prices are subject to change without notice. **POSTMASTER:** Send address changes to *Medical Clinics of North America*, Elsevier Health Sciences Division, Subscription Customer Service, 3251 Riverport Lane, Maryland Heights, MO 63043. **Customer Service: Telephone: 1-800-654-2452** (U.S. and Canada); **1-314-447-8871** (outside U.S. and Canada). **Fax: 314-447-8029. E-mail: journalscustomerserviceusa@elsevier.com** (for print support); **journalsonlinesupport-usa@elsevier.com** (for online support).

Reprints. For copies of 100 or more of articles in this publication, please contact the Commercial Reprints Department, Elsevier Inc., 360 Park Avenue South, New York, NY 10010-1710. Tel.: 212-633-3874; Fax: 212-633-3820; E-mail: reprints@elsevier.com.

Medical Clinics of North America is also published in Spanish by McGraw-Hill Interamericana Editores S. A., P.O. Box 5-237, 06500 Mexico, D.F., Mexico.

Medical Clinics of North America is covered in *MEDLINE/PubMed (Index Medicus), Current Contents, ASCA, Excerpta Medica, Science Citation Index,* and *ISI/BIOMED.*

PROGRAM OBJECTIVE
The goal of the *Medical Clinics of North America* is to keep practicing physicians up to date with current clinical practice by providing timely articles reviewing the state of the art in patient care.

TARGET AUDIENCE
All practicing physicians and other healthcare professionals.

LEARNING OBJECTIVES
Upon completion of this activity, participants will be able to:
1. Review the principles of nutrition assessment in primary care.
2. Discuss nutrition recommendations in children, adolescents, adults, and elderly populations.
3. Recognize nutrition guidelines for chronic conditions such as kidney disease, liver disease, and cancers, among others.

ACCREDITATION
The Elsevier Office of Continuing Medical Education (EOCME) is accredited by the Accreditation Council for Continuing Medical Education (ACCME) to provide continuing medical education for physicians.

The EOCME designates this enduring material for a maximum of 15 *AMA PRA Category 1 Credit*(s)™. Physicians should claim only the credit commensurate with the extent of their participation in the activity.

All other health care professionals requesting continuing education credit for this enduring material will be issued a certificate of participation.

DISCLOSURE OF CONFLICTS OF INTEREST
The EOCME assesses conflict of interest with its instructors, faculty, planners, and other individuals who are in a position to control the content of CME activities. All relevant conflicts of interest that are identified are thoroughly vetted by EOCME for fair balance, scientific objectivity, and patient care recommendations. EOCME is committed to providing its learners with CME activities that promote improvements or quality in healthcare and not a specific proprietary business or a commercial interest.

The planning committee, staff, authors and editors listed below have identified no financial relationships or relationships to products or devices they or their spouse/life partner have with commercial interest related to the content of this CME activity:
Cheryl A.M. Anderson, PhD, MPH, MS; Jamy D. Ard, MD; Hope Barkoukis, PhD, RDN, LD; Edward R. Bollard, MD, DDS, FACP; Mark R. Corkins, MD, CNSC, SPR, FAAP; Stephen R. Daniels, MD, PhD; Janet M. de Jesus, MS, RD; Robert H. Eckel, MD; Anjali Fortna; Neville H. Golden, MD; David Heber, MD, PhD; Ryan T. Hurt, MD, PhD; Scott Kahan, MD, MPH; Ruth W. Kimokoti, MD, MA, MPH; Michelle A. Kominiarek, MD, MS; Robert F. Kushner, MD; Michelle Lai, MD, MPH; Zhaoping Li, MD, PhD; Sheela N. Magge, MD, MSCE; Stephen A. McClave, MD; Jessica McCool; Jeffrey I. Mechanick, MD, FACP, FACE, FACN; Gary Miller, PhD; Premkumar Nandhakumar; Hoang Anh Nguyen, MD, MPH; Carolina Frade Magalhaes Girardin Pimentel, MD, PhD; Priya Rajan, MD; Dena E. Rifkin, MD, MS; Sarah Jane Schwarzenberg, MD; Megan Suermann; Michael A. Via, MD.

The planning committee, staff, authors and editors listed below have identified financial relationships or relationships to products or devices they or their spouse/life partner have with commercial interest related to the content of this CME activity:
Sarah D. de Ferranti, MD, MPH receives royalties/patents from UpToDate, Inc.
Jae H. Kim, MD, PhD is on the speakers' bureau for Abbott; Medela; Nestlé Health Science; Mead Johnson & Company, LLC; and Nutricia Advanced Medical Nutrition, is a consultant/advisor for Medela, and has stock ownership in PediaSolutions.
Barbara E. Millen, DrPH, RD, FADA has stock ownership in, and an employment affiliation with, Millennium Prevention, Inc and Boston Nutrition Foundation Inc.

UNAPPROVED/OFF-LABEL USE DISCLOSURE
The EOCME requires CME faculty to disclose to the participants:
1. When products or procedures being discussed are off-label, unlabelled, experimental, and/or investigational (not US Food and Drug Administration [FDA] approved); and
2. Any limitations on the information presented, such as data that are preliminary or that represent ongoing research, interim analyses, and/or unsupported opinions. Faculty may discuss information about pharmaceutical agents that is outside of FDA-approved labelling. This information is intended solely for CME

and is not intended to promote off-label use of these medications. If you have any questions, contact the medical affairs department of the manufacturer for the most recent prescribing information.

TO ENROLL

To enroll in the *Medical Clinics of North America* Continuing Medical Education program, call customer service at 1-800-654-2452 or sign up online at http://www.theclinics.com/home/cme. The CME program is available to subscribers for an additional annual fee of USD $295.

METHOD OF PARTICIPATION

In order to claim credit, participants must complete the following:

1. Complete enrolment as indicated above.
2. Read the activity.
3. Complete the CME Test and Evaluation. Participants must achieve a score of 70% on the test. All CME Tests and Evaluations must be completed online.

CME INQUIRIES/SPECIAL NEEDS

For all CME inquiries or special needs, please contact elsevierCME@elsevier.com.

MEDICAL CLINICS OF NORTH AMERICA

THE CLINICS ARE AVAILABLE ONLINE!
Access your subscription at:
www.theclinics.com

Contributors

CONSULTING EDITORS

DOUGLAS S. PAAUW, MD, MACP
Professor of Medicine, Division of General Internal Medicine, Rathmann Family Foundation Endowed Chair for Patient-Centered Clinical Education; Medicine Student Programs, Professor of Medicine, University of Washington School of Medicine, Seattle, Washington

EDWARD R. BOLLARD, MD, DDS, FACP
Professor of Medicine, Associate Dean of Graduate Medical Education, Designated Institutional Official, Department of Medicine, Penn State–Hershey Medical Center, Penn State University College of Medicine, Hershey, Pennsylvania

EDITORS

SCOTT KAHAN, MD, MPH
Johns Hopkins Bloomberg School of Public Health; Director, National Center for Weight and Wellness; Medical Director, Strategies To Overcome and Prevent (STOP) Obesity Alliance; Professorial Lecturer, Milken Institute School of Public Health, George Washington University, Washington, DC

ROBERT F. KUSHNER, MD
Professor of Medicine, Northwestern Comprehensive Center on Obesity, Northwestern University Feinberg School of Medicine, Chicago, Illinois

AUTHORS

CHERYL A.M. ANDERSON, PhD, MPH, MS
Associate Professor of Preventive Medicine, Department of Family Medicine and Public Health, UC San Diego School of Medicine, La Jolla, California

JAMY D. ARD, MD
Professor, Department of Epidemiology and Prevention, Wake Forest School of Medicine, Winston Salem, North Carolina

HOPE BARKOUKIS, PhD, RDN, LD
Interim Chair, Associate Professor, Department of Nutrition, School of Medicine, Case Western Reserve University, Cleveland, Ohio

MARK R. CORKINS, MD, CNSC, SPR, FAAP
Division Chief, Pediatric Gastroenterology, Professor of Pediatrics, University of Tennessee Health Sciences Center, Memphis, Tennessee

STEPHEN R. DANIELS, MD, PhD
Professor and Chair, Department of Pediatrics, Pediatrician-in-Chief and L. Joseph Butterfield Chair in Pediatrics, Children's Hospital Colorado, University of Colorado School of Medicine, Aurora, Colorado

SARAH D. DE FERRANTI, MD, MPH
Director, Preventive Cardiology Clinic, Department of Cardiology, Children's Hospital Boston, Assistant Professor of Pediatrics, Harvard University Medical School, Boston, Massachusetts

JANET M. DE JESUS, MS, RD
Public Health Advisor, Center for Translation Research and Implementation Science (CTRIS), National Heart, Lung, and Blood Institute, National Institutes of Health, Bethesda, Maryland

ROBERT H. ECKEL, MD
Professor of Medicine, Divisions of Endocrinology, Metabolism, and Diabetes; Cardiology, University of Colorado Denver Anschutz Medical Campus, Aurora, Colorado

NEVILLE H. GOLDEN, MD
Chief, Division of Adolescent Medicine, Department of Pediatrics, Lucile Packard Children's Hospital Stanford, Stanford University School of Medicine, Palo Alto, California

DAVID HEBER, MD, PhD
Center for Human Nutrition, David Geffen School of Medicine at UCLA, Los Angeles, California

RYAN T. HURT, MD, PhD
Divisions of General Internal Medicine, Gastroenterology and Hepatology, Associate Professor of Medicine, Mayo Clinic, Rochester, Minnesota; Assistant Clinical Professor of Medicine, Division of Gastroenterology, Hepatology and Nutrition, University of Louisville, Louisville, Kentucky

SCOTT KAHAN, MD, MPH
Johns Hopkins Bloomberg School of Public Health; Director, National Center for Weight and Wellness; Medical Director, Strategies To Overcome and Prevent (STOP) Obesity Alliance; Professorial Lecturer, Milken Institute School of Public Health, George Washington University, Washington, DC

JAE H. KIM, MD, PhD
Professor of Clinical Pediatrics, Program Director, Neonatal-Perinatal Medicine Fellowship, Nutrition Director, Supporting Premature Infant Nutrition Program, Rady Children's Hospital of San Diego, University of California San Diego Health, San Diego, California

RUTH W. KIMOKOTI, MD, MA, MPH
Research Assistant Professor, Department of Nutrition, Simmons College, Boston, Massachusetts

MICHELLE A. KOMINIAREK, MD, MS
Division of Maternal-Fetal Medicine, Associate Professor, Department of Obstetrics and Gynecology, Northwestern University Feinberg School of Medicine, Chicago, Illinois

ROBERT F. KUSHNER, MD
Professor of Medicine, Northwestern Comprehensive Center on Obesity, Northwestern University Feinberg School of Medicine, Chicago, Illinois

MICHELLE LAI, MD, MPH
Gastroenterology, Liver Center, Beth Israel Deaconess Medical Center, Harvard University, Boston, Massachusetts

ZHAOPING LI, MD, PhD
Center for Human Nutrition, David Geffen School of Medicine at UCLA, Los Angeles, California

SHEELA N. MAGGE, MD, MSCE
Division of Endocrinology and Diabetes, Director of Research, Center for Translational Science, Director, Patient and Clinical Interactions (formerly CRC), CTSI, Children's National Health System, Associate Professor of Pediatrics, The George Washington University School of Medicine and Health Sciences, Washington, DC

STEPHEN A. McCLAVE, MD
Division of Gastroenterology, Hepatology and Nutrition, Professor of Medicine, University of Louisville School of Medicine, Louisville, Kentucky

JEFFREY I. MECHANICK, MD, FACP, FACE, FACN
Clinical Professor of Medicine; Director, Metabolic Support, Division of Endocrinology, Diabetes and Bone Disease, Icahn School of Medicine at Mount Sinai, New York, New York

BARBARA E. MILLEN, DrPH, RD, FADA
Millennium Prevention, Inc, Westwood, Massachusetts

GARY MILLER, PhD
Associate Professor, Department of Health and Exercise Science, Wake Forest University, Winston Salem, North Carolina

HOANG ANH NGUYEN, MD, MPH
Nephrology Fellow, Department of Nephrology and Hypertension, UCSD Medical Center, San Diego, California

CAROLINA FRADE MAGALHAES GIRARDIN PIMENTEL, MD, PhD
Gastroenterology, Liver Center, Beth Israel Deaconess Medical Center, Harvard University, Boston, Massachusetts

PRIYA RAJAN, MD
Division of Maternal-Fetal Medicine, Assistant Professor, Department of Obstetrics and Gynecology, Northwestern University Feinberg School of Medicine, Chicago, Illinois

DENA E. RIFKIN, MD, MS
Associate Professor of Nephrology, Department of Nephrology and Hypertension, VA San Diego Healthcare System, San Diego, California

SARAH JANE SCHWARZENBERG, MD
Director, Pediatric Gastroenterology, Hepatology and Nutrition, Executive Medical Director, Masonic Children's Hospital, University of Minnesota, Minneapolis, Minnesota

MICHAEL A. VIA, MD
Assistant Professor of Medicine; Associate Fellowship Director, Division of Endocrinology and Metabolism, Mount Sinai Beth Israel Medical Center, Icahn School of Medicine at Mount Sinai, New York, New York

Contents

> Provision of dietary counseling in the office setting is enhanced by using team-based care and electronic tools. Effective provider-patient communication is essential for fostering behavior change: the key component of lifestyle medicine. The principles of communication and behavior change are skill-based and grounded in scientific theories and models. Motivational interviewing and shared decision making, a collaboration process between patients and their providers to reach agreement about a health decision, is an important process in counseling. The stages of change, self-determination, health belief model, social cognitive model, theory of planned behavior, and cognitive behavioral therapy are used in the counseling process.

> Alterations in nutritional status are common and can be associated with increased morbidity and mortality. However, for healthcare providers, the definition of malnutrition is vague, insensitive, and poorly standardized. In contrast, nutrition risk is more easily defined, and recognizes that both poor nutritional status and disease severity contribute to increased morbidity and mortality. Clinicians need to identify patients who may already have evidence of nutrient deficiencies or have disease processes that affect nutrition risk. This article reviews risk assessment tools and provides practical tips to screen patients and identify those whose nutrition risk warrants specialized nutrition therapy.

> Chronic non-communicable diseases (NCDs) are the leading causes of morbidity and mortality in the United States and globally, and are attributable largely to poor nutrition and suboptimal lifestyle behaviors. The 2015–2020 *Dietary Guidelines for Americans* promote healthy eating and lifestyle patterns across the lifespan to reduce risk of NCDs. Physicians are well positioned to provide lifestyle preventive interventions that are personalized to their patients' biological needs and cultural preferences through multidisciplinary team activities or referral to professional nutrition and

Cheryl A.M. Anderson, Hoang Anh Nguyen, and Dena E. Rifkin

Dietary modification is recommended in the management of chronic kidney disease (CKD). Individuals with CKD often have multiple comorbidities, such as high blood pressure, diabetes, obesity, and cardiovascular disease, for which dietary modification is also recommended. As CKD progresses, nutrition plays an important role in mitigating risk for cardiovascular disease and decline in kidney function. The objectives of nutrition interventions in CKD include management of risk factors, ensuring optimal nutritional status throughout all stages of CKD, preventing buildup of toxic metabolic products, and avoiding complications of CKD. Recommended dietary changes should be feasible, sustainable, and suited for patients' food preferences and clinical needs.

Michael A. Via and Jeffrey I. Mechanick

For individuals at risk for type 2 diabetes mellitus or the metabolic syndrome, adherence to an idealized dietary pattern can drastically alter the risk and course of these chronic conditions. Target levels of carbohydrate intake should approximate 30% of consumed calories. Healthy food choices should include copious fruits, vegetables, and nuts while minimizing foods with high glycemic indices, especially processed foods.

Carolina Frade Magalhaes Girardin Pimentel and Michelle Lai

The progressively increasing rates of obesity have led to a worldwide epidemic of nonalcoholic fatty liver disease (NAFLD), the hepatic manifestation of the metabolic syndrome. It is currently the most common cause of liver disease worldwide and projected to be the leading indication for liver transplantation in the United States by 2020. NAFLD is associated with both liver-related and overall mortality. Undoubtedly, nutrition interventions are key in the treatment of NAFLD, to reverse the disease, and prevent disease progression, complications, and associated comorbidities, including cardiovascular disease and diabetes.

David Heber and Zhaoping Li

Malnutrition in advanced cancer patients continues to be a vexing problem that contributes to morbidity and mortality. Nutrition interventions have traditionally been used to support patients with malnutrition secondary to cancer and cancer treatments. More recently it has been utilized in the primary and secondary prevention of common forms of cancer in patients undergoing cancer treatment and in cancer survivors respectively. During the emotional stress of dealing with cancer at any stage, patients derive increased quality of life and a sense of control over their lives as the result of receiving supportive advice on diet and lifestyle.

Obesity is a common disorder with complex causes. The epidemic has spurred significant advances in the understanding of nutritional approaches to treating obesity. Although the primary challenge is to introduce a dietary intake that creates an energy deficit, clinicians should also consider targeted risk factor modification with manipulation of the nutrient profile of the weight-reducing diet. These strategies produce significant weight loss and improvements in cardiometabolic risk factors. Future research is needed to better understand how to personalize nutrient prescriptions further to promote optimal risk modification and maintenance of long-term energy balance in the weight-reduced state.

Foreword
Practice-Based Nutrition Care

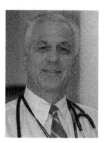

Edward R. Bollard, MD, DDS, FACP
Consulting Editor

It is rare that a patient seen in a primary care office today for any chronic illness does not have as a part of their care plan some type of nutritional recommendation or counseling. Yet, how often are we able to provide the appropriate amount of time and/or expertise necessary to truly educate and engage our patients to understand as well as engage in dietary changes that will impact their health?

Our patients are exposed to information related to the size of their soft drinks in order to limit the amount of simple carbohydrates they consume, removal of "trans fats" from the products they purchase because they are "bad," and recommendations to consider an increase in their daily intake of antioxidants in order to protect against free radical damage. But, do they truly understand the impact this will have on their diabetes management, secondary prevention for their coronary artery disease, or potential reduction in their risk of certain malignancies? Likely not.

In this issue of *Medical Clinics of North America*, Drs Kahan and Kushner lead an impressive list of authors who provide evidence-based medicine to enhance our knowledge of nutrition as it pertains to various medical conditions in our patients. More importantly, however, they provide what they have titled a "practice-based" approach that takes it beyond the nutritional sciences to the practical application that one can incorporate in the busy clinical setting.

Med Clin N Am 100 (2016) xv–xvi
http://dx.doi.org/10.1016/j.mcna.2016.09.002
0025-7125/16/© 2016 Published by Elsevier Inc.

medical.theclinics.com

So, grab a bag of chips and pretzels—I mean walnuts and raisins—and take advantage of this exceptional collection of articles directed at "Practice-Based Nutrition Care."

Edward R. Bollard, MD, DDS, FACP
Department of Medicine
Penn State–Hershey Medical Center
Penn State University College of Medicine
500 University Drive
PO Box 850 (Mail Code H039)
Hershey, PA 17033-0850, USA

E-mail address:
ebollard@hmc.psu.edu

Preface

Nutrition in Clinical Medicine: A Core Competency for Healthcare Providers

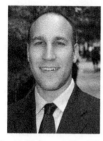 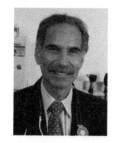

Scott Kahan, MD, MPH   Robert F. Kushner, MD

Editors

Health is influenced by five general determinants: genetics, social circumstances, environmental exposures, medical care, and behavioral patterns. The single greatest opportunity to improve health and function, reduce disability and premature deaths, and increase quality of life is by improving health behaviors, which account for nearly 50% of all deaths in the United States.[1] Health behaviors play a central role in the risk for, development of, and treatment and management of the most common causes of disease, disability, and death in the modern world. In one landmark study, those with the poorest of four key health behaviors (tobacco use, alcohol use, fruit and vegetable intake, and physical activity) had more than four times higher risk of death over a decade, compared with those exhibiting the most healthful of these behaviors; this resulted in a chronological difference of 14 years in life expectancy![2] Incredibly, fewer than 1% of 20,244 adults included in the study regularly achieved all four of these behaviors; 70% achieved none or just one.

While behavioral patterns drive much of the development and propagation of chronic diseases, poor nutrition is a particularly integral driver of morbidity and mortality in the United States and throughout the world. The most common scourges of modern society are nutrition-related, including cardiovascular disease, diabetes, renal disease, liver disease, and many cancers.[3] Poor diet may be the primary "cause of the cause," underlying much of what ails us, and on par with tobacco smoking as the most common actual causes of death in the United States and beyond.[4] As an example, increasing dietary intake of trans fats by just 2%—about a teaspoon a day—doubles the risk for coronary artery disease.[5]

The nineteenth century has been called the "Century of Hygiene," due to vast improvements in understanding of microbes and prevention of infectious disease, leading to an "epidemiologic transition," in which mortality related to acute and infectious

Med Clin N Am 100 (2016) xvii–xx
http://dx.doi.org/10.1016/j.mcna.2016.09.001
0025-7125/16/© 2016 Published by Elsevier Inc.

diseases began to wane and chronic disease burden began to increase. The twentieth century has been called the "Century of Medicine," due to the vast improvements in clinical care and medical treatment options, which led to substantial declines in premature mortality associated with chronic diseases, such as cardiovascular disease. However, the "nutrition transition"—rapid shifts in diet as societies develop toward increased processed foods, refined grains, outside-of-home intake, greater use of edible oils and added sugars—has led to an epidemic increase in chronic and nutrition-related health conditions. We are now in the midst of a "Century of Behavior Change," in which diseases related to preventable behaviors represent the largest healthcare burden.[6] But where there is crisis, there is also opportunity. Preventable, nutrition-related health conditions are just that: preventable.

Relatively moderate interventions—at both broad community and societal levels, as well as individual levels—can reap large rewards. Primary prevention interventions, such as iodination of salt and folate fortification of cereal grain products, which combined have prevented countless cases of mental retardation and neural tube defects, respectively, have also prevented numerous deaths.[7,8] Bans on trans fats have similar potential for public health benefit.[9] Clinical nutrition interventions can be similarly impressive, albeit on a different scale. The Diabetes Prevention Program (DPP) showed a moderate diet and lifestyle intervention led to 58% decreased development of diabetes, compared with placebo, and community adaptation of DPP provided in YMCA and similar group settings has been nearly as effective.[10,11] The PREDIMED study showed a Mediterranean diet intervention lowered cardiovascular events by 30%, compared with a basic control diet.[12]

Continued progress on primary prevention and policy to improve nutrition environments is important, but it will also be essential to equip clinicians with the knowledge and know-how to counsel and support patients to improve diet and lifestyle behaviors. In preparing this article, we referred back to the first issue of *Medical Clinics of North America* that focused on nutrition—published in 1993—which stated on the opening page: "...teaching of Clinical Nutrition is still lacking from many medical school curricula and, when studied, it is often in a fragmented form...." Unfortunately, we haven't made much progress in the intervening quarter century. Nutrition is covered inadequately or unevenly at all levels of medical training, including undergraduate, postgraduate, fellowship, licensing, board certification, and continuing education.[13–15] Few medical schools reach the 30 hours of nutrition education recommended by the National Academy of Sciences.[16] Worse, nutrition education appears to be on the decline: The percentage of medical schools offering a dedicated nutrition course declined from 35% in 2000 to 25% in 2008, and the average hours devoted to nutrition in US medical schools declined from 22.3 hours in 2004 to 19.6 hours in 2008-2009.[17] Less than one in four physicians feel they received adequate training in nutrition and lifestyle counseling.[18] Less than one in eight medical visits include counseling for nutrition.[19] Just 4% of medical visits are related to obesity, despite the nearly 40% obesity prevalence in the United States.[20]

Nutrition and health behavior change must become a core competency for anyone working with patients with chronic diseases in clinical medicine, which is virtually everyone. In deciding which articles to include in the issue, we purposely sought to identify topics that represent a wide spectrum of conditions or states in which diet and nutrition have a vital role. Similarly, we chose authors that are experts in their respective fields. As few of us have had the opportunity to engage in formal nutrition education during medical training, we hope this issue of *Medical Clinics of North America* focused on practice-based nutrition will be a valuable resource for clinicians.

Scott Kahan, MD, MPH
Johns Hopkins Bloomberg School of Public Health
National Center for Weight and Wellness
Strategies To Overcome and Prevent (STOP)
Obesity Alliance
1020 19th Street NW, Suite 450
Washington, DC 20036, USA

Robert F. Kushner, MD
Northwestern University
Feinberg School of Medicine
750 North Lake Shore Drive, Rubloff 9-976
Chicago, IL 60611, USA

E-mail addresses:
kahan@gwu.edu (S. Kahan)
rkushner@northwestern.edu
Website: http://www.drrobertkushner.com (R.F. Kushner)

REFERENCES

1. Schroeder SA. We can do better—improving the health of the American people. New Engl J Med 2007;357:1221–8.
2. Khaw KT, Wareham N, Bingham S, et al. Combined impact of health behaviours and mortality in men and women: the EPIC-Norfolk prospective population study. PLoS Med 2008;5(1):e12, 39–46.
3. Minino AM, Arias E, Kochanek KD, et al. Deaths: final data for 2000. Natl Vital Stat Rep 2002;50(15):1–120.
4. Mokdad AH, Marks JS, Stroup DF, et al. Actual causes of death in the United States, 2000. JAMA 2004;291(10):1238–46.
5. Hu FB, Stampfer MJ, Manson JA, et al. Dietary fat intake and the risk of coronary heart disease in women. New Engl J Med 1997;337(21):1491–9.
6. Kahan S, Fagan P, Gielen A. Health behavior change in populations. Baltimore (MD): Johns Hopkins University Press; 2015.
7. Available at: http://www.unicef.org/publications/files/Sustainable_Elimination_of_Iodine_Deficiency.pdf.
8. Available at: http://www.cdc.gov/ncbddd/folicacid/global.html.
9. Angell SY, Cobb LK, Curtis CJ, et al. Change in trans fatty acid content of fast-food purchases associated with New York City's restaurant regulation: a pre-post study. Ann Intern Med 2012;157(2):81–6.
10. Knowler WC, Barrett-Connor E, Fowler SE, et al. Reduction in the incidence of type 2 diabetes with lifestyle intervention or metformin. New Engl J Med 2002; 346:393–403.
11. Ackermann RT, Finch EA, Brizendine E, et al. Translating the Diabetes Prevention Program into the community. Am J Prev Med 2008;35(4):357–63.
12. Estruch R, Ros E, Salas-Salvado J, et al. Primary prevention of cardiovascular disease with a Mediterranean diet. New Engl J Med 2013;368:1279–90.
13. Adams KM, Kohlmeier M, Zeisel SH. Nutrition education in U.S. medical schools: latest update of a national survey. Acad Med 2013;85(9):1537–42.
14. Kushner RF, Butsch WS, Kahan S, et al. Obesity coverage on medical licensing examinations in the United States. What is being tested? Oral presentation at The Obesity Society National Meeting. Los Angeles, November, 2015.

15. Hark LA, Iwamoto C, Melnick DE, et al. Nutrition coverage on medical licensing examinations in the United States. Am J Clin Nutr 1997;65:568–71.
16. National Research Council. Nutrition Education in U.S. Medical Schools. Washington, DC: The National Academies Press; 1985.
17. Adams KM, Kohlmeier M, Zeisel SH. Nutrition education in U.S. medical schools: latest update of a national survey. Acad Med 2010;85(9):1537–42.
18. Howe M, Leidel A, Krishnan SM, et al. Patient-related diet and exercise counseling: do providers' own lifestyle habits matter? Prevent Cardiol 2010;12(4): 180–5.
19. Healthy People 2020. Washington, DC: U.S. Department of Health and Human Services, Office of Disease Prevention and Health Promotion. Available at: http://www.healthypeople.gov/2020/Data/SearchResult.aspx?topicid=29&topic= Nutrition%20and%20Weight%20Status&objective=NWS-6.3&anchor=152176.
20. Talwalkar A, McCarty F. Characteristics of physician office visits for obesity by adults aged 20 and over: United States, 2012. NCHS Data Brief 2016;237:1–8.

Providing Nutritional Care in the Office Practice

Teams, Tools, and Techniques

Robert F. Kushner, MD

KEYWORDS

- Communication • Behavior change • Counseling • Motivational interviewing
- Shared decision making

KEY POINTS

- Provision of dietary counseling in the office setting will be enhanced by using team-based care and electronic tools.
- Effective provider-patient communication is essential for fostering behavior change: the key component of lifestyle medicine.
- The principles of communication and behavior change are skill-based and grounded in scientific theories and models.
- Motivational interviewing and shared decision making, a collaboration process between patients and their providers to reach agreement about a health decision, is an important process in counseling.
- The 5 A's also can be used as an organizational construct for the clinical encounter.
- The behavioral principle stages of change, self-determination, health belief model, social cognitive model, theory of planned behavior, and cognitive behavioral therapy are used in the counseling process.

INTRODUCTION

Providing dietary counseling in the office setting is challenging because of multiple barriers that include time restraints, limited resources, inadequate reimbursement, and low physician confidence.[1,2] However, changes in practice management that include formation of practice-based teams, incorporation of electronic tools, and more skillful communication and counseling techniques should lessen some of these barriers.

PROVIDING DIETARY CARE IN THE OFFICE SETTING
Team Approach

Although still emerging, the patient-centered medical home and accountable care organizations (ACO) are intended to provide collaborative patient-centered, team-based

Northwestern Comprehensive Center on Obesity, Northwestern University Feinberg School of Medicine, 750 North Lake Shore Drive, Rubloff 9-976, Chicago, IL 60611, USA
E-mail address: rkushner@northwestern.edu

Med Clin N Am 100 (2016) 1157–1168
http://dx.doi.org/10.1016/j.mcna.2016.06.002
0025-7125/16/$ – see front matter © 2016 Elsevier Inc. All rights reserved.

health care for a defined population of patients.[3] Within this infrastructure, each member of the team can use their unique skills to provide optimal long-term care, including dietary and physical activity counseling by trained interventionists. Another example that emphasizes teamwork is the Chronic Care Model (CCM), an innovative health systems approach to deliver collaborative chronic disease management.[4] The CCM calls for creation of multidisciplinary teams to create both cooperation and a division of labor to improve the care of patients with chronic diseases.[5,6] Such teams ensure that key elements of care that physicians may not have the training or time to do well are competently performed.[4,7] Another integrative model is to colocate or embed advanced practice nurses[8–10] and mental or behavioral-health providers into the medical setting.[11] Multidisciplinary teams have been implemented in the treatment of several chronic diseases, including diabetes[12] and hypertension,[13] 2 common comorbid conditions that are diet-related. Regardless of how the workload is distributed, the physician is generally considered the team leader and the source of a common philosophy of care. The key to success is physician commitment and a supportive organizational structure.

Tools and Resources

A significant portion of time spent in evaluation and treatment can be reduced by the use of tools, protocols, and procedures. Tools assist in patient risk assessment, prompting and tracking of counseling and referral, and education.[14] According to the CCM, optimal clinical encounters occur when an informed, activated patient interacts with a prepared, proactive team.[6] Two "paper-and-pen" tools previously developed to assist in dietary assessment and counseling are the WAVE (Weight, Activity, Variety, and Excess) and REAP (Rapid Eating and Activity Assessment for Patients).[15] However, with passage of the Affordable Care Act (ACA) and widespread use of Electronic Health Records (EHR), work is under way on developing electronic Health Risk Assessments (HRAs) that incorporate pertinent, patient-centered social and behavioral risk factors to be used for improving and monitoring health status.[16] My Own Health Report (MOHR) is one such tool that collects information on 8 sociodemographic elements and 13 specific health risk factors, including items on consumption of fruits and vegetables, fast food, and sugary beverages.[17]

Other tools, such as Web-based technologies, mobile devices, wearables, and electronic apps for smartphones or tablets, have emerged that facilitate self-monitoring and behavioral counseling.[18] The benefits to the patient are increased awareness of dietary intake, education regarding the quantity and quality of food consumed, and improved motivation and adherence. Provider benefits include a better understanding of patients' diets and more data to measure and analyze. Perhaps most importantly, self-monitoring is integral to managing chronic diseases and has been shown to be an essential initial step in promoting behavior change.[19] Routine incorporation of electronic tools into the office practice facilitates another key component of the CCM: self-management support. With the utilization of team-based care and electronic-based assessment and treatment resources, the provision of dietary care should be more practical and achievable in the ambulatory care setting.

COMMUNICATION

The cornerstone of effective dietary counseling and behavior change is grounded in skillful and empathetic provider-patient communication. This vital interaction is affirmed by Balint's[20] assertion that "the most frequently used drug in medical practice is the doctor himself." In a review of the literature, Stewart[21] found that the quality of communication between the physician and patient directly influenced patient health outcomes. Because the primary aim of dietary counseling is to influence what the patient does *outside* the office, the time spent *in* the office needs to be structured and effective.

Depending on the patient's course of treatment, various strategies and techniques are used during the visit. The interaction is directed toward supporting patients' motivation and sense of control, which boosts patient empowerment. Patient empowerment is often defined as a process by which people gain mastery over their lives.[22] A fundamental objective in dietary counseling is for patients to take increased responsibility for and a more active role in decision making regarding their own health.

STRUCTURING THE ENCOUNTER: USING THE 5 A'S

The 5 A's is an organizational construct for clinical counseling that has been used for smoking cessation, alcohol dependence, and weight management among other lifestyle behaviors. It provides a structured framework for the clinician when engaging a patient in behavior change. The 5 A's are *Assess, Advise, Agree, Assist*, and *Arrange*. An example of how to apply the 5 A's for dietary counseling is shown in **Table 1**. An abbreviated version of the 5 A's (*Ask, Advise*, and *Refer*)[23] can be used for the busy clinician who does not have the time or resources to implement dietary counseling

Table 1
Application of the 5 A's to dietary assessment and counseling

5 A's	Purpose	Example Dialogue
Assess	Assess the patient's diet and diet-related comorbidities	"I am interested in knowing more about your diet. Can you please take me through a typical day, starting first thing in the morning?" "Have you ever tried to change your diet in the past?"
Advise	Provide feedback and information about the patient's diet and the benefits of making selected changes	"The excess sodium in your diet is likely contributing to your elevated blood pressure." "Reducing the saturated fat in your diet is an important step in helping to bring down your blood cholesterol."
Agree	Appraise readiness and decide with patient where to begin making changes and which behaviors to focus on	"How confident are you that you can tackle your weight at this time?" "Do you think you can add a serving of vegetables with your lunch and dinner meal?"
Assist	Decide with patient where to begin making changes and which behaviors to focus on	"Tracking your diet using an electronic program will allow you to monitor your diet and caloric intake."
Arrange	Arrange for a follow-up appointment; make referrals to other resources	"I would like to schedule an appointment for you to see our registered dietitian." "A good option for you is to sign up for the Weight Watchers class at your work site."

in the office. An example would be to *ask* about the importance and impact of dietary choices in the patient's life or role in presenting symptoms, *advise* the patient that adopting a healthier diet would help improve the patient's health, and *refer* the patient to a registered dietitian in the community.

MOTIVATIONAL INTERVIEWING

How do clinicians assess motivation and facilitate lifestyle behavior change? Simply asking patients "Are you motivated to make a change?" is likely to yield mixed results, ranging from "yes, no, or maybe," which is difficult to interpret. Motivational Interviewing, or MI, is a client-centered, directive method for enhancing intrinsic motivation to change by exploring and resolving ambivalence.[24] It focuses on what the patient wants and how the patient thinks and feels. According to MI, motivation to change is viewed as something that is evoked in the patient rather than imposed. It is the patient's task (not the clinician's) to articulate and resolve his or her own ambivalence.[25] Readiness is viewed as the balance of 2 opposing forces: motivation or the patient's desire to change, and resistance or the patient's resistance to change.[26] Readiness for change is seen as the extent to which the patient has contemplated the need for change, having considered the pros and cons of change.

Intrinsic to this model is the concept that most patients are ambivalent about changing long-standing lifestyle behaviors, fearing that change will be difficult, uncomfortable, or depriving. The result of initiating a change plan when the patient is not ready often leads to frustration and disappointment. Patients frequently misattribute their lack of success to either a failure of effort (low willpower) or a poorly conceived diet. Patients who are ready and have thought about the benefits and difficulties of changing their diet are more likely to succeed. One helpful, simple, and rapid method to begin a readiness assessment is to 'anchor' the patient's interest and confidence to change on a 10-point numerical scale.

To assess readiness, simply ask the patient, *"On a scale from 0 to 10, with 0 being not important and 10 being very important, how important is it for you get your diabetes under control at this time?"* and *"Also on a scale from 0 to 10, with 0 being not confident and 10 being very confident, how confident are you that you get your diabetes under control at this time?."*[27]

Patients will frequently respond with a higher importance score compared with confidence score. In this case, the clinician would point out the discrepancy as follows: *"It is interesting that you rate the importance as an '8' and confidence as a '5.' What needs to happen or what can I do to help bring your confidence score up to an '8'?."* This technique allows patients to freely express the perceived or real barriers that have hindered their ability to be more successful.

MI uses 4 general principles to explore and resolve ambivalence[24]:

- Express empathy. Empathy refers to understanding the patient's feelings and perspectives without judging, criticizing, or blaming.
- Develop discrepancy. The second principle is to create and amplify the discrepancy between present behavior and the patient's broader goals and values. Discrepancy has to do with the importance of change and the distance that the patient's behavior would need to travel to reach the desired level. This is called the "behavioral gap." The general approach is one that results in the patient reflecting on the actions and reasons for change. The following dialogue illustrates this principle.
- Support self-efficacy. Self-efficacy refers to a person's belief in his or her ability to carry out and succeed with a specific task. Other common terms are hope and

faith. A general goal of MI is to enhance the patient's confidence in his or her capacity to cope with obstacles and to succeed in change. The confidence scale used previously quickly assesses the patient's level of confidence for a particular behavioral change.

- Roll with resistance. Although reluctance to change is to be expected in lifestyle behaviors, resistance (denial, arguing, putting up objections, yes-but statements) arises from the interpersonal interaction between the clinician and patient. In this case, the therapeutic relationship is endangered and the counseling process becomes dysfunctional. It is a signal that the patient-clinician rapport is damaged. If this occurs, the clinician's task is to double back, understand the reason for resistance behavior, and redirect counseling. Rolling with resistance means not to confront patients but allow them to express themselves. Using a reflective response serves to acknowledge the person's feelings or perceptions.

Multiple systematic reviews and meta-analyses have been published on the use of MI as an interventional behavior change strategy. Moderate levels of evidence have been established on the benefit of using MI for several chronic health conditions, including change in physical activity,[28] body weight,[29] alcohol, tobacco use,[30,31] and some dietary behaviors in patients with type 2 diabetes.[32]

SHARED DECISION MAKING

The concept of shared decision making (SDM) is stipulated in the ACA to ensure that medical care better aligns with patients' preferences and values.[33] SDM describes a collaboration process between patients and their clinicians to reach agreement about a health decision that may involve multiple treatment options and targets or therapy.[34,35] Clinicians and patients work together to clarify the patients' values and concerns, select a preference-sensitive decision, and agree on a follow-up plan. This process is consistent with the "agree" and "arrange" components of the 5 A's model described previously. Intrinsic to SDM is the use of patient decision aids (which are written materials, videos, or interactive electronic presentations) designed to inform patients about care options.[33] An example of SDM using a patient decision aid is weight management. The pros and cons of joining a commercial weight loss program, Internet support group, or referral to a registered dietitian can be discussed along with the options of which treatment to choose based on time, cost, and effectiveness.

BEHAVIOR CHANGE THEORIES AND PRINCIPLES

Whereas the 5 A's construct and motivational interviewing are counseling frameworks to use for structuring the patient encounter, behavior change theories and principles are used to facilitate targeted changes. The theories that are discussed in the following sections are intended to explain the biological, cognitive, behavioral, psychological, environmental, and motivational determinants of patient behavior. They also provide interventions to produce changes in knowledge, attitudes, motivation, self-confidence, skills, and social support required for behavior change and maintenance. Although this article focuses on dietary changes, the theories are generalizable to all health behaviors.

Self-Determination Theory

One of the most frustrating and distressing situations in clinical care is when a patient seems to lack motivation for change. Even after the clinician has addressed all of the benefits and obstacles to change and has laid out specific strategies to take action, the patient appears to be stuck in inertia (the inability or unwillingness to move or act). It is therefore not surprising that one of the most frequently asked questions by clinicians is, *"How do I motivate my patient?"* Self-Determination Theory and the counseling process of Motivational Interviewing (discussed previously) are particularly useful for these patients who seem to lack motivation for change.

According to Self-Determination Theory, people are motivated to act by different types of factors, either because they value a particular activity (internal motivation) or because there is external coercion (external motivation).[36] People will be internally motivated only when a change holds personal interest for them, that is enjoyment, satisfaction, and intrinsic reward.

Although powerful in its own right, intrinsic motivation requires supportive conditions (eg, people and an environment that are positive influences on behavior change, as intrinsic motivation can be readily disrupted by various less-supportive conditions). For example, consider a patient who wants to reduce the size of his dinner meal but whose wife serves family style (all food is presented in large serving dishes on the table), uses large plates, and encourages him to finish the food so there are no leftovers. In this case, the nonsupportive condition (the way dinner meals are served) will trump intrinsic motivation. Therefore, patients must not only be ready, willing, and able to make change, there must also be a supportive condition. At the other end of the spectrum are nonmotivated patients who do not see any value in changing, do not feel competent to change, or are not expecting the change to yield a desired outcome. The basic skill of the clinician is to identify whether patients' motivation is internal or external and to help patients find supportive conditions for health behavior change.

Between these 2 extremes is a continuum of externally motivated patients who are prompted to change by their significant others or their need to feel a connectedness with or valued by others. The more one is externally motivated, the less he or she shows interest, value, and movement toward achievement of change and the more he or she tends to blame others for a negative outcome. One end of this continuum is the patient who presents himself for changing a particular behavior, for example, cigarette smoking, solely based on the prompting of his physician or wife. He will likely just "go through the motions" to satisfy these external demands. The other end of the continuum is an externally motivated patient who makes changes to avoid guilt or anxiety or to achieve pride in oneself. An example would be a binge eater who feels bad about herself whenever she binges alone. Although an externally motivated patient can make positive behavior changes, the ultimate goal is to help patients become self-determined, that is to internalize and assimilate the changes to the self so that they experience greater autonomy in their action.

According to Watson and Tharp,[37] all behaviors pass through the following sequence: control by others, control by self, and automatization. When the patient achieves internal motivation, changes become more automatic and patients are authentic to their own goals. For example, a patient gains the assertiveness to say "no" to many of the peripheral demands asked of her and learns to prioritize her time to exercise on a regular schedule. This new acquired sense of autonomy and control reinforces her internal motivation to carve out precious time for herself.

STAGES OF CHANGE

When counseling patients, it is also important to assess whether the patient is ready to make changes in his or her behavior. One model, the Transtheoretical or Stages of Change (SOC) Model, clarifies this process. It proposes that at any specific time, patients change problem behaviors by moving through a series of stages representing several levels of readiness to change. There are 5 discreet stages of change: precontemplation, contemplation, preparation, action, and maintenance.[38,39] Patients move from one stage to the next in the process of change and it is likely that they may repeat stages several times before lasting change occurs. Within the stages of change model, the clinician's tasks include both assessing the patient's stage of change and using behavioral counseling strategies to help advance the patient from one stage to the next.

It is important to remember that stages of change often reflect discrete behaviors. For instance, a patient may be in the preparation stage for making changes to his or her diet, for example, adding more fruits and vegetables to each meal, but in the precontemplation stage for engaging in more physical activity. In this case, you would praise the patient and provide specific advice about adding more fruits and vegetables while encouraging the patient to think about how to add small bouts of physical activity in the course of the day.

The SOC model incorporates 10 specific processes of change that are activities and experiences that individuals engage in when they attempt to modify problem behaviors. Successful changers use different processes at each particular stage of change. The basic skill for the clinician is to listen for these experiential verbal statements to determine where a patient is in the 5 stages of change. Four of the most useful processes of change are consciousness raising (patients actively seek new information and gain understanding and feedback about behavior change), environmental reevaluation (patients consider and assess how diet, physical activity, and coping are affected by their physical and social environments), helping relationships (patients trust, accept, and use the support of others in their attempts to change behavior), and self-reevaluation (patients conduct emotional and cognitive reappraisal of individual values with respect to their behavior change goals).[40]

Many of these processes are embedded in other behavior change models. The role of the clinician is to guide the patient through these behavioral or thought processes, depending on their particular stage of change for a specific behavior.

Part of the decision for individuals to move from one stage to the next is based on the relative weight given to the *pros* and *cons* of changing behavior. The pros represent positive aspects of changing behavior, whereas the cons represent negative aspects of changing behavior, which may be thought of as barriers to change.[41]

HEALTH BELIEF MODEL

What about the patient who does not seem to understand the need to change a health behavior? This is another situation that can arise when counseling patients. The model that describes this, the Health Belief Model, holds the principle that health behavior change is a function of the individual's perceptions regarding his or her vulnerability to illness and perceived effectiveness of treatment.[42,43] Behavior change is determined by individuals who

- Perceive themselves to be susceptible to a particular health problem
- See the problem as serious
- Are convinced that treatment/prevention is effective and not overly costly with regard to money, effort, or pain
- Are exposed to a cue to take health action
- Have confidence that they can perform a specific behavior (self-efficacy)

The basic skill for the clinician is to help patients understand these behavioral change factors. This model is particularly useful when a patient is perceived to be in the precontemplation stage.

When using the Health Belief Model for behavior change, it is important to give feedback to the patient and to continuously link the patient's behavior changes to positive internal cues of health by pointing out that the changes the patient is making are directly leading to improved physical or mental well-being. These positive attributions are intended to strengthen the "cause-and-effect" relationship between behavior and health and reinforce motivation.

SOCIAL COGNITIVE THEORY/ECOLOGICAL MODELS

It is important to know the supportive resources and barriers patients have to changing their behaviors. Social Cognitive Theory emphasizes the interactions between the person and his or her environment. Behavior, therefore, is a function of aspects of both the environment and the person, all of which are in constant reciprocal interaction.[44] The behavioral choices we make regarding what we eat or what we do are determined, in part, by accessibility, affordability, and available resources. Ecological models expand our definition of environmental influences to include interpersonal relationships, family, community, and city. The "built environment," meaning the environment that humans built, is an important concept in viewing behavior.[45] For example, our patients may be more likely (or less likely) to take a walk depending on neighborhood safety, lighting, sidewalks, traffic, and if there is an enjoyable route. Diet may be determined, in part, by whether the patient has access to neighborhood grocery stores versus large supermarkets, fast-food chains versus sit-down restaurants, fresh versus processed foods, and the price of food. These are essential questions to ask the patient before establishing behavior-change goals.

Two central concepts of social learning theory are self-efficacy and outcome expectations:

- Self-efficacy or confidence, previously mentioned under the Health Belief Model and Motivational Interviewing, refers to a patient's belief in his or her ability to change or maintain a specific behavior under a variety of circumstances. It is not a general belief about oneself, but a specific belief that is tied to a particular task.[35] Higher levels of self-efficacy are predictive of improved treatment outcomes.[46] Low self-efficacy may be due to either perceived or actual deficits in personal knowledge, skills, resources, or environmental supports.[47]
- Outcome expectancies are the degree to which a patient believes that a given course of action will lead to a particular outcome. This is also a central feature of the Health Belief Model. Outcome expectations must be favorable for behavior change to occur. Expectations are typically described as an individual's anticipation of the effects of future experiences.

THEORY OF PLANNED BEHAVIOR

Considering the patient's perceived control over behavioral change is also important. This is where the theory of planned behavior (TPB) comes in (**Fig. 1**). According to the TPB, the intention to act is guided by 3 belief considerations: behavioral beliefs, normative beliefs, and control beliefs.[48] Behavioral beliefs refer to the patient's perceived outcomes (benefits and rewards) and attitudes toward engaging in the behavior. Normative beliefs refer to the subjective norms or pressure of others in the family or community regarding the behavioral change. Control beliefs refer to the presence of factors that may facilitate or impede performance of the behavior and the perceived power of these factors. In combination, these 3 beliefs lead to the formation of a behavioral *intention* to take action, similar to the support provided

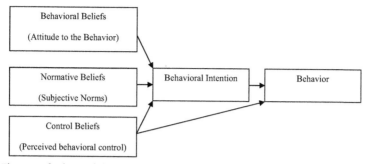

Fig. 1. Theory of planned behavior (TPB). (*Adapted from* Aizen I. Theory of planned behavior. Available at: http://people.umass.edu/aizen/. Accessed December 25, 2015.)

by a 3-legged stool. A key principle of TPB is that behavioral change (an observed action) is immediately preceded by intention. Applying this model, the more favorable the attitude and subjective norm, and the greater the perceived control, the stronger should be the patient's intention to change behavior.

But intention may not be enough. Behavioral change will only occur if the patient has a sufficient degree of perceived AND actual control over the behavior. Multiple studies have identified the importance of the TPB in explaining intended behavior change.[49–52]

COGNITIVE BEHAVIORAL THERAPY

When it comes to helping patients take action, cognitive behavioral therapy (CBT) is a common behavioral therapy that is used. It incorporates various strategies intended to help change and reinforce new dietary and physical activity behaviors as well as thoughts and attitudes.[53,54] Rather than exploring the psychological underpinning for behavior that may be rooted in childhood (the past), CBT focuses on short-term, problem-oriented treatments that address the present and future. The primary aim of CBT is to produce cognitive change: attention to inner thoughts, attitudes, and emotions, as well as to the events that both trigger and result from our actions.[55]

Behavior is a function of the person in interaction with the environment; this is in contrast to "willpower," which implies that some entity, inner strength, or psychological makeup is all that is needed to lose weight. CBT is based on the need to cultivate skills that are developed through knowledge and practice versus just needing good intentions to succeed. Patients may present for treatment interested to cut down on their alcohol intake (Contemplation Stage of Change) but need to consciously apply learned techniques and strategies to make something happen. The key traditional cognitive behavior therapy techniques are self-monitoring, stimulus control, problem solving, stress management, social support, and cognitive restructuring.

SUMMARY

With the advent of team-based care and a myriad of electronic tools, the barriers to provide dietary counseling should be lessened. Good communication between the provider and patient is paramount in eliciting behavior change. Rather than simply educating and instructing patients on what to do, behavior change counseling should be a guiding and collaborative process. Behavior change theories are intended to explain the multiple determinants of human behavior. They also provide interventions to produce changes in multiple domains, including knowledge, attitudes, motivation, self-confidence, skills, and social support required for behavior change and maintenance. A skilled clinician mixes and matches all of these behavior change principles, strategies, and techniques during counseling. Often, several methods are used with the same patient depending on the targeted behavior and course of treatment.

REFERENCES

1. Kushner RF. Barriers to providing nutrition counseling by physicians: a survey of primary care practitioners. Prev Med 1995;24(6):546–52.
2. Kolasa KM, Rickett K. Barriers to providing nutrition counseling cited by physicians: a survey of primary care practitioners. Nutr Clin Pract 2010;25:502–9.
3. Arena R, Lavie CJ. The healthy lifestyle team is central to the success of accountable care organizations. Mayo Clin Proc 2015;90(5):572–6.
4. Wagner EH, Austin BT, Davis C, et al. Improving chronic illness care: translating evidence into action. Health Aff (Millwood) 2001;20(6):64–78.
5. Casalino LP. Disease management and the organization of physician practice. JAMA 2005;293(4):485–8.
6. Bodenheimer T, Wagner EH, Grumbach K. Improving primary care for patients with chronic illness. JAMA 2002;288(14):1775–9.
7. Milani RV, Lavie CJ. Health care 2020: reengineering health care delivery to combat chronic disease. Am J Med 2015;128(4):337–43.
8. Campbell DL, Asselin J, Osunlana AM, et al. Implementation and evaluation of the 5As framework of obesity management in primary care: design of the 5As Team (5AsT) randomized control trial. Implement Sci 2014;9:78.
9. Osunlana AM, Asselin J, Anderson R, et al. 5As Team obesity intervention in primary care: development and evaluation of shared decision-making weight management tools. Clin Obes 2015;5:219–25.
10. Asselin J, Osunlana AM, Ogunleye AA, et al. Missing an opportunity: the embedded nature of weight management in primary care. Clin Obes 2015;5(6): 325–32.
11. Manderscheid R, Kathol R. Fostering sustainable, integrated medical and behavioral health services in medical settings. Ann Intern Med 2014;160:61–5.
12. Bratcher CR, Bellow E. Traditional or centralized models of diabetes care: the multidisciplinary diabetes team approach. J Fam Pract 2011;60(11 Suppl):S6–11.
13. Houle SK, Chatterley T, Tsuyuki RT. Multidisciplinary approaches to the management of high blood pressure. Curr Opin Cardiol 2014;29(4):344–53.
14. Dickey LL, Gemson DH, Carney P. Office system interventions supporting primary care-based health behavior change counseling. Am J Prev Med 1999;17: 299–308.
15. Gans KM, Ross E, Barner CW, et al. REAP and WAVE: new tools to rapidly assess/discuss nutrition with patients. J Nutr 2003;133:556S–62S.
16. Institute of Medicine. Capturing social and behavioral domains and measures in electronic health records: phase 2. Available at: http://www.nap.edu/catalog/18951/capturing-social-and-behavioral-domains-and-measures-in-electronic-health-records. Accessed December 31, 2015.
17. Phillips SM, Glasgow RE, Bello G, et al. Frequency and prioritization of patient health risks from a structured health risk assessment. Ann Fam Med 2014; 12(6):505–13.

18. Bonilla C, Brauer P, Royall D, et al. Use of electronic dietary assessment tools in primary care: an interdisciplinary perspective. BMC Med Inform Decis Mak 2015; 15:14.
19. Yu Z, Sealey-Potts C, Rodriguez J. Dietary self-monitoring in weight management: current evidence on efficacy and adherence. J Acad Nutr Diet 2015; 115(12):1931–8.
20. Balint M. The doctor, his patient, and the illness. New York: International University Press; 1972.
21. Stewart MA. Effective physician-patient communication and health outcomes: a review. Can Med Assoc J 1995;152:1423–33.
22. Schulz PJ, Nakamoto K. Health literacy and patient empowerment in health communication: the importance of separating conjoined twins. Patient Educ Couns 2013;90:4–11.
23. Fiore MC, Balley WC, Cohen SJ, et al. Treating tobacco use and dependence: clinical practice guideline. Rockville (MD): US Dept of Health and Human Services (USDHHS); Public Health Service (PHS); 2000. Report 1-58763-007-9.
24. Miller WR, Rollnick S, editors. Motivational interviewing. Preparing people for change. 3rd edition. New York: The Guilford Press; 2002. p. 25.
25. Britt E, Hudson SM, Blampied NM. Motivational interviewing in health settings: a review. Patient Educ Couns 2004;53:147–55.
26. Katz DL. Behavior modification in primary care: the pressure system model. Prev Med 2001;32:66–72.
27. Rollnick S, Mason P, Butler C. Health behavior change: a guide for practitioners. London: Churchill Livingstone; 1999.
28. O'Halloran PD, Blackstock F, Shields N, et al. Motivational interviewing to increase physical activity in people with chronic health conditions: a systematic review and meta-analysis. Clin Rehabil 2014;28:1159–71.
29. Barnes RD, Ivezaj V. A systematic review of motivational interviewing for weight loss among adults in primary care. Obes Rev 2015;16:304–18.
30. Lundahl B, Moleni T, Burke BL, et al. Motivational interviewing in medical care settings: a systematic review and meta-analysis of randomized controlled trials. Patient Educ Couns 2013;93:157–68.
31. Lee WW, Choi KC, Yum RW, et al. Effectiveness of motivational interviewing on lifestyle modification and health outcomes of clients at risk or diagnosed with cardiovascular diseases: a systematic review. Int J Nurs Stud 2016;53:331–41.
32. Ekong G, Kavookjian J. Motivational interviewing and outcomes in adults with type 2 diabetes: a systematic review. Patient Educ Couns 2016;99(6):944–52.
33. Oshima Lee E, Emanuel EJ. Shared decision making to improve care and reduce costs. N Engl J Med 2013;368:6–8.
34. Politi MC, Wolin KY, Legarie F. Implementing clinical practice guidelines about health promotion and disease prevention through shared decision making. J Gen Intern Med 2013;28:838–44.
35. Sonntag U, Wiesner J, Fahrenkrog S, et al. Motivational interviewing and shared decision making in primary care. Patient Educ Couns 2012;87:62–6.
36. Ryan RM, Deci EL. Self-determination theory and the facilitation of intrinsic motivation, social development, and well-being. Am Psychol 2000;55(1):68–78.
37. Watson DL, Tharp RG, editors. Self-directed behavior. Self-modification for personal adjustment. 8th edition. Belmont (CA): Wadsworth Group Publ; 2002.
38. Prochaska J, DiClemente C. Stages and processes of self-change of smoking. Toward an integrative model of change. J Consult Clin Psychol 1983;51:390–5.

39. Prochaska JO, DiClimente CC. Toward a comprehensive model of change. In: Miller WR, editor. Treating addictive behaviors. New York: Plenum Press; 1986. p. 3–27.

40. Prochaska JO, Velicer WF. The transtheoretical model of health behavior change. Am J Health Promot 1997;12(1):38–48.

41. Levenson W, Cohen MS, Brandy D, et al. To change or not to change: "Sounds like you have a dilemma". Ann Intern Med 2001;135(5):386–90.

42. Becker MH. The health belief model and sick-role behavior. Health Ed Monographs 1974;2:409–19.

43. Janz NK, Champion VL, Strecher VJ. The health belief model. In: Glanz K, Rimer BK, Lewis FM, editors. Health behavior and health education: theory, research, and practice. 3rd edition. San Francisco (CA): Jossey-Bass; 2002. p. 45–66.

44. Barnanowski T, Cullen KW, Nicklas T, et al. Are current health behavioral change models helpful in guiding prevention of weight gain efforts? Obes Res 2003; 11(Suppl):23S–43S.

45. Booth KM, Pinkston MM, Poston WS. Obesity and the built environment. J Am Dent Assoc 2005;105:S110–7.

46. Witkiewitz K, Marlatt GA. Relapse prevention for alcohol and drug problems. That was zen, this is tao. Am Psychol 2004;59(4):224–35.

47. Rosal MC, Ebbeling CB, Lofgren I, et al. Facilitating dietary change: the patient-centered counseling model. J Am Diet Assoc 2001;101:332–41.

48. Aizen I. Theory of planned behavior. Available at: http://people.umass.edu/aizen/. Accessed December 25, 2015.

49. Brickell TA, Chatzisarantis NL, Pretty GM. Autonomy and control: augmenting the validity of the theory of planned behaviour in predicting exercise. J Health Psychol 2006;11:51–63.

50. Rhodes RE, Bianchard CM, Matheson DH. A multicomponent model of the theory of planned behaviour. Br J Health Psychol 2006;11(Pt 1):119–37.

51. Brug J, De Vet E, de Nooijer J, et al. Predicting fruit consumption; cognitions, intention, and habits. J Nutr Educ Behav 2006;38:73–81.

52. Armitage CJ, Conner M. Efficacy of the theory of planned behaviour: a meta-analytic review. Br J Soc Psychol 2001;40:471–99.

53. Foreyt JP, Poston WS. What is the role of cognitive-behavior therapy in patient management? Obes Res 1998;6(Suppl 1):18S–22S.

54. Wadden TA, Foster GD. Behavioral treatment of obesity. Med Clin North Am 2000; 84:441–6.

55. Williamson DA, Perrin LA. Behavioral therapy for obesity. Endocrinol Metab Clin North Am 1996;25(4):943–54.

Nutritional Assessment in Primary Care

Ryan T. Hurt, MD, PhD[a,b,c], Stephen A. McClave, MD[c],*

KEYWORDS

- Malnutrition • Obesity • Nutrition assessment • Nutritional state • Nutrition risk

KEY POINTS

- Malnutrition is not well understood and thus is poorly defined. Signs of deterioration of nutritional status are subtle, especially in the setting of obesity.
- Both nutritional status and disease severity contribute to each patient's nutrition risk.
- A careful nutrition screen based on patient history, anthropometric measures, and physical examination help differentiate high from low probability of micronutrient/macronutrient deficiencies and deterioration of nutritional status.
- Patients whose initial screen is of high predictive value should go on to have further imaging or laboratory testing, leading to targeted management strategies and appropriate nutrition therapy.

INTRODUCTION

Clinicians receive limited training during medical school and residency in nutrition and obesity.[1] Nutritional assessment in primary care is essential, because it provides physicians with the needed tools to evaluate nutritional status and eventually treat individuals over a wide body mass index (BMI) range who may be at risk for macronutrient or micronutrient deficiencies. Evidence of poor nutritional state occurs at both ends of the BMI spectrum. It is said that obesity often hide in plain sight on a typical medical examination.[2] A minority of patients are in the healthy BMI (18.5–24.9 kg/m^2) category, with more than 70% being classified as either underweight (<18.5 kg/m^2), overweight (25.0–29.9 kg/m^2), or having obesity (>30.0 kg/m^2).[3] Evidence of poor nutritional status is more subtle in the setting of obesity, but still common. Surprisingly, patients with BMI greater than 30 kg/m^2 have an odds ratio of 1.5 for having evidence of malnutrition, compared with those with BMI less than 30 kg/m^2.[4] There are several conditions

Disclosure: The authors have nothing to disclose.
[a] Division of General Internal Medicine, Mayo Clinic, Rochester, MN, USA; [b] Division of Gastroenterology and Hepatology, Mayo Clinic, 200 First Street SW, Rochester, MN 55905, USA; [c] Division of Gastroenterology, Hepatology and Nutrition, University of Louisville School of Medicine, 550 South Jackson Street, Louisville, KY 40292, USA
* Corresponding author.
E-mail address: samcclave@louisville.edu

that predispose patients to deterioration of nutritional status and low BMI, such as chronic obstructive pulmonary disease (COPD), short bowel syndrome, cancer, eating disorders, substance abuse, inflammatory bowel disease, and older age.[2]

This article identifies conditions in which the nutritional state may be compromised. Clinicians need to know which laboratory, clinical, and radiologic studies are appropriate to identify poor nutritional status and provide assistance in directing therapy for patients at high nutrition risk. Clinicians need the skills to screen patients for risk of nutrient abnormalities, learning to differentiate those factors that have high versus low predictive value for detecting further deterioration of nutritional status.

DIFFICULTY DEFINING MALNUTRITION

Despite poor nutritional status being associated with increased morbidity and mortality in a wide range of medical conditions, malnutrition is not well understood, and thus remains poorly defined. Malnutrition has been defined broadly as a nutritional imbalance involving those patients who lack an adequate combination of macronutrients (fat, glucose, and protein), and micronutrients (minerals, trace elements, and vitamins) to repair and maintain tissues.[5] The American Society for Parenteral and Enteral Nutrition (ASPEN) and the Academy of Nutrition and Dietetics (AND) developed guidelines and a consensus statement on the definition of malnutrition that are applicable to a wide range of clinical settings.[5] The definition is based on several causal factors (social and environmental), and takes acute and chronic illness into consideration. Because no specific parameter has been highly predictive of malnutrition, the guidelines recommend a diagnosis of malnutrition if 2 of 6 characteristics are met.[5] These characteristics are insufficient energy intake, weight loss, loss of muscle mass, loss of subcutaneous fat, localized or generalized fluid accumulation, and diminished functional status determined by handgrip dynometry (**Table 1**).[5] Malnutrition is categorized as moderate or severe, with the consensus statement recognizing the difficulty in differentiating mild from moderate degrees of malnutrition.

Despite the consensus efforts of ASPEN and AND, the definition of malnutrition remains nonspecific, vague, and not universally accepted. In contrast, nutrition risk is more easily defined, and recognizes that both nutritional status and severity of disease contribute to the patient's overall risk. There are several tools that have been developed to help stratify the patients who are at nutrition risk and who may benefit from aggressive nutrition delivery. The Nutrition Risk in Critically Ill (NUTRIC) scoring system uses 6 variables to calculate the score: age, Acute Physiology and Chronic Health Assessment (APACHE) II, Sepsis-related Organ Failure Assessment, number of comorbidities, days from hospital to intensive care unit (ICU) admission, and interleukin-6 (IL-6) level.[6] The NUTRIC score ranges from 0 to 10. Those patients having scores between 6 and 10 have higher risk for adverse clinical outcomes (mainly mortality), and are more likely to see improvement in outcomes in response to aggressive nutrition therapy (compared with patients with low scores of 0–5). The NUTRIC score has been validated without using IL-6, because this test is not readily available at many hospitals.[6] In a revised and updated validation study of the NUTRIC score, a total of 1199 ICU patients with an overall 28-day mortality of 29% and a mean NUTRIC score of 5.5 were evaluated to determine whether the score correlated with mortality and whether adequate nutrition therapy would have a clinical impact on patient outcomes. The odds ratio of mortality at 28 days was multiplied by 1.4 for every point increase in the NUTRIC score. There were positive associations in 28-day survival and

Table 1
ASPEN and AND guidelines for the definition of malnutrition

Clinical Characteristic	Malnutrition in the Context of Acute Illness or Injury		Malnutrition in the Context of Chronic Illness		Malnutrition in the Context of Social or Environmental Circumstances	
	Nonsevere (Moderate) Malnutrition	Severe Malnutrition	Nonsevere (Moderate) Malnutrition	Severe Malnutrition	Nonsevere (Moderate) Malnutrition	Severe Malnutrition
(1) Energy Intake	<75% of estimated energy requirement for >7 d	≤50% of estimated energy requirement for ≥5 d	<75% of estimated energy requirement for ≥1 mo	≤75% of estimated energy requirement for ≥1 mo	<75% of estimated energy requirement for ≥3 mo	≤50% of estimated energy requirement for ≥1 mo
(2) Interpretation of Weight Loss	% / Time: 1–2 / 1 wk, 5 / 1 mo, 7.5 / 3 mo	% / Time: >2 / 1 wk, >5 / 1 mo, >7.5 / 3 mo	% / Time: 5 / 1 mo, 7.5 / 3 mo, 10 / 6 mo, 20 / 1 y	% / Time: >5 / 1 wk, >7.5 / 3 mo, >10 / 6 mo, >20 / 1 y	% / Time: 5 / 1 mo, 7.5 / 3 mo, 10 / 6 mo, 20 / 1 y	% / Time: >5 / 1 wk, >7.5 / 3 mo, >10 / 6 mo, >20 / 1 y
Physical Findings						
(3) Body Fat	Mild	Moderate	Mild	Severe	Mild	Severe
(4) Muscle Mass	Mild	Moderate	Mild	Severe	Mild	Severe
(5) Fluid Accumulation	Mild	Moderate to severe	Mild	Severe	Mild	Severe
(6) Reduced Grip Strength	NA	Measurably reduced	NA	Measurably reduced	NA	Measurably reduced

Abbreviation: NA, not available.
From White JV, Guenter P, Jensen G, et al. Consensus statement: Academy of Nutrition and Dietetics and American Society for Parenteral and Enteral Nutrition: characteristics recommended for the identification and documentation of adult malnutrition (undernutrition). J Parenter Enteral Nutr 2012;36(3):278; with permission.

6-month mortality for patients with a high NUTRIC score who received adequate nutrition.[6]

The Nutritional Risk Score (NRS)-2002, another nutrition risk assessment tool, has been evaluated in several patient populations, including hospitalized geriatric patients and those with head and neck cancer.[7–10] The NRS-2002 focuses on 4 initial screening factors: BMI less than 20 kg/m^2, loss of weight in the previous 3 months, decreased nutritional intake, and severe illness. If any of these factors are present, then a final screening assessment is performed. The final screen has 2 components: impaired nutritional status and severity of disease.[9] An evaluation of nutritional status assigns a score (0–3) based on recent weight loss, decreased oral intake, and low BMI. Determination of disease severity assigns a score (0–3) based on examples of increasingly severe disease processes such as hip fracture, presence of COPD, or critical illness (APACHE II score >10). The NRS-2002 adds a point for age more than 70 years. A total score greater than or equal to 3 suggests that the patient is at nutritional risk and should undergo implementation of a nutrition plan.[9] Both the NRS-2002 and NUTRIC scoring systems were developed and validated for hospitalized patients requiring artificial nutrition support.

Although several other assessment tools have been developed to evaluate nutritional status, none measure the impact of disease severity.[11] However, one of these, the Mini Nutritional Assessment (MNA), can be useful in an ambulatory outpatient practice.[12] The MNA is a simple assessment that does not require a nutrition specialist to implement and can be applied to ambulatory outpatient, home, or intermediate care settings.[11,13,14] The MNA was tested almost exclusively in the geriatric population, being validated in several chronic medical conditions such as Parkinson disease, COPD, and cancer.[15–17] The full MNA version evaluates factors pertaining to mobility, amount of nutrition intake, weight loss, and social interaction (eg, independent living and stress level).[18] There is a validated short form of the MNA (the MNA-SF), which focuses on the 6 issues of food intake, weight loss, presence of psychological stress, dementia/depression, mobility, and BMI.[19–21] If BMI is not available, calf circumference can be substituted, with a low measurement being suggestive of malnutrition (<33 cm).[21]

FINDINGS ON PATIENT HISTORY

There are several so-called red flags obtained from a detailed history and physical examination and these should alert clinicians that nutritional status may be in jeopardy. Initially, the historical findings typically focus on changes in body weight. Both weight loss and weight gain should be carefully evaluated, because increased nutrition risk can be associated with either. Sarcopenia (low muscle mass) has been associated with deterioration of nutritional status from such conditions as cancer and obesity.[22] A temporal time frame for the weight loss or gain should be established. Weight loss even as low as 5% over a 3-year period in nursing home patients (>65 years old) has been shown to be an independent predictor of mortality.[23] Documenting accurate weights from either ambulatory clinic visits or from a reliable scale in the home can help establish the amount of weight loss and the time frame over which it occurred.

Reasons for involuntary weight changes need to be evaluated. Decreased oral intake is a primary cause for involuntary weight loss, and the differential needs to be explored. Among the elderly the reasons for reduced oral intake may include social isolation, financial limitations, and depression.[24] Isolation can be a significant cause of decreased oral intake in the elderly, with one study showing that meals eaten in groups were 75% larger compared with those meals consumed alone. Financial limitations are often a barrier to both adequacy of nutrient intake and the quality of calories consumed.[25,26] Depression is commonly associated with weight loss, but may in some cases lead to weight gain and obesity.[27,28]

There are also many disease processes that cause weight loss. Some common examples include inflammatory bowel disease, human immunodeficiency virus/acquired immunodeficiency syndrome, alcohol abuse, COPD, multiple sclerosis, rheumatoid arthritis, and cancer. Most of these conditions are associated with systemic inflammation. One specific condition associated with the systemic inflammatory response syndrome is cachexia. Cachexia is distinct from starvation, malabsorption, age-associated muscle loss (sarcopenia), or endocrine causes of weight loss (hyperthyroidism or new onset diabetes).[29] Cachexia has been defined as a complex metabolic condition associated with inflammation from an underlying illness, characterized by loss of muscle with or without loss of fat mass.[29] Clinical features of cachexia include weight loss in adults, growth failure in children, anorexia, insulin resistance, and increased muscle breakdown.[30] The exact inflammatory mechanism for cachexia is not clear, but the role of increased circulating levels of IL-6 and tumor necrosis factor (TNF) have been implicated.[31-33] Cachexia is common in patients with cancer (50%–80%) and is associated with 20% mortality.[31,34] Several treatments, including fish oil, nonsteroidal antiinflammatory drugs, thalidomide, and anti-TNF agents have been tried to reverse or improve cachexia with limited success.[35]

Gastrointestinal causes of weight loss are important aspects to evaluate in patients with deteriorating nutritional status. Short bowel syndrome is an important cause of weight loss typically associated with diarrhea.[36] When the length of small bowel remaining is less than one-third that of the normal gut, the diarrhea can lead to weight loss and a wide range of micronutrient and macronutrient deficiencies.[36] The malabsorption of nutrients, increased transit time, gastric acid hypersecretion, and intestinal bacterial overgrowth all can contribute to the diarrhea. Chronic diarrhea in any other condition, such as infectious colitis, inflammatory bowel disease (IBD), or enterocutaneous fistulas can lead to poor nutritional state. Patients who have had bariatric surgery, which by design is an operation that leads to malabsorption, reduced caloric intake, and long-term micronutrient deficiencies, should be followed closely for signs of deterioration of nutritional status.

Elderly patients often have poor dentition, which can compromise the ability to swallow and lead subsequently to nutrient deficiencies. A recent cross-sectional study assessed 343 (mean age, 83 years) assisted living residents in 3 groups: those without teeth, those with removable dentures, and those with teeth.[37] MNA screening showed that there was an overall 22% rate of malnourishment in this population. Residents without teeth had the poorest nutritional status and lower intake of protein compared with those with dentures or natural teeth.[37]

Upper gastrointestinal symptoms such as nausea, vomiting, abdominal distention, and bloating can be signs that an underlying disease process is contributing to deterioration of nutritional status. Chemotherapy-induced nausea and vomiting in addition to cancer-associated cachexia can contribute to impaired nutritional status in this high-risk patient population.[38] Gastrointestinal cancer may present with nausea and vomiting as the result of a partial or complete intestinal obstruction resulting in decreased nutrient absorption. Dysphagia, present in approximately 10% of the elderly population, warrants a full investigation, because such symptoms cannot be attributed solely to the physiologic changes associated with aging.[39,40] Dysphagia can be present in numerous conditions, such as amyotrophic lateral sclerosis, Parkinson disease, stroke, achalasia, diffuse esophageal spasm, scleroderma, and malignancy.[40]

Anorexia (a decrease in appetite) is an important red-flag symptom that needs to be thoroughly evaluated in patients being screened for nutrition risk. In addition to the association with cachexia, cancer and the treatments for cancer may lead to anorexia through mechanisms that are not well understood.[41] With aging, intake of nutrients may gradually diminish and this may be caused by several physiologic factors, including diminished taste and smell.[42] The anorexia of aging is thought to be caused by increased levels of satiety hormones such as cholecystokinin and decreases in hunger neuromediators such as neuropeptide Y.[43] Careful screening for the presence of an eating disorder should occur in patients who appear malnourished. The decrease in appetite associated with anorexia nervosa is distinctly different from anorexia of aging or the cachexia of cancer.[41] Anorexia nervosa is a condition associated with low body weight and an intense fear of gaining weight in the setting of a distorted body image. Initiating nutrition therapy in patients with anorexia nervosa who are severely malnourished has led to refeeding syndrome and cardiac arrest.[44] Anorexia nervosa needs to be considered especially in young patients who have poor nutritional status.

Medications can be responsible for both weight gain and loss, contributing respectively to overnutrition and undernutrition.[45] The side effect of weight loss can be used to the patient's advantage, because several new medications with such a profile have been approved by the US Food and Drug Administration for the treatment of obesity.[46] Weight loss is seen predictably with the use of some antidepressant agents (bupropion) and drugs to treat diabetes (eg, liraglutide, exenatide, pramlintide, and metformin).[47] In contrast, several medications have been associated with weight gain and obesity.[45,47] First-generation (eg, thioridazine) and second-generation (eg, risperidone, olanzapine, clozapine, and quetiapine) antipsychotic agents have long been associated with weight gain.[47] Numerous psychiatric medications have been associated with weight gain (eg, paroxetine, amitriptyline, imipramine, mirtazapine, lithium).[47] Likewise, several antidiabetes medications are associated with weight gain (eg, insulin, sulfonylureas, thiazolidinediones).[47] Other classes of medications, such as glucocorticoids, are also associated with potentially significant weight gain.[45,47] Clinicians should carefully evaluate the medication history, scrutinizing the duration, dosing, and potential side effects when patients present with obesity or unexplained weight loss.

FINDINGS ON PHYSICAL EXAMINATION

Use of self-reported height and weight should be avoided, because these values have been shown in a prospective cohort of 508 ambulatory internal medicine patients to be consistently inaccurate compared with clinician measurements.[48] All patients being evaluated for deterioration of nutritional status should have height and weight measured, and BMIs calculated from these values. The World Health Organization and the National Institutes of Health provide a standardized classification scheme for BMI: underweight, BMI less than or equal to 18.49 kg/m^2; healthy weight, BMI greater than or equal to 18.5 to 24.9 kg/m^2; overweight, BMI greater than or equal to 25.0 to 29.9 kg/m^2; obesity class I, BMI greater than or equal to 30 to 34.9 kg/m^2; obesity class II, BMI greater than or equal to 35 to 39.9 kg/m^2; and obesity class III, BMI greater than or equal to 40 kg/m^2.[49] Both low BMI (<20 kg/m^2) and high BMI (>30 kg/m^2) have been shown to be associated with increased all-cause mortality compared with BMI in the normal range.[50]

Waist circumference (WC) is an important anthropometric measure used to evaluate health risk, and is a surrogate marker for visceral adipose tissue.[51] WC is most useful for persons who have a BMI between 25 and 35 kg/m^2. Persons who have an increased BMI in combination with an increased WC (men, >102 cm; women, >88 cm), have a greater risk of obesity comorbidities than if the BMI alone is increased.[52] BMI values greater than 35 kg/m^2 are associated with increased risk of comorbidities, so, in that BMI range, WC adds no additional predictive power. There is no prognostic value and thus no role for measuring WC in underweight BMI.[52] Although there are several other anthropometric measures that can be used clinically, such as waist/hip ratio and skin fold thickness, the amount of staff training needed to make them reliable in the ambulatory setting and the unproven superiority to WC in many conditions makes them a lower priority. Patients are usually interested in determining their ideal weight. Although ideal body weight can easily be calculated, it may have some limitations in certain disease processes or when dealing with patients of tall or short stature.[53]

The clinician's first impression of patient appearance (eg, older than stated age) may be the primary reason to initiate screening for nutrition risk. Although physical examination findings of undernutrition may be obvious, poor nutritional status in the setting of obesity may be more difficult to detect on general appearance. The clinician may miss that a patient's BMI of 44 kg/m^2 on examination day was 50 kg/m^2 several weeks before, and that the patient has a new desquamative rash over the chest and abdomen. Obesity may hide in plain sight on physical examination, as highlighted by studies in which clinicians fail to diagnose obesity in an ambulatory clinic.[2,3] In a large cohort study of 2543 patients with obesity, only 19.9% received a diagnosis of obesity, and only 22.6% had a treatment plan initiated for obesity.[3] Thus, it is important that, before the history and physical examination portion of a patient encounter, anthropometrics should be obtained and made available for the clinician to review.

There are several specific findings on physical examination that should raise red flags for clinicians as to the presence of poor nutritional status. However, most of these findings have non–nutrition-related causes as well. Changes in hair are common early findings associated with deterioration of nutritional status. Hair loss can be associated with inadequate protein or deficiencies of vitamin B$_{12}$ and folate.[54] Dry or coiled hair is a potential sign of vitamin A or E deficiency.[54] Temporal atrophy is a classic sign that is associated with poor nutritional state, as is generalized muscle wasting. Ocular examination findings such as Bitot spots, xerosis, and night blindness are suggestive of vitamin A deficiency, whereas angular palpebritis has been associated with riboflavin deficiency.[54] On oral examination, poor dentition (including missing teeth) can be a sign of general macronutrient deficiencies or specific micronutrient losses such as vitamins C, D, or B$_{12}$.[54–57] Low vitamin C intake has been associated with specific oral disorder, that of bleeding gums. Glossitis and angular cheilosis have been linked to low vitamin B complex intake.[58–60] Peripheral edema has long been associated with poor nutritional status, and edema has been noted specifically in thiamine deficiency. However, edema associated with hypoproteinemia may be the result of the negative acute phase response of serum proteins to inflammation.[61,62] Decreased hand/grip strength has been associated with decreased muscle mass, although the use of hand/grip dynometry has not been widely adopted in clinical practice.[63,64]

Dermatologic abnormalities are also common early findings associated with poor nutritional status. Poor wound healing in general or the development of pressure sores can be associated with macronutrient deficiencies, and should be considered, especially in the elderly. Desquamation can be caused by low levels of riboflavin.[54] Petechiae, perifollicular hemorrhage, and ecchymosis are examination findings that have been associated with vitamin C deficiency. Petechiae, acneiform keratosis, follicular keratosis, and xerosis can be signs of vitamin A deficiency.[54] Dry, scaly skin has been associated with deficiencies of vitamin A, biotin, protein, niacin, and essential fatty acid.[54]

Neurologic abnormalities may reflect macronutrient or micronutrient deficiencies. Short neurologic examinations can identify cognition problems commonly associated with poor nutritional status, and can then be used to monitor patients as nutrition therapy is implemented to see whether the cognitive function returns.[65] Severe thiamine deficiency can lead to Wernicke encephalopathy (WE) and is the acute syndrome that, if left untreated, may progress to the chronic Korsakoff syndrome (KS). The WE diagnostic triad includes encephalopathy, oculomotor dysfunction, and gait ataxia. Emergence of these symptoms in an undernourished patient makes early immediate thiamine replacement imperative, to prevent progression to the usually irreversible KS.[66] Thiamine deficiency can be responsible for something as subtle as foot drop. Vitamin B_{12} and/or thiamine deficiency have been associated with paresthesias and hyporeflexia.[66] Vitamin B_{12} deficiency has been associated with cognitive impairment, proprioceptive abnormalities, and depressed vibratory sense.[54] Functional assessment importantly complements neurologic testing and the physical examination for patients at high nutritional risk. Function tests such as the 30-second chair stand, the stair climb test, the 4 × 10 m fast-paced walk, the timed up-and-go test, and the 6-minute walk test can be used to assess physical function in patients with compromised nutritional status and to gauge improvement following implementation of nutrition therapy.[67]

PATIENTS WITH INITIAL SCREEN OF LOW PREDICTIVE VALUE

Patients whose initial screen is of low predictive value are those who are at low nutrition risk and have no red flags detected on historical or physical examination. Such patients have stable weight and oral intake. Additional testing is likely to be of low predictive value. These patients should have continued age-appropriate screening, routine preventive health measures, and should be given reinforcement regarding principles of healthy lifestyle. If a few positive findings are identified on patient history or physical examination (in the absence of high nutrition risk or overt signs of poor nutritional status), then more frequent screening should be considered. Clinicians need to scrutinize positive examination findings to see whether nonnutritional causes should be evaluated (eg, edema and heart failure).

PATIENTS WITH INITIAL SCREEN OF HIGH PREDICTIVE VALUE

Patients whose initial screen is of high predictive value are those determined to be at higher nutrition risk who should go on to have further evaluation as indicated. Such patients may be overweight or have obesity, be significantly underweight, or simply have been shown to have multiple red flags on initial examination. One of the difficult aspects of nutritional assessment is that there is no single test that evaluates comprehensive nutritional status. An important starting point in the subsequent evaluation of these patients is the dietary assessment, which can be used to detect inadequate intake, excessive food consumption, or imbalances with the ingestion of macronutrients (eg, low protein, high fat, high carbohydrates). Dietary records can be obtained in several different ways. Two common dietary assessments are the 24-hour recall and the 7-day diet record. Patients who perform a 24-hour recall are asked to recall the exact food and beverages they consumed in the previous 24-hour period. Although the benefits are that specific food portions are recalled, the drawbacks are that 1 day may not reflect true long-term eating patterns. Recall even after 1 day may be problematic. The 7-day diet record is prospective and does not rely on recall.

However, the act of self-monitoring (recording) may influence intake. Although this may be beneficial in obesity, it may be problematic in weight loss and undernutrition.[68]

With the advent of online and smartphone applications, monitoring programs have become available to more quickly and efficiently record dietary intake.[69,70] A recent study of a mobile phone application for dietary assessment showed that it was as effective as the 24-hour recall in estimating 24-hour energy intake.[70] A study involving subjects with obesity evaluated similar technology with or without feedback components compared with hand-written dietary logs.[71] Energy intake and measured WC were decreased in both technology groups, compared with the group randomized to hand-written dietary logs (suggesting that technologic advances increased accountability and improved success of the weight loss program).[71] In addition to being useful for management of weight loss in obesity, some of these applications can be used for patients with undernutrition to calculate the amount of macronutrients consumed. Because of the widespread availability of these technologies and access to the Internet, recording dietary intake using one of these novel tools can be valuable in patients who are both malnourished and have obesity. For those patients who do not have access to computer or phone applications, paper logs and recall can still be used.

Patients at high risk should have further laboratory testing. A basic panel of laboratory tests includes a complete blood count with differential, electrolytes (including calcium, phosphorus, and magnesium), blood urea nitrogen (BUN), creatinine, fasting glucose, lipid panel, albumin, prealbumin, transferrin, and liver enzymes. Although lacking sensitivity and specificity as a marker of nutritional status in most populations, albumin levels are predictive of morbidity and mortality in several surgical populations.[61,62,72] Low BUN levels can be suggestive of decreases in lean body mass, but are primarily used as a marker of renal function.[73,74] Anemia may reflect micronutrient deficiencies. Any disease state associated with low-grade inflammation will cause levels of acute phase proteins such as albumin and transferrin to be altered, making them less reliable.[61,75] Lipid levels, including total cholesterol and triglycerides, can be low in a malnourished state, or high in obesity.[76,77] Electrolyte shifts (potassium, phosphorus, magnesium) are seen when refeeding high-risk individuals.[78]

If the basic laboratory panel, patient history, or physical examination findings suggest increased nutritional risk (especially from the standpoint of poor nutritional status), then a process should be initiated to evaluate specific micronutrient deficiencies (**Table 2**). Depending on the findings and degree of risk, micronutrient levels that should be evaluated, including the fat-soluble vitamins (A, D, E, K), zinc, copper, selenium, iron, thiamine, vitamin B_{12}, folate, and iron. It is appropriate to order the entire panel on patients who are high risk. Clinicians may need to consult nutrition specialists about replacement strategies for some micronutrient or vitamin deficiencies, because repletion of stores may be complicated (eg, low therapeutic window of vitamin A). In addition, there are several different pharmaceutical preparations, such as microsphere-encapsulated fat-soluble vitamins or intramuscular injections, that may help facilitate delivery or absorption of the micronutrient.

Imaging and other measurement tools may be helpful in assessing body composition beyond what is provided by the basic anthropometric measurements. Handgrip dynometry and skin fold thickness are typically used for research purposes, but have little clinical applicability at this time. Because weight gain or loss alone may not accurately reflect changes in body compartments (eg, muscle), imaging tests can assist in the assessment of these patients.[79] Body composition studies can estimate loss of fat-free mass (FFM), which has been associated with sarcopenic obesity, decreased quality of life, and mortality.[80,81] The relationship between loss of FFM and

Table 2
Micronutrient panel

Micronutrient	Normal Range
Vitamin A retinoic acid	19–83 μg/dL
Vitamin D-25	30–60 ng/mL
Vitamin E alpha-tocopherol	3.0–15.8 mg/L
Vitamin K PT	9.3–11.2 s
Vitamin B_1 thiamine	9–44 ng/L (66–200 nmol/L)
Folate	3.0–16.0 ng/mL
Vitamin B_{12} cobalamin	211–946 pg/mL
Homocysteine Methylmalonic Acid (24 h Urine)	—
Vitamin B_6 pyridoxine	5–24 ng/mL (20–125 nmol/L)
Copper	70–155 μg/dL
Selenium	79–326 μg/L
Zinc	70–150 μg/dL
Manganese	79–336 μg/L
Serum Iron	50–212 μg/dL
% Iron Saturation	15%–55%
Ferritin	13–150 ng/mL
Biotin	221.0–3004.0 pg/mL

Abbreviation: PT, prothrombin time.

mortality has been documented in several patient populations involving cancer, older age, hemodialysis, and COPD.[81] Dual-energy x-ray absorptiometry (DXA) is an imaging modality commonly used for direct measurement of body composition.[80] DXA is often used to evaluate metabolic bone disease, but can be used for measurement of soft tissue compartments such as fat, muscle, and FFM.[81] Although DXA measurements are easily reproducible, some limitations to its use exist, such as low accessibility, x-ray exposure, high cost, and inability to be performed at bedside.[81]

Bioelectrical impedance analysis (BIA) is another modality used to determine body composition. Newer multifrequency BIA techniques have correlated well with DXA measurements.[82] In a study evaluating FFM in healthy adults, there was a small difference in FFM (4%) in DXA versus BIA.[83] It has been validated against DXA in several chronic disease states as well.[81] The advantages of BIA include that it is easy to use, noninvasive, has limited interobserver variation, and is fairly inexpensive.[78] Disadvantages of this technology include variations of measurement caused by hydration status (overhydration or dehydration) and that it has not been validated in patients with cancer.[78]

Computed tomography (CT) has also been used as an imaging modality to measure FFM. The CT assessment of FFM uses computerized software to acquire colorized quantification of fat, muscle, and other tissue compartments, standardized at the level of the third lumbar vertebra.[78] The software can be applied retrospectively to CT scans done previously on the patient.

SUMMARY

Evidence of deterioration of nutritional status can be subtle, especially in the setting of obesity. A modified and practical nutritional assessment can be performed by clinicians in an office-based practice. Recognition of red flags in both the history and physical examination can lead to targeted laboratory and imaging testing. Referral to a nutrition specialist may be required to assist in complex treatment strategies to replete nutrient stores. Failure to recognize early signs of a compromised nutritional state or to identify patients at high nutritional risk can lead to increased incidence of complications and adverse patient outcomes.

REFERENCES

1. Kiraly LN, McClave SA, Neel D, et al. Physician nutrition education. Nutr Clin Pract 2014;29(3):332–7.
2. Hurt RT, Frazier TH, McClave SA, et al. Obesity epidemic: overview, pathophysiology, and the intensive care unit conundrum. JPEN J Parenter Enteral Nutr 2011; 35(5 Suppl):4S–13S.
3. Flegal KM, Carroll MD, Kit BK, et al. Prevalence of obesity and trends in the distribution of body mass index among US adults, 1999-2010. JAMA 2012;307(5):491–7.
4. Kee AL, Isenring E, Hideman I, et al. Resting energy expenditure of morbidly obese patients using indirect calorimetry: a systematic review. Obes Rev 2012; 13(9):753–65.
5. White JV, Guenter P, Jensen G, et al. Consensus statement: Academy of Nutrition and Dietetics and American Society for Parenteral and Enteral Nutrition: characteristics recommended for the identification and documentation of adult malnutrition (undernutrition). JPEN J Parenter Enteral Nutr 2012;36(3):275–83.
6. Rahman A, Hasan RM, Agarwala R, et al. Identifying critically-ill patients who will benefit most from nutritional therapy: further validation of the "modified NUTRIC" nutritional risk assessment tool. Clin Nutr 2016;35(1):158–62.
7. Orell-Kotikangas H, Osterlund P, Saarilahti K, et al. NRS-2002 for pre-treatment nutritional risk screening and nutritional status assessment in head and neck cancer patients. Support Care Cancer 2015;23(6):1495–502.
8. Gur AS, Atahan K, Aladag I, et al. The efficacy of Nutrition Risk Screening-2002 (NRS-2002) to decide on the nutritional support in general surgery patients. Bratisl Lek Listy 2009;110(5):290–2.
9. Kondrup J, Rasmussen HH, Hamberg O, et al. Nutritional Risk Screening (NRS 2002): a new method based on an analysis of controlled clinical trials. Clin Nutr 2003;22(3):321–36.
10. Drescher T, Singler K, Ulrich A, et al. Comparison of two malnutrition risk screening methods (MNA and NRS 2002) and their association with markers of protein malnutrition in geriatric hospitalized patients. Eur J Clin Nutr 2010;64(8): 887–93.
11. Koren-Hakim T, Weiss A, Hershkovitz A, et al. Comparing the adequacy of the MNA-SF, NRS-2002 and MUST nutritional tools in assessing malnutrition in hip fracture operated elderly patients. Clin Nutr 2015. [Epub ahead of print].
12. Winter J, Flanagan D, McNaughton SA, et al. Nutrition screening of older people in a community general practice, using the MNA-SF. J Nutr Health Aging 2013; 17(4):322–5.
13. Sieber CC. Nutritional screening tools–how does the MNA compare? Proceedings of the session held in Chicago May 2-3, 2006 (15 Years of Mini Nutritional Assessment). J Nutr Health Aging 2006;10(6):488–92 [discussion: 492–84].
14. Rubenstein LZ, Harker JO, Salva A, et al. Screening for undernutrition in geriatric practice: developing the short-form mini-nutritional assessment (MNA-SF). J Gerontol A Biol Sci Med Sci 2001;56(6):M366–72.

15. Fereshtehnejad SM, Ghazi L, Sadeghi M, et al. Prevalence of malnutrition in patients with Parkinson's disease: a comparative study with healthy controls using Mini Nutritional Assessment (MNA) questionnaire. J Parkinsons Dis 2014;4(3): 473–81.

16. Hsu MF, Ho SC, Kuo HP, et al. Mini-Nutritional Assessment (MNA) is useful for assessing the nutritional status of patients with chronic obstructive pulmonary disease: a cross-sectional study. COPD 2014;11(3):325–32.

17. Gioulbasanis I, Georgoulias P, Vlachostergios PJ, et al. Mini nutritional assessment (MNA) and biochemical markers of cachexia in metastatic lung cancer patients: interrelations and associations with prognosis. Lung Cancer 2011;74(3): 516–20.

18. Vellas B, Guigoz Y, Garry PJ, et al. The mini nutritional assessment (MNA) and its use in grading the nutritional state of elderly patients. Nutrition 1999;15(2): 116–22.

19. Nourhashemi F, Guyonnet S, Ousset PJ, et al. Mini nutritional assessment and Alzheimer patients. Nestle Nutr Workshop Ser Clin Perform Programme 1999;1: 87–91 [discussion: 91–2].

20. de Luis DA, Lopez Mongil R, Gonzalez Sagrado M, et al. Evaluation of the Mini-Nutritional Assessment Short-Form (MNA-SF) among institutionalized older patients in Spain. Nutr Hosp 2011;26(6):1350–4.

21. Kaiser MJ, Bauer JM, Ramsch C, et al. Validation of the mini Nutritional Assessment Short-Form (MNA-SF): a practical tool for identification of nutritional status. J Nutr Health Aging 2009;13(9):782–8.

22. Prado CM, Cushen SJ, Orsso CE, et al. Sarcopenia and cachexia in the era of obesity: clinical and nutritional impact. Proc Nutr Soc 2016;75(2):188–98.

23. Newman AB, Yanez D, Harris T, et al. Weight change in old age and its association with mortality. J Am Geriatr Soc 2001;49(10):1309–18.

24. Sullivan DH, Martin W, Flaxman N, et al. Oral health problems and involuntary weight loss in a population of frail elderly. J Am Geriatr Soc 1993;41(7):725–31.

25. Brinkman HJ, de Pee S, Sanogo I, et al. High food prices and the global financial crisis have reduced access to nutritious food and worsened nutritional status and health. J Nutr 2010;140(1):153S–61S.

26. Klesges LM, Pahor M, Shorr RI, et al. Financial difficulty in acquiring food among elderly disabled women: results from the Women's Health and Aging Study. Am J Public Health 2001;91(1):68–75.

27. Fabricatore AN, Wadden TA, Higginbotham AJ, et al. Intentional weight loss and changes in symptoms of depression: a systematic review and meta-analysis. Int J Obes 2011;35(11):1363–76.

28. Ozsoy S, Besirli A, Unal D, et al. The association between depression, weight loss and leptin/ghrelin levels in male patients with head and neck cancer undergoing radiotherapy. Gen Hosp Psychiatry 2015;37(1):31–5.

29. Evans WJ, Morley JE, Argiles J, et al. Cachexia: a new definition. Clin Nutr 2008; 27(6):793–9.

30. Dewys WD, Begg C, Lavin PT, et al. Prognostic effect of weight loss prior to chemotherapy in cancer patients. Eastern Cooperative Oncology Group. Am J Med 1980;69(4):491–7.

31. de Matos-Neto EM, Lima JD, de Pereira WO, et al. Systemic inflammation in cachexia - is tumor cytokine expression profile the culprit? Front Immunol 2015; 6:629.

32. Barton BE. IL-6-like cytokines and cancer cachexia: consequences of chronic inflammation. Immunol Res 2001;23(1):41–58.

33. Cerami A. Tumor necrosis factor as a mediator of shock, cachexia and inflammation. Blood Purif 1993;11(2):108–17.
34. Ryan AM, Power DG, Daly L, et al. Cancer-associated malnutrition, cachexia and sarcopenia: the skeleton in the hospital closet 40 years later. Proc Nutr Soc 2016; 75(2):199–211.
35. Rolland Y, Onder G, Morley JE, et al. Current and future pharmacologic treatment of sarcopenia. Clin Geriatr Med 2011;27(3):423–47.
36. Kumpf VJ. Pharmacologic management of diarrhea in patients with short bowel syndrome. JPEN J Parenter Enteral Nutr 2014;38(1 Suppl):38S–44S.
37. Saarela RK, Lindroos E, Soini H, et al. Dentition, nutritional status and adequacy of dietary intake among older residents in assisted living facilities. Gerodontology 2016;33(2):225–32.
38. Marx W, Kiss N, McCarthy AL, et al. Chemotherapy-induced nausea and vomiting: a narrative review to inform dietetics practice. J Acad Nutr Diet 2016; 116(5):819–27.
39. Logemann JA, Curro FA, Pauloski B, et al. Aging effects on oropharyngeal swallow and the role of dental care in oropharyngeal dysphagia. Oral Dis 2013;19(8):733–7.
40. Achem SR, Devault KR. Dysphagia in aging. J Clin Gastroenterol 2005;39(5): 357–71.
41. Cooper C, Burden ST, Cheng H, et al. Understanding and managing cancer-related weight loss and anorexia: insights from a systematic review of qualitative research. J Cachexia Sarcopenia Muscle 2015;6(1):99–111.
42. Donini LM, Poggiogalle E, Piredda M, et al. Anorexia and eating patterns in the elderly. PLoS One 2013;8(5):e63539.
43. Morley JE. Anorexia of aging: physiologic and pathologic. Am J Clin Nutr 1997; 66(4):760–73.
44. Garber AK, Sawyer SM, Golden NH, et al. A systematic review of approaches to refeeding in patients with anorexia nervosa. Int J Eat Disord 2016;49(3):293–310.
45. Medici V, McClave SA, Miller KR. Common medications which lead to unintended alterations in weight gain or organ lipotoxicity. Curr Gastroenterol Rep 2015;18(1):2.
46. Hurt RT, Edakkanambeth Varayil J, Ebbert JO. New pharmacological treatments for the management of obesity. Curr Gastroenterol Rep 2014;16(6):394.
47. Tsai AG, Wadden TA. In the clinic: obesity. Ann Intern Med 2013;159(5):ITC3-1, ITC3-15; [quiz: ITC13–16] Available at: http://annals.org/article.aspx?article id=1733379.
48. Mueller KG, Hurt RT, Abu-Lebdeh HS, et al. Self-perceived vs actual and desired weight and body mass index in adult ambulatory general internal medicine patients: a cross sectional study. BMC Obes 2014;1:26.
49. Kuczmarski RJ, Flegal KM. Criteria for definition of overweight in transition: background and recommendations for the United States. Am J Clin Nutr 2000;72(5): 1074–81.
50. de Hollander EL, Van Zutphen M, Bogers RP, et al. The impact of body mass index in old age on cause-specific mortality. J Nutr Health Aging 2012;16(1):100–6.
51. Rankinen T, Kim SY, Perusse L, et al. The prediction of abdominal visceral fat level from body composition and anthropometry: ROC analysis. Int J Obes Relat Metab Disord 1999;23(8):801–9.
52. Chan JM, Rimm EB, Colditz GA, et al. Obesity, fat distribution, and weight gain as risk factors for clinical diabetes in men. Diabetes Care 1994;17(9):961–9.
53. Hirche TO, Hirche H, Jungblut S, et al. Statistical limitations of percent ideal body weight as measure for nutritional failure in patients with cystic fibrosis. J Cyst Fibros 2009;8(4):238–44.

54. Jensen GL, Binkley J. Clinical manifestations of nutrient deficiency. JPEN J Parenter Enteral Nutr 2002;26(5 Suppl):S29–33.
55. Lowe G, Woodward M, Rumley A, et al. Total tooth loss and prevalent cardiovascular disease in men and women: possible roles of citrus fruit consumption, vitamin C, and inflammatory and thrombotic variables. J Clin Epidemiol 2003; 56(7):694–700.
56. Zong G, Holtfreter B, Scott AE, et al. Serum vitamin B12 is inversely associated with periodontal progression and risk of tooth loss: a prospective Cohort Study. J Clin Periodontol 2016;43(1):2–9.
57. Millen AE. Adequate vitamin D status may prevent subsequent tooth loss. J Evid Based Dent Pract 2014;14(4):197–9.
58. Stoopler ET, Kuperstein AS. Glossitis secondary to vitamin B12 deficiency anemia. CMAJ 2013;185(12):E582.
59. Lehman JS, Bruce AJ, Rogers RS. Atrophic glossitis from vitamin B12 deficiency: a case misdiagnosed as burning mouth disorder. J Periodontol 2006;77(12): 2090–2.
60. Thongprasom K, Youngnak P, Aneksuk V. Folate and vitamin B12 levels in patients with oral lichen planus, stomatitis or glossitis. Southeast Asian J Trop Med Public Health 2001;32(3):643–7.
61. Giovannini I, Chiarla C, Giuliante F, et al. The relationship between albumin, other plasma proteins and variables, and age in the acute phase response after liver resection in man. Amino Acids 2006;31(4):463–9.
62. Kalender B, Mutlu B, Ersoz M, et al. The effects of acute phase proteins on serum albumin, transferrin and haemoglobin in haemodialysis patients. Int J Clin Pract 2002;56(7):505–8.
63. McLean RR, Mangano KM, Hannan MT, et al. Dietary protein intake is protective against loss of grip strength among older adults in the Framingham Offspring Cohort. J Gerontol A Biol Sci Med Sci 2016;71(3):356–61.
64. Windsor JA, Hill GL. Grip strength: a measure of the proportion of protein loss in surgical patients. Br J Surg 1988;75(9):880–2.
65. Chen LY, Liu LK, Hwang AC, et al. Impact of malnutrition on physical, cognitive function and mortality among older men living in veteran homes by minimum data set: a prospective Cohort Study in Taiwan. J Nutr Health Aging 2016; 20(1):41–7.
66. Latt N, Dore G. Thiamine in the treatment of Wernicke encephalopathy in patients with alcohol use disorders. Intern Med J 2014;44(9):911–5.
67. Russell MK. Functional assessment of nutrition status. Nutr Clin Pract 2015;30(2): 211–8.
68. Olendzki B, Hurley TG, Hebert JR, et al. Comparing food intake using the dietary risk assessment with multiple 24-hour dietary recalls and the 7-day dietary recall. J Am Diet Assoc 1999;99(11):1433–9.
69. Svensson A, Larsson C. A mobile phone app for dietary intake assessment in adolescents: an evaluation study. JMIR Mhealth Uhealth 2015;3(4):e93.
70. Rangan AM, O'Connor S, Giannelli V, et al. Electronic dietary intake assessment (e-DIA): comparison of a mobile phone digital entry app for dietary data collection with 24-hour dietary recalls. JMIR Mhealth Uhealth 2015;3(4):e98.
71. Burke LE, Conroy MB, Sereika SM, et al. The effect of electronic self-monitoring on weight loss and dietary intake: a randomized behavioral weight loss trial. Obesity (Silver Spring) 2011;19(2):338–44.
72. Slattery E, Patchett S. Albumin as a marker of nutrition: a common pitfall. Ann Surg 2011;254(4):667–8 [author reply: 668].

73. Shavit L, Lifschitz M, Galperin I. Influence of enteric nutrition on blood urea nitrogen (BUN) in very old patients with chronic kidney disease (CKD). Arch Gerontol Geriatr 2012;54(1):228–31.

74. Roggero P, Gianni ML, Morlacchi L, et al. Blood urea nitrogen concentrations in low-birth-weight preterm infants during parenteral and enteral nutrition. J Pediatr Gastroenterol Nutr 2010;51(2):213–5.

75. Nielsen OM, Thunedborg P, Jorgensen K. Albumin administration and acute phase proteins in abdominal vascular surgery. A randomised study. Dan Med Bull 1989;36(5):496–9.

76. Goichot B, Schlienger JL, Grunenberger F, et al. Low cholesterol concentrations in free-living elderly subjects: relations with dietary intake and nutritional status. Am J Clin Nutr 1995;62(3):547–53.

77. Feingold KR, Grunfeld C. Obesity and dyslipidemia. In: De Groot LJ, Beck-Peccoz P, Chrousos G, et al, editors. Endotext. South Dartmouth (MA): MDText.com, Inc; 2000.

78. Miller SJ. Death resulting from overzealous total parenteral nutrition: the refeeding syndrome revisited. Nutr Clin Pract 2008;23(2):166–71.

79. Mattar L, Godart N, Melchior JC, et al. Underweight patients with anorexia nervosa: comparison of bioelectrical impedance analysis using five equations to dual X-ray absorptiometry. Clin Nutr 2011;30(6):746–52.

80. Thibault R, Pichard C. The evaluation of body composition: a useful tool for clinical practice. Ann Nutr Metab 2012;60(1):6–16.

81. Thibault R, Genton L, Pichard C. Body composition: why, when and for who? Clin Nutr 2012;31(4):435–47.

82. Anderson LJ, Erceg DN, Schroeder ET. Utility of multifrequency bioelectrical impedance compared with dual-energy x-ray absorptiometry for assessment of total and regional body composition varies between men and women. Nutr Res 2012;32(7):479–85.

83. Leahy S, O'Neill C, Sohun R, et al. A comparison of dual energy x-ray absorptiometry and bioelectrical impedance analysis to measure total and segmental body composition in healthy young adults. Eur J Appl Physiol 2012;112(2):589–95.

Nutrition for the Prevention of Chronic Diseases

Ruth W. Kimokoti, MD, MA, MPH[a],*, Barbara E. Millen, DrPH, RD[b]

KEYWORDS

- Chronic • Diet • *Dietary Guidelines for Americans* • Dietary patterns • Lifestyle
- Noncommunicable diseases • Physicians • Prevention

KEY POINTS

- Chronic noncommunicable diseases (NCDs) are the leading cause of morbidity and mortality in the United States and globally.
- Suboptimal nutrition is the single leading modifiable cause of NCDs in the United States and globally.
- Healthy dietary and lifestyle patterns, as advocated in the 2015 to 2020 *Dietary Guidelines for Americans*, protect against NCDs.
- Physicians have a vital unique role in promoting a healthy lifestyle at both the individual and the population levels.

INTRODUCTION

Chronic noncommunicable diseases (NCDs) are the leading cause of morbidity and mortality in the United States and globally, accounting for 70% of all deaths worldwide,[1,2] and are a major priority for intervention by the United Nations and the World Health Organization (WHO).[3,4] They are projected to cost US$47 trillion over the next 20 years.[5] The NCD epidemic and concerning levels of their metabolic risk factors are driven by the nutrition transition as populations adopt Western-style lifestyles, including unhealthful dietary patterns, physical inactivity, tobacco use, and excess alcohol consumption.[6] Thus, international health experts have called for public policies and preventive interventions at both individual and population levels to reverse these trends and promote well-being.

Disclosure: The authors have no conflict of interest.
Dr B.E. Millen is President of Millennium Prevention, Inc, a life sciences company with a public health mission. It develops Web and mobile platforms on prevention including www.HealthMain.com and www.my.healthmain.com.
[a] Department of Nutrition, Simmons College, 300 The Fenway, Boston, MA 02115, USA;
[b] Millennium Prevention, Inc, PO Box 311, Westwood, MA 02090, USA
* Corresponding author.
E-mail address: ruth.kimokoti@simmons.edu

Med Clin N Am 100 (2016) 1185–1198
http://dx.doi.org/10.1016/j.mcna.2016.06.003
0025-7125/16/$ – see front matter © 2016 Elsevier Inc. All rights reserved.

In this report an overview is provided of NCDs and their modifiable risk factors, and the 2015 to 2020 *Dietary Guidelines for Americans* (DGAs),[7] the public policy framework that guides the far-reaching programs, services, and research priority areas of the US Departments of Health and Human Services (HHS) and Agriculture (USDA), is highlighted. The DGAs may considerably impact the US health care and public health systems, the National Institutes of Health, and Centers for Disease Control and Prevention, as well as the elaborate networks of school and community nutrition and health programs under HHS and USDA jurisdiction. There are also many opportunities for impact across sectors relating to food product formulation and food retail as well as the health- and wellness-related industries and the settings they influence, such as corporate and other work sites. Examined are the clinical applications of the DGAs and opportunities to promote prevention-oriented services and programs by physicians and other medical professionals in health care, public health, and community settings, including evidence-based Web and mobile technology. In addition, other recent expert guidelines are summarized on the prevention and management of obesity and the lifestyle management of cardiovascular disease (CVD) risk in the United States.

TRENDS IN CHRONIC DISEASE RATES AND LIFESTYLE FACTORS
Chronic Diseases

Globally, deaths due to chronic NCDs have increased by 42% in the last 2 decades.[1] In the United States, 117 million American men and women—about half of adults— have one or more NCDs and use 86% of health care expenditure[8] for hospitalizations and treatment. CVDs, diabetes, and lung, colorectal, breast, and prostate cancers disproportionately affect older individuals and minority populations.[8–10] Emerging NCDs of significance include osteoporosis and low bone mass, spina bifida without anencephaly, congenital heart defects, Alzheimer disease, and depression and are likewise commonest in minorities.[8]

Lifestyle Factors

Suboptimal nutrition ranks highest among lifestyle risk factors for NCDs globally and in the United States and has been identified as the most important preventable NCD risk factor.[11,12] Worldwide, despite increased overall intake of healthful foods during the last 2 decades, this was surpassed by higher consumption of less healthful foods.[13]

The 2015 Dietary Guidelines Advisory Committee (DGAC)[8] found that several nutrients, which it characterized as shortfall nutrients, were underconsumed in the United States; conversely, other nutrients were identified as overconsumed. When these nutrients could be linked to adverse health outcomes or prevalent metabolic risk factors, they were classified as *nutrients of public health concern*.

- Vitamins A, D, E, and C, folate, calcium, magnesium, fiber, and potassium are shortfall nutrients in the general population; iron is a shortfall nutrient among adolescent and premenopausal women.
- Calcium, vitamin D, fiber, and potassium are *underconsumed nutrients of public health concern*.
- Saturated fat and sodium are *overconsumed nutrients of public health concern*.

Consistent with the nutrient intake, most Americans have low intakes of key food groups that are important sources of the shortfall nutrients, including vegetables, fruits, whole grains, and dairy. In addition, they overconsume refined grains and added sugars. Consequently, overall dietary quality remains generally poor,[8,9,13,14] and

Americans score on average about 58% (of 100 points) on the Healthy Eating Index, a composite measure of nutritional quality that comprises total fruit, whole fruit, total vegetables, greens and beans, whole grains, dairy, total protein foods, seafood and plant proteins, fatty acids, refined grains, and sodium.[15]

Factors relating to dietary intakes and quality

Dietary intake in the healthy population varies by race/ethnicity, pregnancy status, age, sex, acculturation, and level of household food insecurity. Particularly vulnerable segments of the population with regard to low intakes of shortfall nutrients are African Americans and pregnant women, recent immigrant populations, and very young children (especially those in low-income households). In addition, individual and family behaviors known to influence dietary intake and quality include timing of food intake (eg, patterns of meals and snacks, meal and snack frequency), meal skipping, social and food environments, and sedentary behavior (such as TV viewing, computer and electronic device use, or driving). Experts recommend that these factors provide insight on ways to target the delivery of nutrition services and design interventions to improve nutrient intake and quality, particularly in vulnerable populations.[8]

Lifestyle factors tend to cluster together as well as with body mass index (BMI).[11,16–19] Concomitantly with unhealthful dietary intakes, sedentariness[6,20,21] and alcohol use have increased,[14,22] but smoking rates have declined[9,14,23] globally and in the United States. Physical activity has declined globally[24] but somewhat improved in the United States.[9,14] Overweight and obesity rates have risen and currently affect about one-third of adults globally[25] and more than two-thirds (68.5%) of adults in the United States.[26] In addition, more than half (54%) of US adults have abdominal obesity.[27,28] Given their association with other cardiometabolic risk factors (CMRFs; hypertension, dyslipidemia, hyperglycemia, insulin resistance), overweight and obesity are key priorities for both preventive measures and clinical treatment.[8,29] About 70% of overweight adults and 75% of those who have obesity have multiple CMRFs. Notably, even normal weight adults (approximately half) have at least one CMRF, attributable largely to poor diet and physical inactivity.[8] Physical inactivity and excess weight are most common in Hispanics and African Americans, with highest prevalence of obesity in African American women.[9,14,26]

According to the US Behavioral Risk Factor Surveillance System data,[30] just 7.7% of US adults have a low-risk lifestyle, defined by consuming fruits and vegetables 5 times or more a day, not smoking, engaging in physical activity, and BMI less than 25 kg/m^2. Women and whites are more likely to meet all 4 criteria, but their profiles are not optimal. Notably, the European Prospective Investigation into Cancer and Nutrition–Norfolk study[31] demonstrated a 14-year difference in life expectancy between individuals with 4 healthy lifestyle factors compared with those with fewer healthful behaviors. Promoting a healthy lifestyle is thus vital in achieving the 2015 to 2020 US Dietary Guidelines and the global Sustainable Development Goals, in particular, the target of reducing by one-third worldwide premature mortality from NCDs by 2030.[32] There is abundant evidence from epidemiologic studies showing moderate to strong relationships between dietary patterns and wide-ranging disease outcomes, and from randomized clinical trials (RCTs) on the efficacy of clinical interventions to reduce disease risk and adverse metabolic profiles.[7,8,29,33] Therefore, the DGAC and DGAs and other expert groups strongly advocated for a paradigm shift in public health and health care systems toward prevention with greater focus on healthy nutrition and other modifiable lifestyle behaviors.

GLOBAL GUIDELINES ON NUTRITION, HEALTH, AND CHRONIC DISEASE PREVENTION ACROSS THE LIFESPAN

In recognition of the importance of diet and related lifestyle factors in the cause of NCDs, the Food and Agriculture Organization and WHO issued expert dietary recommendations aimed at lowering disease risk by promoting healthy lifestyles across the lifespan.[34,35] They emphasize food-based rather than nutrient-based guidelines,[36] in particular, higher consumption of healthful foods. To supplement the scientific guidelines, countries publish food guides usually in the form of visual graphics, such as food pyramids or food plates to improve understanding and adoption of the recommendations.[36]

The USDA[37] in conjunction with the Department of HHS[38] led US policy development of the DGAs and its companion educational tool, *My Plate*. Since 1985, the DGAs have been informed by the science-based conclusions and recommendations of expert DGAC, which conduct thorough, independent, and transparent reviews of current scientific evidence on nutrition and health to be translated by USDA and HHS into the DGA public policies. As part of the 2015 DGAC process, high-quality literature on 5 major thematic areas was critically reviewed, including food and nutrient intakes and health; current status and trends; dietary patterns, foods and nutrients, and health outcomes; individual diet and physical activity behavior change; food environment and setting (to promote population level lifestyle behavior changes); and food sustainability and safety. Where there was sufficiently strong and consistent evidence on the relationships between dietary patterns and selected nutrients and wide-ranging health outcomes and the efficacy and effectiveness of nutrition interventions, the DGAC drew conclusions and made recommendations. Each of these statements was graded using recognized expert criteria on the quality of evidence. Where otherwise appropriate, the DGAC presented its original research findings and made relevant recommendations. The DGAC process and its conclusions and recommendations are extensively discussed in the Scientific Report of the DGAC (http://health.gov/dietaryguidelines/2015-scientific-report/).

2015–2020 DIETARY GUIDELINES FOR AMERICANS

The central messages of the 2015–2020 DGAs[7] are summarized as (http://health.gov/dietaryguidelines/2015/guidelines/):

- Follow a healthy eating pattern across the lifespan.
- Focus on variety, nutrient density, and amount.
- Limit calories from added sugars and saturated fats and reduce sodium intake.
- Shift to healthier food and beverage choices.
- Support healthy eating patterns for all.

These overall guidelines are complemented by key quantitative policy recommendations:

- Consume less than 10% of calories per day from added sugars.
- Consume less than 10% of calories per day from saturated fats.
- Consume less than 2300 mg per day of sodium.
- If alcohol is consumed, it should be consumed in moderation, up to 1 drink per day for women and up to 2 drinks per day for men, and only by adults of legal drinking age.
- Meet the *Physical Activity Guidelines for Americans*.

The 2015 to 2020 guidelines and recommendations are extensively discussed in the DGA policy document (http://health.gov/dietaryguidelines/2015/guidelines/). To understand these guidelines completely, it is important for clinicians to delve into the evidence base that supports the summary recommendations and to clarify details on how they can be applied in clinical settings to improve individual health.

EVIDENCE BASE ON NUTRITION AND PREVENTION OF MAJOR CHRONIC DISEASES AND DISABILITY

A major goal of the DGAC was to describe the common characteristics of healthy dietary patterns. Thus, the Committee focused primarily on evaluating overall dietary patterns, that is, the totality of food and nutrient intake, rather than specific nutrients or foods, and the evidence for the associations of such patterns with health outcomes. Dietary patterns are defined as "the quantities, proportions, variety or combinations of different foods and beverages in diets, and the frequency with which they are habitually consumed."[8] The methods used are extensively discussed in the DGAC report (http://health.gov/dietaryguidelines/2015-scientific-report/07-chapter-2/).[8] Differences in methodological approaches may complicate comparisons of studies and limit reproducibility. Nonetheless, given the strength of current evidence, the DGAC and DGAs emphasize dietary patterns in the development of expert, science-based recommendations to improve population diet and health.

Healthy Dietary Patterns

Common characteristics
Based on the totality of research, the DGAC identified the common characteristics of a healthy dietary pattern across wide-ranging health outcomes and recommended that individuals consume patterns that are rich in vegetables, fruit, whole grains, seafood, legumes, and nuts; moderate in low-fat and nonfat dairy products and alcohol (among adults); lower in red and processed meat; and low in sugar-sweetened foods and beverages and refined grains. Targets were also set to limit intakes of saturated fat, added sugars, and sodium. Three alternative dietary patterns were modeled to achieve these patterns of food intake and to be rich in essential nutrients, particularly those deemed to be of public health concern. The modeled patterns are presented in the DGAC report and detailed by calorie increments in the DGA (Composition of Healthy Patterns: http://health.gov/dietaryguidelines/2015-scientific-report/15-appendix-E3/e3-7.asp; Nutrients in the 3 USDA Food Patterns: http://health.gov/dietaryguidelines/2015-scientific-report/06-chapter-1/d1-10.asp#table-d1-33).

Types of patterns
The healthy patterns include the Healthy US–style Pattern (based on the Dietary Guidelines), the Healthy Mediterranean-style Patterns (take into account food group intakes from studies using a Med-diet index), and the Healthy Vegetarian Pattern (based on food choices of self-identified vegetarians). These patterns are higher in healthful foods and lower in less healthful foods as described above. The patterns were presented in the 2015 to 2020 DGAs as the basis for achieving the first 3 of the overall guidelines (http://health.gov/dietaryguidelines/2015/guidelines/). The DGAs also provide reference tables for each of the dietary patterns by 200-calorie increments (1000–3200 calories). Once an individual patient's calorie needs are determined, these patterns can be used for creating personalized nutrition interventions and implementing nutrition counseling and education programs that address the biological needs and preferences of individuals. Furthermore, they can be used to guide public health initiatives.

Association Between Dietary Patterns and Health Outcomes

The evidence base used by the DGAC to draw its conclusions and recommendations on the relationships between dietary patterns and health outcomes is derived from large prospective cohort studies in adults, RCTs, and systematic reviews of current high-quality literature using a combination of such studies (**Table 1**; Description of the dietary patterns: http://health.gov/dietaryguidelines/2015-scientific-report/07-chapter-2/d2-6.asp).[8]

Dietary patterns and cardiovascular diseases

Evidence from prospective cohort studies and RCTs consistently shows that greater adherence to Mediterranean-style patterns and US Dietary Guidelines–related patterns is associated with a lower risk for CVDs (22%–59% and 20%–44% lower risk, respectively).

Vegetarian dietary patterns may confer lower risk (12%–29%) for CVDs but evidence is limited.

Dietary patterns and body weight

Prospective cohort studies and RCTs provide strong evidence that healthy dietary patterns as part of a comprehensive lifestyle intervention result in weight loss and its maintenance. However, evidence for the association of healthy dietary patterns per se with healthy body weight and lower risk for developing overweight and obesity is moderate. RCTs demonstrate that levels of weight reduction of 4 to 12 kg can be achieved in the near term, up to 6 months, 4 to 10 kg up to 1 year, with clinically meaningful levels of 3 to 4 kg maintained over periods of up to 2 years. Although some weight regain occurs, the overall level of weight loss is sufficient to achieve important reductions in metabolic risk factors. For example, in the Diabetes Prevention Program trial, a moderate weight loss intervention with targets of 7% body weight loss over 6 months led to 58% decrease in development of diabetes over 3 to 4 years.[39] The American Heart Association/American College of Cardiology/The Obesity Society guidelines[29] report that a 5% weight loss in overweight adult individuals with varying metabolic risk factors is sufficient to achieve meaningful improvements in CVD risk factors (including blood pressure and lipids) and diabetes outcomes (such as fasting blood glucose and hemoglobin A1c levels). Weight losses of 2% to 5% have also been shown effective at improving fasting blood glucose levels in overweight and obese adults with type 2 diabetes.

Dietary patterns and type 2 diabetes

Prospective cohort studies and RCTs also provide moderately strong evidence of benefits of healthy dietary patterns and reductions in diabetes risk (21% lower risk vs 44% higher risk with an unhealthy pattern).

Dietary patterns and cancer

Scientific literature on the relationships between dietary patterns and cancer is most robust for the 4 most common malignancies in the United States: lung, breast, colon/rectal, and prostate. Evidence from prospective cohort studies and RCTs is moderately strong for colorectal cancer, postmenopausal breast cancer, and premenopausal breast cancer, and limited for lung cancer. The DGAC grade for prostate cancer was deemed not assignable based on current research evidence.

Dietary patterns and bone health

Limited evidence from prospective studies and RCTs suggests that healthy patterns may protect against fracture and osteoporosis as well as improve bone mineral density.

Table 1

Association of dietary patterns with overweight and obesity and priority noncommunicable diseases

Dietary Patterns	Overweight and Obesity		CVDs		Type 2 Diabetes		Diet-Related Cancers	
	Strength of Evidence	Conclusion	Strength of Evidence	Conclusion	Strength of Evidence	Conclusion	Strength of Evidence	Conclusion
A priori								
US Dietary Guidelines–related pattern HEI-2005[a]; HEI-2010[b] AHEI[c]; AHEI-2010[d] RFS[e]	Moderate	Beneficial	Strong	Beneficial	Moderate	Beneficial	Moderate Breast: postmenopausal	Beneficial
DASH[f]	Evidence not available		Strong	Beneficial	Moderate	Beneficial	Moderate Colon/rectal	Beneficial
Mediterranean-style patterns	Moderate	Beneficial	Strong	Beneficial	Moderate	Beneficial	Moderate Breast: postmenopausal Colon/rectal	Beneficial
A posteriori								
Healthy/prudent	Moderate	Beneficial	Evidence not available		Moderate	Beneficial	Moderate Breast: postmenopausal	Beneficial
Unhealthy/western	Moderate	Harmful	Evidence not available		Moderate	Harmful	Moderate Breast: postmenopausal	Harmful
Vegetarian	Evidence not available		Limited evidence		Evidence not available		Evidence not available	

[a] HEI-2005: Healthy Eating Index–2005.
[b] HEI-2010: Healthy Eating Index–2010.
[c] Alternate Healthy Eating Index (AHEI).
[d] Alternate Healthy Eating Index–2010 (AHEI-2010).
[e] RFS: Recommended Foods Score.
[f] DASH: Dietary Approaches to Stop Hypertension.
Data from Scientific report of the 2015 Dietary Guidelines Advisory Committee (advisory report). Available at: http://health.gov/dietaryguidelines/2015-scientific-report/. Accessed November 6, 2015.

Dietary patterns and congenital anomalies
Evidence is emerging, but data are limited. Case-control studies provide limited evidence that healthy maternal dietary patterns may confer benefits for neural tube defects in infants. For congenital heart defects, the DGAC grade was not assignable.

Dietary patterns and neurologic and psychological illnesses
There is limited evidence from prospective cohort studies and RCTs that healthy dietary patterns may lower risk of age-related cognitive impairment, dementia, and/or Alzheimer disease as well as depression in men and nonperinatal women.

Healthy dietary patterns can be achieved in many ways using the dietary pattern options discussed above (Composition of Healthy Patterns: http://health.gov/dietaryguidelines/2015-scientific-report/15-appendix-E3/e3-7.asp). The DGAC did reach consensus on the healthy dietary pattern characteristics across diverse outcomes as summarized above. The consistency of evidence is discussed in greater detail in the DGAC report.

STRATEGIES FOR CHRONIC DISEASE PREVENTION AND RISK REDUCTION AT INDIVIDUAL AND POPULATION LEVELS

The 2 main strategies for NCD prevention are the individual, including high-risk (clinical) interventions, and population approaches.[40] At the individual level, physicians should ideally work in multidisciplinary teams that include registered dietitians/nutritionists, behaviorists, exercise specialists, and/or other relevant providers to promote adoption of healthy eating patterns, smoking cessation or abstinence, moderate alcohol consumption if consumed (by adults), increased physical activity, and weight control.[10,29,33,41] Where appropriate, these interventions may combine pharmacotherapy and medical nutrition therapies and target people at high risk for chronic disease.

The DGAs emphasize that clinicians should personalize their approaches to nutrition and lifestyle interventions. This personalization entails working collaboratively with individual patients and clients to *tailor* dietary patterns and other behavioral approaches to the individual's biological needs, lifestyle characteristics, and personal preferences. It is important for clinicians to understand that the DGA recommendations for healthy dietary patterns are supported by a sufficiently strong evidence base to guide practice, particularly in light of RCTs, which demonstrate the efficacy and effectiveness of individual, preventive nutrition, lifestyle interventions, and counseling when implemented by professional multidisciplinary teams. Furthermore, the DGAC points out that individuals and populations may be motivated to adopt these healthy nutrition and lifestyle practices because healthier dietary patterns are additionally environmentally friendly. They contain food products whose production is more sustainable (that is, use fewer land, energy, and water resources and produce lower greenhouse gas emissions when produced in environmentally sound ways). More on these topics can be found in the DGAC report at http://health.gov/dietaryguidelines/2015-scientific-report/10-chapter-5/.

Regrettably, preventive nutrition and lifestyle modification for weight management and chronic disease risk reduction are not widely available in US health care and public health systems. Lack of preventive lifestyle interventions is due in part to insufficient training of health care providers in nutrition, limited reimbursement for nutrition counseling and prevention-oriented lifestyle interventions, and relatively few available multidisciplinary teams to provide comprehensive preventive care.

It is critical that recent expert guidelines on the Prevention and Management of Overweight and Obesity,[29] the Lifestyle Management of CVD,[33] and the US DGAs[7] call for a much greater focus on expanding clinical and public health services to promote healthy nutrition and lifestyle. Treatment guidelines include preventive lifestyle interventions across the lifespan to promote health and prevent disease as well as targeted intervention for those at high risk. In addition, population approaches advocate for healthy lifestyles in the general public for risk reduction. The combination of individual and population strategies has great potential to improve the health of the public.

Preventive Interventions at Individual Levels

Physicians play a vital role in the health of their patients; hence, they are uniquely positioned to help patients achieve a healthy lifestyle. It is important to note that physicians, nutritionists, and public health and other professionals are the intended primary audiences of the DGAs.[7] Accordingly, physicians need to take the lead particularly in promoting healthy lifestyles in their patients and making preventive services more widely accessible. In addition, their leadership roles are critical to making as many resources as possible available in their practice settings that make adoption of healthy lifestyle behaviors easier and normative, including healthy dietary patterns, physical activity, smoking abstinence, and alcohol moderation (if consumed by adults). This public health approach is advocated in the DGAs and other recent expert guidelines.

Comprehensive lifestyle intervention and nutrition counseling through a multidisciplinary approach to achieve and maintain a healthy weight are outlined in the guidelines for the management of overweight and obesity.[29] Most American adults meet the clinical guidelines to be candidates for clinical weight reduction intervention, based on excess weight status and concomitant CMRFs. It is also important to acknowledge that half or more of healthy weight American adults have at least 1 CMRF that would benefit from nutrition and lifestyle interventions that address poor diet and limited physical activity. It is recommended that primary care physicians (PCPs) assess and monitor patients' weight and lifestyle risk profiles, proactively provide counseling and education, or where applicable, refer patients for further preventive interventions and specialized management, such as medical nutrition therapy (MNT), intensive behavioral counseling, multidisciplinary intervention, and/or clinical obesity treatments.

- *Assessment* of risk profiles involves assessing weight status to determine presence of overweight or obesity followed by evaluation of other CMRFs.
- Regular *monitoring* of the risk factors is essential to assess need for further management.
- Physicians should assess a patient's readiness to make lifestyle changes and identify barriers to success. DGAs and other expert guidelines recommend that physicians *tailor* services and programs to the individual's biological and health needs, sociocultural preferences and profile, and lifestyle habits and refer to qualified professionals in their practice settings.
- For intervention to be truly *personalized* and targeted, *best practices* have clinicians conducting, or referring their patients for not only medical and health risk assessments and metabolic risk factor screening (biometric screening) but also comprehensive lifestyle risk assessments. These assessments provide a sound basis for prevention-oriented lifestyle interventions and disease management. In some settings, electronic health record systems have begun to incorporate and monitor such preventive components of patient care.
- Comprehensive lifestyle interventions are ideally offered on-site in the PCP's offices or practice settings by multidisciplinary teams; however, if these programs

are unavailable, experts recommend referral to a nutrition professional for dietary counseling, weight management, and MNT, as appropriate.

Use of Web and mobile health (m-health) and "wearable" technologies (pedometers, heart rate monitors, and others) are emerging areas that might potentially improve nutrition, dietary and weight-related and physical activity outcomes, and risk factor interventions. However, most of these advanced technologies, including mobile "apps" and "wearables," are neither validated nor sufficiently accurate for clinical settings. Physicians can guide their patients to sound resources and tools and caution the use of substandard technologies and "gadgets." HHS and USDA are anticipating the development of resources to complement their Web-based DGAs and the *MyPlate* framework. In addition, corporate health and wellness resource platforms are emerging, but, as yet, are largely information-based and incomplete in terms of evidence-based health risk assessment and monitoring tools.

Best practices would *similarly* have clinicians be aware of and use sound, evidence-based resources to guide disease prevention and health promotion activities in their clinical practice settings.

HealthMain (www.healthmain.com)[42] is an entirely evidence-based Web and mobile platform that is HIPAA-compliant and designed for clinician use with patients and clients. It provides a *Lifestyle GPS* in a secure "cloud" framework. HealthMain offers the research-driven resources for comprehensive lifestyle assessment and monitoring and interactive tools to support physician and health care professionals in providing their patients and clients with preventive interventions and disease management. The lifestyle risk assessment incorporates key demographic features, lifestyle assessment including food and beverage intake and nutrient profiles, physical activity, tobacco and alcohol use, and an array of other behavioral characteristics associated with health (seatbelt and helmet use, health and disease risk screening, stress and mental health, and so forth). Patients receive a *Personalized Lifestyle Profile* based on this comprehensive, evidence-based lifestyle and behavioral-oriented health risk assessment. The report pinpoints areas in which the individual has already met expert guideline benchmarks for health promotion and disease prevention and discusses where targeted and effective behavioral changes can be considered and made. Personalized lifestyle interventions can be guided by this tool and the accompanying additional Web and mobile reports and cloud-based resources. They will guide patients and health care professionals to the most effective, evidence-based strategies for lifestyle changes to promote better health outcomes and reduce disease risk profiles. The platforms also integrate tools to enhance communications between providers and their patients and to enable individuals to take greater control of their health by changing key lifestyle behaviors that are known to be associated with improved health outcomes and reduced chronic disease and metabolic profile risks.

Environmental Strategies to Promote Healthy Dietary Patterns and Lifestyle Behaviors

Effecting healthy nutrition and related lifestyle changes requires access to healthy and affordable foods. Thus, physicians, likewise, need to be leaders in advocating for environmental changes at the population level. *Best practices for population behavior change*, as described by the DAGC, are essentially environmental and policy approaches that complement efforts at individual patient and client levels such as improving access to and availability of healthy food in health care, public health and other community settings (such as schools, day care, and work sites), and retails outcomes, particularly in underserved neighborhoods. Multicomponent approaches are more effective than single-component interventions in improving dietary intakes and weight status.

An impediment to achieving individual and population level lifestyle changes consistent with the DGAC and DGAs is the lack in the US health system of preventive nutrition services that consider individual and social determinants of health. Nevertheless, physicians should attempt to become leaders in their health care environment and advocate that preventive services be made available to health care staff and other employees and that initiatives are mounted to improve environments there and locally to make adoption of healthy dietary patterns and physical activity more feasible.

SUMMARY AND RECOMMENDATIONS
Summary

- Approximately half of American adults, mainly minority and low-income populations, have multiple NCDs and use more than three-quarters of health care expenditure for treatment.
- Suboptimal nutrition is the leading cause of NCDs: calcium, vitamin D, fiber, and potassium are underconsumed nutrients of public health concern, whereas saturated fat and sodium are overconsumed nutrients of public health concern.
- The overall quality of the US population's dietary patterns is suboptimal. Low-income, minority and immigrant populations, pregnant women and children, particularly those in low-income households, are at particular risk of food insecurity and poor-quality dietary patterns.
- Sedentary behavior, physical activity, and alcohol use also show negative trends. Owing to clustering of lifestyle factors together and with BMI, overweight and obesity rates have increased substantially: only 7.7% of US adults have a low-risk lifestyle.
- The 2015 to 2020 DGAs recommend following a healthy eating pattern across the lifespan and regular physical activity to reduce risk of NCDs. The healthy dietary pattern is rich in vegetables, fruit, whole grains, seafood, legumes, and nuts; moderate in low-fat and nonfat dairy products and alcohol (among adults); lower in red and processed meat; and low in sugar-sweetened foods and beverages and refined grains; and lower in saturated fat, added sugars, and sodium. The DGAC and DGA modeled 3 dietary pattern options to achieve targeted food and nutrient goals.
- The DGAs emphasize the roles played by all, but particularly health care professionals, in creating "cultures of health" that make the adoption of healthy lifestyle behaviors easier for, and more normative among, individuals and community populations. They make adoption of preventive interventions and treatments for reducing disease risks much easier (DGAC 2015 Recommendations for action: http://health.gov/dietaryguidelines/2015-scientific-report/04-integration.asp).[8]
- Initiatives emphasized in the DGAs are complemented by those advocated in the Guidelines for Management and Treatment of Overweight and Obesity[29] and Lifestyle Management of Cardiovascular Disease[33] and are elaborated in other articles in this issue.

Recommendations

Physicians are well positioned to promote lifestyle preventive interventions for their patients by providing these multidisciplinary services or making referrals to professional experts and to advocate for environmental changes at the population level.

They can innovate with evidence-based Web and mobile applications to personalize nutrition and lifestyle preventative intervention. They can also take leadership roles toward shifting the paradigms in health care and public health toward a greater focus on prevention with a focus on effective, research-driven lifestyle changes.

REFERENCES

1. Global Burden of Disease Study 2013 Collaborators. Global, regional, and national incidence, prevalence, and years lived with disability for 301 acute and chronic diseases and injuries in 188 countries, 1990-2013: a systematic analysis for the Global Burden of Disease Study 2013. Lancet 2015;386:743–800.

2. GBD 2013 Mortality and Causes of Death Collaborators. Global, regional, and national age-sex specific all-cause and cause-specific mortality for 240 causes of death, 1990-2013: a systematic analysis for the Global Burden of Disease Study 2013. Lancet 2015;385:117–71.

3. United Nations. Political declaration of the high-level meeting of the general assembly on the prevention and control of non-communicable diseases. Available at: http://www.un.org/en/ga/ncdmeeting2011/index.shtml. Accessed November 6, 2015.

4. World Health Organization. Global action plan for the prevention and control of noncommunicable diseases 2013-2020. Available at: http://www.who.int/nmh/publications/en/. Accessed November 6, 2015.

5. Bloom DE, Cafiero ET, Jané-Llopis E, et al. The global economic burden of noncommunicable diseases. Geneva (Switzerland): World Economic Forum; 2011. Available at: http://www.weforum.org/reports/global-economic-burden-non-communicable-diseases. Accessed November 6, 2015.

6. Shetty P, Schmidhuber J, UN Department of Economic and Social Affairs. Expert paper No. 2011/3. Nutrition, lifestyle, obesity and chronic disease. New York: United Nations; 2011. Available at: http://www.un.org/en/development/desa/population/publications/expert/index.shtml. Accessed November 8, 2015.

7. U.S. Department of Health and Human Services and U.S. Department of Agriculture. 2015–2020 Dietary guidelines for Americans. 8th edition. 2015. Available at: http://health.gov/dietaryguidelines/2015/guidelines/. Accessed January 10, 2016.

8. Scientific Report of the 2015 Dietary Guidelines Advisory Committee (Advisory Report). Available at: http://health.gov/dietaryguidelines/2015-scientific-report/. Accessed November 6, 2015.

9. Mozaffarian D, Benjamin EJ, Go AS, et al. Heart disease and stroke statistics—2016 update: a report from the American Heart Association. Circulation 2016; 133:e38–360.

10. Kushi LH, Doyle C, McCullough M, et al. American Cancer Society Guidelines on nutrition and physical activity for cancer prevention: reducing the risk of cancer with healthy food choices and physical activity. CA Cancer J Clin 2012;62:30–67.

11. GBD 2013 Risk Factors Collaborators. Global, regional, and national comparative risk assessment of 79 behavioural, environmental and occupational, and metabolic risks or clusters of risks in 188 countries, 1990-2013: a systematic analysis for the Global Burden of Disease Study 2013. Lancet 2015;386:2287–323.

12. Marczak L, O'Rourke K, Shepard D. When and why people die in the United States, 1990-2013. JAMA 2016;315:241.

13. Imamura F, Micha R, Khatibzadeh S, et al. Dietary quality among men and women in 187 countries in 1990 and 2010: a systematic assessment. Lancet Glob Health 2015;3:e132–42.

14. National Center for Health Statistics. Health, United States, 2014: with special feature on adults aged 55–64. Hyattsville (MD); 2015. Available at: http://www.cdc.gov/nchs/hus.htm. Accessed November 6, 2015.

15. Guenther PM, Kirkpatrick SI, Reedy J, et al. The Healthy Eating Index-2010 is a valid and reliable measure of diet quality according to the 2010 Dietary Guidelines for Americans. J Nutr 2014;144:399–407.

16. Kimokoti RW, Newby PK. Dietary patterns, smoking, and cardiovascular diseases: a complex association. Curr Nutr Rep 2013;2:113–25.

17. Chiolero A, Faeh D, Paccaud F, et al. Consequences of smoking for body weight, body fat distribution, and insulin resistance. Am J Clin Nutr 2008;87:801–9.

18. Noble N, Paul C, Turon H, et al. Which modifiable health risk behaviours are related? A systematic review of the clustering of Smoking, Nutrition, Alcohol and Physical activity ('SNAP') health risk factors. Prev Med 2015;81:16–41.

19. Leech RM, McNaughton SA, Timperio A. The clustering of diet, physical activity and sedentary behavior in children and adolescents: a review. Int J Behav Nutr Phys Act 2014;11:4.

20. Church TS, Thomas DM, Tudor-Locke C, et al. Trends over 5 decades in U.S. occupation-related physical activity and their associations with obesity. PLoS One 2011;6:e19657.

21. Bassett DR, John D, Conger SA, et al. Trends in physical activity and sedentary behaviors of United States youth. J Phys Act Health 2015;12:1102–11.

22. WHO. Global status report on alcohol and health 2014. Geneva: World Health Organization; 2014. Available at: http://www.who.int/substance_abuse/publications/global_alcohol_report/en/. Accessed November 8, 2015.

23. Ng M, Freeman MK, Fleming TD, et al. Smoking prevalence and cigarette consumption in 187 countries, 1980-2012. JAMA 2014;311:183–92.

24. Hallal PC, Andersen LB, Bull FC, et al. Global physical activity levels: surveillance progress, pitfalls, and prospects. Lancet 2012;380:247–57.

25. Ng M, Fleming T, Robinson M, et al. Global, regional, and national prevalence of overweight and obesity in children and adults during 1980-2013: a systematic analysis for the Global Burden of Disease Study 2013. Lancet 2014;384:766–81.

26. Ogden CL, Carroll MD, Kit BK, et al. Prevalence of childhood and adult obesity in the United States, 2011-2012. JAMA 2014;311:806–14.

27. Ford ES, Maynard LM, Li C. Trends in mean waist circumference and abdominal obesity among US adults, 1999-2012. JAMA 2014;312:1151–3.

28. Kimokoti RW, Newby PK, Gona P, et al. Patterns of weight change and progression to overweight and obesity differ in men and women: implications for research and interventions. Public Health Nutr 2013;16:1463–75.

29. Jensen MD, Ryan DH, Apovian CM, et al. 2013 AHA/ACC/TOS guideline for the management of overweight and obesity in adults: a report of the American College of Cardiology/American Heart Association Task Force on Practice Guidelines and The Obesity Society. Circulation 2014;129(25 Suppl 2):S102–38.

30. Ford ES, Li C, Zhao G, et al. Trends in low-risk lifestyle factors among adults in the United States: findings from the Behavioral Risk Factor Surveillance System 1996-2007. Prev Med 2010;51:403–7.

31. Khaw KT, Wareham N, Bingham S, et al. Combined impact of health behaviours and mortality in men and women: the EPIC-Norfolk prospective population study. PLoS Med 2008;5:e12.

32. UN Department of Economic and Social Affairs. Sustainable Development Goals. Available at: https://sustainabledevelopment.un.org/sdgs. Accessed November 6, 2015.

33. Eckel RH, Jakicic JM, Ard JD, et al. 2013 AHA/ACC guideline on lifestyle management to reduce cardiovascular risk: a report of the American College of Cardiology/American Heart Association Task Force on Practice Guidelines. Circulation 2014;129(25 Suppl 2):S76–99.

34. WHO. Diet, nutrition and the prevention of chronic diseases: report of the joint WHO/FAO Expert Consultation. WHO Technical Report Series, No. 916 (TRS 916). World Health Organization; 2003. Available at: http://www.who.int/nutrition/publications/nutrientrequirements/en/. Accessed November 8, 2015.

35. Nishida C, Uauy R, Kumanyika S, et al. The joint WHO/FAO expert consultation on diet, nutrition and the prevention of chronic diseases: process, product and policy implications. Public Health Nutr 2004;7:245–50. Available at: http://www.who.int/nutrition/publications/nutrientrequirements/en/. Accessed November 8, 2015.

36. FAO. Food-based dietary guidelines. Available at: http://www.fao.org/nutrition/education/food-dietary-guidelines/home/en/. Accessed November 8, 2015.

37. USDA. Center for Nutrition Policy and Promotion. Dietary Guidelines. Available at: http://www.cnpp.usda.gov/dietaryguidelines/. Accessed November 6, 2015.

38. U.S. Department of Health and Human Services. Dietary Guidelines. Available at: http://health.gov/dietaryguidelines/. Accessed November 6, 2015.

39. Knowler WC, Barrett-Connor E, Fowler SE, et al. Reduction in the incidence of type 2 diabetes with lifestyle intervention or metformin. N Engl J Med 2002;346: 393–403.

40. WHO. Global status report on noncommunicable diseases 2010. World Health Organization; 2011. Available at: http://www.who.int/nmh/publications/en/. Accessed November 6, 2015.

41. American Diabetes Association. Standards of medical care in diabetes—2016. Available at: http://professional.diabetes.org/content/clinical-practice-recommendations/?loc=rp-slabnav. Accessed November 8, 2015.

42. HealthMain. Available at: https://www.healthmain.com/. Accessed November 8, 2015.

Nutrition Recommendations in Pregnancy and Lactation

Michelle A. Kominiarek, MD, MS*, Priya Rajan, MD

KEYWORDS

- Nutrition • Pregnancy • Lactation • Gestational weight gain

KEY POINTS

- Energy, macronutrient, and micronutrient requirements increase during both pregnancy and lactation.
- Gestational weight gain goals vary according to the prepregnancy body mass index. Weight gain within the recommended guidelines is associated with improved perinatal outcomes.
- Special attention is required in the nutritional management of multiple gestations, obesity, and pregnancies after bariatric surgery.

INTRODUCTION

Nutrition counseling is a cornerstone of prenatal care for all women during pregnancy. A woman's nutritional status not only influences her health but also pregnancy outcomes and the health of her fetus-neonate. Physicians and other health care providers need to be cognizant of nutritional needs during pregnancy because they differ significantly compared with nonpregnant populations. Furthermore, an individualized approach to nutritional counseling that considers a woman's access to food, socioeconomic status, race-ethnicity and cultural food choices, and body mass index (BMI) is recommended. In addition, many of the recommendations are geared for uncomplicated pregnancies, so adjustments need to be made when complications, such as gestational diabetes, arise. A nutritionist or registered dietitian can help facilitate dietary counseling and interventions. In this article, the maternal physiologic adaptations

The authors have no conflicts of interest related to the material in this article to disclose.
This work was supported by the Eunice Kennedy Shriver National Institute of Child Health & Human Development of the National Institutes of Health under award number K23HD076010 (M.A. Kominiarek).
Division of Maternal-Fetal Medicine, Department of Obstetrics and Gynecology, Northwestern University Feinberg School of Medicine, 250 East Superior Street, Suite 05-2175, Chicago, IL 60611, USA
* Corresponding author.
E-mail address: mkominia@nm.org

as well as macronutrient and micronutrient requirements during pregnancy and lactation are reviewed. Other discussions on these topics include multiple gestations, obesity in pregnancy, pregnancies after bariatric surgery, special diets, and common exposures during pregnancy.

PREGNANCY
Energy Expenditure During Pregnancy

Caloric intake should increase by approximately 300 kcal per day during pregnancy. This value is derived from an estimate of 80,000 kcal needed to support a full-term pregnancy and accounts not only for increased maternal and fetal metabolism but for fetal and placental growth. Dividing the gross energy cost by the mean pregnancy duration (250 days after the first month) yields the 300 kcal per day estimate for the entire pregnancy.[1,2] However, energy requirements are generally the same as nonpregnant women in the first trimester and then increase in the second trimester, estimated at 340 kcal and 452 kcal per day in the second and third trimesters, respectively. Furthermore, energy requirements vary significantly depending on a woman's age, BMI, and activity level. Caloric intake should, therefore, be individualized based on these factors.

Laboratory Testing During Pregnancy

Physiologic changes during pregnancy alter the normal ranges of several laboratory values. Both total red blood cell mass and plasma volume increase, but plasma volume increases to a greater extent, resulting in hemodilution and anemia during pregnancy. Consequently, a hemoglobin less than 10.5 g/dL or a hematocrit less than 32% is considered anemic during the second trimester (**Table 1**). Serum total protein and albumin also decrease by approximately 30% compared with nonpregnant values.[3] Additionally, because estrogen increases the hepatic production of certain proteins, there is greater protein binding of corticosteroids, sex steroids, thyroid hormones, and vitamin D during pregnancy, resulting in lower free levels.

Nutrients

Macronutrients
Recommended protein intake during pregnancy is 60 g per day, which represents an increase from 46 g/d in nonpregnant states. This increase reflects a change to 1.1 g of protein/kg/d during pregnancy from 0.8 g of protein/kg/d for nonpregnant states.[2] Carbohydrates should make up 45% to 64% of daily calories and this includes approximately 6 to 9 servings of whole grain daily. Total fat intake should make up 20% to 35% of daily calories, similar to nonpregnant women.

Micronutrients
The recommendations for daily micronutrient intake for a pregnant woman are determined by the Recommended Dietary Allowance (RDA) data. In general, RDA refers to

Table 1 Definitions of anemia during pregnancy		
Trimester	Hemoglobin (g/dL)	Hematocrit (%)
First	<11.0	<33
Second	<10.5	<32
Third	<11.0	<33
Normal values for nonpregnant women	12.1–15.1	37–48

the levels of intake of essential nutrients that are judged by the Food and Nutrition Board of the Institute of Medicine (IOM) to be adequate to meet the known nutrient needs of practically all healthy persons. The RDAs have been modified for pregnant women. **Table 2** shows the dietary allowances for most vitamins and minerals during pregnancy (see later discussion).

A daily prenatal multivitamin is generally recommended before conception and during pregnancy. **Table 3** describes the typical composition of a prenatal vitamin. The critical difference compared with other multivitamins is the folic acid dose, which is necessary to support rapid cell growth, cell replication, cell division, and nucleotide synthesis for fetal and placental development. Although there are data to support additional folic acid and iron supplementation during pregnancy, there is no high quality evidence demonstrating that all women require the increased levels of nutrients in a prenatal vitamin.

Folic acid is the synthetic form of the naturally occurring B vitamin, folate. Folic acid is the form used in most vitamin supplements and food fortification. As mandated by the Food and Drug Administration (FDA), commonly fortified foods include bread, cereal, and pasta. Folate-rich food sources are citrus fruits, dark-green leafy vegetables, nuts, and liver. Folate requirements increase during pregnancy as a result of rapidly dividing cells related to fetal growth. Notably, folic acid supplements (400–800 µg daily) taken before conception can reduce the risk for neural tube defects in the fetus.[4] Since the FDA mandate, blood folate levels have increased and neural tube defects have declined.[4] To reduce the risk for neural tube defects in their offspring, it is recommended that women take folic acid from fortified food or daily supplements in addition to consuming a diet rich in food sources of folate.[5] Women with a history of a neural tube defect in a prior pregnancy should take a higher dose (4 mg) of folic acid daily for subsequent pregnancies. Deficiencies in folate have

Table 2
Recommended daily dietary allowances for pregnant and lactating women

Nutrient	Nonpregnant	Pregnant[a]	Lactation[a]
Vitamin A (µg/d)	700	770	1300
Vitamin D (µg/d)	5	15	15
Vitamin E (mg/d)	15	15	19
Vitamin K (µg/d)	90	90	90
Folate (µg/d)	400	600	500
Niacin (mg/d)	14	18	17
Riboflavin (mg/d)	1.1	1.4	1.6
Thiamine (mg/d)	1.1	1.4	1.4
Vitamin B_6 (mg/d)	1.3	1.9	2
Vitamin B_{12} (µg/d)	2.4	2.6	2.8
Vitamin C (mg/d)	75	85	120
Calcium (mg/d)	1000	1000	1000
Iron (mg/d)	18	27	9
Phosphorus (mg/d)	700	700	700
Selenium (µg/d)	55	60	70
Zinc (mg/d)	8	11	12

[a] Applies to women older than 18 years old.
Data from Otten JJ, Pitzi Hellwig J, Meyers LD, editors. Dietary reference intakes. The essential guide to nutrient requirements. Washington, DC: National Academies Press; 2006.

Table 3
Typical composition of micronutrients in a prenatal vitamin

Component	Amount	% Daily Value for Pregnant and Lactating Women
Vitamin A	4000 IU as beta carotene	50
Vitamin D$_3$	400 IU as cholecalciferol	100
Vitamin E	11 IU as dl-alpha-tocopheryl acetate	37
Folic acid	800 µg	100
Niacin	18 mg as niacinamide	90
Riboflavin	1.7 mg as thiamine mononitrate	85
Thiamine	1.5 mg	88
Vitamin B$_6$	2.6 mg as pyridoxine hydrochloride	104
Vitamin B$_{12}$	4 µg as cyanocobalamin	50
Vitamin C	100 mg as ascorbic acid	167
Calcium	150 mg as calcium carbonate	12
Iron	27 mg as ferrous fumarate	150
Zinc	25 mg as zinc oxide	167

been associated with megaloblastic anemia in pregnancy, though not with other pregnancy outcomes such as preterm birth or stillbirths.[6]

Iron supplements have routinely been recommended in pregnancy because iron needs nearly double during pregnancy. A standard prenatal vitamin contains 27 mg of elemental iron. Vitamin C supplements can assist with iron absorption, whereas milk and tea can inhibit iron supplementation. Women with iron deficiency, defined by a ferritin level less than 15 µg/L, can increase their hemoglobin by 2 g/dL over a 1 month period with a daily replacement of 60 to 120 mg of elemental iron. Common side effects of iron, such as stomach pain, constipation, nausea, and vomiting, are often reasons why women are not compliant with iron supplementation. Iron-rich foods include red meat, pork, fish, and eggs.

Vitamin D is a fat-soluble vitamin that is primarily found in fortified milk or juice; natural sources include eggs and fish such as salmon. The skin also manufactures vitamin D when it is exposed to sunlight. Regardless of the source, oral ingestion or skin absorption, further processing in the liver and then the kidney is required to create the active form, 1,25-dihydroxyvitamin D, which promotes calcium absorption from the intestines and thereby allows appropriate bone mineralization and growth. Vitamin D deficiency is common in pregnancy, especially in high-risk groups such as vegetarians, women who live in cold climates, and ethnic minority women with darker skin. Severe vitamin D deficiency has been associated with congenital rickets and fractures, but this is less common in the United States. Although vitamin D levels can be measured via a serum level of 25-hydroxy vitamin D, an optimal level during pregnancy has not been established. Furthermore, there is insufficient evidence to recommend screening all pregnant women for vitamin D deficiency. If vitamin D deficiency is discovered during pregnancy, supplements (1000–2000 IU per day) can be given.[7] Routine vitamin D supplementation during pregnancy to prevent preeclampsia is also not recommended.[8]

Vitamin A is essential for cell differentiation and proliferation, as well as development of the spine, heart, eyes, and ears. Offspring of mothers with vitamin A deficiency, which is rare in the United States, have a higher mortality rate, which may be associated with decreased immune function. Although most micronutrients have a wide safety margin with little concern for teratogenic effects, vitamin A is one exception.[9] Excessive doses of vitamin A (>10,000 IU/d) have been associated with cranial-facial (face, palate, ears) and cardiac birth defects. The maximal supplement in pregnancy is 8000 IU per day. It is the retinol form of vitamin A that is associated with teratogenic effects, not the carotenoid version found in food sources such as carrots.

Studies regarding the risks and benefits of fish during pregnancy can often seem contradictory.[10] This is in part because most fish contain competing benefits and risks in the forms of omega-3 fatty acids and mercury.[11,12] Omega-3 fatty acids are critical for fetal brain development and have been associated with improved vision in preterm infants, as well as better cardiovascular health later in life.[13] Higher mercury levels in children, however, have been associated with deficits in memory, learning, and behavior.[14] Ideally, pregnant women would consume those fish that are low in mercury and high in omega-3 fatty acids such as salmon, sardines, and anchovies (**Box 1**). High mercury fish such as shark, swordfish, tilefish, and king mackerel should be avoided. FDA and the Environmental Protection Agency Web sites offer information regarding local fish and their mercury content.[15] Available data suggest that fish-oil supplements do not confer the same health benefits as consumption of the actual fish.[16]

Gestational Weight Gain

Pregnancy has traditionally been considered a time for weight gain, not weight loss. The obligatory weight gain during pregnancy is approximately 8 kg, which accounts for the fetus, the placenta, amniotic fluid volume, and adaptations to maternal tissues (eg, uterus, breast, blood volume). A weight gain less than this amount implies that existing maternal adipose and protein stores would be mobilized to support the pregnancy. Metabolic changes of women who lose weight during pregnancy are not well described, but ketonemia, increased urinary nitrogen excretion, and decreased gluconeogenic amino acid production result after a period of fasting during pregnancy.[17] Pregnancy is often considered a time of accelerated starvation due to the increase in insulin resistance, with an increased risk for developing ketonuria and ketonemia.[18] This physiologic change is important to consider in the setting of weight loss during pregnancy because maternal ketonemia or ketonuria may subsequently be associated with abnormal fetal growth or later neurocognitive development.[19–21]

A woman's prepregnancy BMI determines the total amount of weight gain and rate of weight gain during pregnancy (**Table 4**).[22] Of note, the guidelines on gestational weight gain that IOM published in 2009 differ from their original 1990 recommendations in that women with a prepregnancy BMI greater than or equal to 30 kg/m² should gain 5 to 9 kg or 11 to 20 lb during pregnancy.[22,23] Women who are overweight or obese have lower ranges for recommended total gestational weight gain compared with women of normal weight, yet greater than 50% of all women exceed the gestational weight gain recommendations.[24] The IOM 2009 guidelines also recommend

Box 1
Fish to avoid during pregnancy and lactation
Shark
Swordfish
Tilefish
King Mackerel

Table 4
Gestational weight gain recommendations

Prepregnancy BMI	Total Weight Gain at Term	Rate of Weight Gain in the 2nd and 3rd Trimester; Mean (Range)
Underweight (<18.5 kg/m^2)	12.5–18 kg 28–40 lb	0.51 (0.44–0.58) kg/wk 1 (1–1.3) lb/wk
Normal weight (18.5–24.9 kg/m^2)	11.5–16 kg 25–35 lb	0.42 (0.35–0.50) kg/wk 1 (0.8–1) lb/wk
Overweight (25.0–29.9 kg/m^2)	7–11.5 kg 15–25 lb	0.28 (0.23–0.33) kg/wk 0.6 (0.5–0.7) lb/wk
Obesity (≥30.0 kg/m^2)	5–9 kg 11–20 lb	0.22 (0.17–0.27) kg/wk 0.5 (0.4–0.6) lb/wk

Data from Institute of Medicine. Weight gain during pregnancy: reexamining the guidelines. Washington, DC: Institute of Medicine; 2009.

that women should conceive at a normal weight so as to achieve optimal maternal and neonatal outcomes.[22] One study found that women who gain weight in the appropriate range for their BMI during pregnancy have fewer adverse perinatal outcomes than those gaining more than the described thresholds.[25]

Special Considerations

Multiple gestations

In twins, the maternal metabolic rate is approximately 10% greater than in single-tons.[26] Furthermore, the physiologic changes in a singleton pregnancy are exacerbated in multiple gestations. This includes an increase in plasma volume, which results in further decreases in hemoglobin, albumin, and water-soluble vitamins.[27] There are no standardized nutritional guidelines for multiple gestations, but they have been inferred from singletons. One recommendation for macronutrient composition is 20% protein, 40% fat, and 40% carbohydrates.[28,29] It is estimated that a 40% higher-calorie diet may maintain a woman's nutritional state during a twin pregnancy. Rates of iron deficiency anemia are 2.4 to 4 times higher in twins than in single-tons.[28] Anemia due to folate deficiency is 8 times more common in twins compared with singletons.[27] As such, a 1 mg folic acid daily supplement has been recommended for twin gestations.[30] Some experts recommend 1000 IU/d of vitamin D and 2000 to 2500 mg/d of calcium for twins.[28] Multiple gestations have a higher risk of complications such as premature birth and low birth weight. The IOM 2009 guidelines for gestational weight gain in twin gestations are presented in **Table 5**. Of note, these guidelines are considered provisional because the evidence to support them is not as strong as it is for singletons. Interestingly, a weight gain of 24 pounds by 24 weeks has been associated with higher rates of birth weights greater than 2500 g.[31,32] Evidence for nutritional management of higher order multiples (eg, triplets, quadruplets) is lacking, but they can be managed similarly to twin gestations.

Obesity

The World Health Organization and the National Institutes of Health define normal weight as a BMI of 18.5 to 24.9 kg/m^2, overweight as a BMI of 25 to 29.9 kg/m^2, and obesity as a BMI of 30 kg/m^2 or greater. Obesity is further categorized by BMI into class I (30–34.9 kg/m^2), class II (35–39.9 kg/m^2), and class III or extreme obesity (≥40 kg/m^2).[33,34] Trends in adult weight over the past couple of decades highlight the escalating role that obesity plays in women's health; 31.8% of reproductive age women (20–39 years) had obesity in 2011 to 2012.[35] Women with a higher

Table 5 Gestational weight gain recommendations for twins	
Prepregnancy BMI	**Total Weight Gain at Term**
Underweight (<18.5 kg/m²)	17–25 kg 37–54 lb
Normal weight (18.5–24.9 kg/m²)	17–25 kg 37–54 lb
Overweight (25.0–29.9 kg/m²)	14–23 kg 31–50 lb
Obesity (≥30.0 kg/m²)	11–19 kg 25–42 lb

Data from Institute of Medicine. Weight gain during pregnancy: reexamining the guidelines. Washington, DC: Institute of Medicine; 2009.

prepregnancy BMI have a greater risk for adverse perinatal outcomes.[36,37] These include both maternal complications such as gestational diabetes, pregnancy-related hypertension, and cesarean deliveries along with adverse fetal effects such as birth defects, stillbirth, and abnormal fetal growth (**Table 6**). As such, weight loss before pregnancy is strongly recommended to reduce the risk of these complications.[38]

Guidelines for the management of obesity during pregnancy differ among countries. Practices endorsed by the American Congress of Obstetricians and Gynecologists are listed below[38]:

- Gestational weight gain recommendations should be individualized by the BMI at the first prenatal visit and based on the IOM 2009 guidelines (11–20 lb).
- Early screening for glucose intolerance (gestational diabetes or overt diabetes) is recommended. If the initial early diabetes screening result is negative repeat diabetes screening generally is performed at 24 to 28 weeks of gestation.
- Behavioral interventions using changes to diet and exercise can improve postpartum weight reduction in contrast to exercise alone.

With respect to health behavior interventions, randomized and nonrandomized studies of interventions to promote optimal gestational weight gain have emphasized combinations of dietary counseling, weight monitoring, and exercise programs. Although a few studies have shown a reduction in gestational weight gain for women with obesity after exposure to a health behavior intervention, most have found no benefit. For example, in one study in which women were randomized to a low glycemic index diet, most women with obesity exceeded the gestational weight gain goals

Table 6 Risks of obesity in pregnancy		
During Pregnancy	**During Labor & Delivery**	**Postpartum Complications**
Spontaneous miscarriage	Difficult fetal monitoring	Postpartum hemorrhage
Birth defects	Cesarean delivery	Wound infection
Limitations to ultrasound	Decreased success of a	Obesity in offspring
Gestational diabetes	vaginal birth after	
Hypertensive disease	cesarean delivery	
Stillbirth	Difficult anesthesia	
Fetal growth abnormalities		

regardless of the study arm (57% control vs 60% intervention, P = .8).[39] When the results of multiple studies have been examined cumulatively in meta-analyses, the interventions for women who are overweight or obese have been shown to have moderate or no influence at all on gestational weight gain or other perinatal outcomes.[40–44] Further research is indicated to determine how to promote adherence to gestational weight gain guidelines with health behavior interventions. Another concern is the influence maternal obesity has on childhood weight, resulting in a propagation of the cycle of obesity. It is likely that environmental and epigenetic influences and not just genetic mechanisms play a role in the obesity epidemic. Several theories suggest that in utero nutrition may impact chronic diseases such as diabetes, hypertension, and other metabolic diseases later in life in the offspring.[45,46] As this research continues to evolve, clinicians should consider that maternal nutrition during pregnancy may have life-long consequences for the offspring.

Pregnancy After Bariatric Surgery

Pregnancy after bariatric surgery is not uncommon because fertility often improves after a bariatric surgery procedure.[47–49] Given that bariatric procedures can create deficiencies of micronutrients and macronutrients, a pregnancy occurring after a bariatric surgery procedure requires particular attention to nutritional status. As stated previously, requirements for calories, vitamins, and minerals increase during pregnancy, so nutritional deficiencies in the bariatric surgery patient can be exacerbated during pregnancy. The most common deficiencies that occur after bariatric surgery are vitamin B_{12}, folate, and iron.[50] Because malabsorptive procedures (eg, Roux-en-Y gastric bypass [RYGB], biliopancreatic diversion) have a higher risk for nutritional deficiencies, closer surveillance in pregnancies that occur after these types of surgeries is appropriate.[51] However, derangements in nutrients can also occur after restrictive-type procedures (eg, laparoscopic adjustable gastric banding), so it may be reasonable to screen all women who are pregnant postbariatric surgery for nutritional deficiencies.[52] Guidelines for screening and management of nutritional deficiencies during pregnancy are adapted from those designed for nonpregnant states and include laboratory testing once a trimester or every 3 months if the levels are normal (**Table 7**).[51,53] Iron deficiency anemia is frequently a long-term complication of bariatric surgery, occurring in 6% to 50% of patients after RYGB.[54–57] In pregnancies after bariatric surgery, iron deficiency anemia can be diagnosed in the usual manner with a low mean corpuscular volume and abnormal iron studies (eg, low serum iron, high total iron-binding capacity, and a low serum ferritin), keeping in mind the physiologic anemia that occurs during pregnancy (see **Table 1**). Treatment of vitamin and mineral deficiencies during pregnancy, in terms of dose and duration, is similar to that of nonpregnant states.

Eating Disorders

For women with either a history of or current eating disorder (eg, anorexia nervosa, bulimia), additional questions regarding their weight should be asked, including how they feel about weight gain, being weighed at every prenatal visit (customary in prenatal care practices in the United States), and the ongoing changes in their body.[58] With respect to weighing, a woman's preference about weighing (ie, whether or not she prefers to see the numbers) should be assessed and documented in the chart. Counseling on gestational weight gain goals is still important for these women because weight influences the growth and development of the fetus. Similar to management before pregnancy, a collaborative team of experts in eating disorders should continue to manage and treat these women during the pregnancy.

Table 7
Diagnostic testing along with prophylaxis and treatment of micronutrient and macronutrient deficiencies in pregnancies after bariatric surgery

Component	Diagnostic Testing (Serum)	Prophylaxis	Treatment if Deficient
Protein	Serum albumin and prealbumin	60g protein/d	Protein supplements
Vitamin A	Vitamin A, if clinically indicated	4000 IU/d in prenatal vitamin	Vitamin A not to exceed 8000 IU/d
Vitamin D	25-hydroxy vitamin D, if clinically indicated	400–800 IU/d in prenatal vitamin	Calcitriol (vitamin D) 1000 IU/d
Vitamin K	Vitamin K_1, if clinically indicated	Not routinely given	Vitamin K_1 1 mg/d Consult with hematologist
Folic acid	Complete blood count, red blood cell folate	600–800 μg/d in prenatal vitamin	Folic acid 1000 μg/d
Vitamin B_{12}	Complete blood cell count, vitamin B_{12}	4 μg/d in prenatal vitamin	Oral vitamin B_{12} 350 μg/d or Intramuscular 1000 μg/month Consult with hematologist
Calcium	Total and ionized calcium	250 mg/d in prenatal vitamin	Calcium citrate 1000 mg/d with vitamin D
Iron	Complete blood count, iron, ferritin, total iron-binding capacity	30 mg/d in prenatal vitamin	Ferrous sulfate 325 mg 2–3 × daily with vitamin C

Data from Mechanick JI, Youdim A, Jones DB, et al. Clinical practice guidelines for the perioperative nutritional, metabolic, and nonsurgical support of the bariatric surgery patient–2013 update: cosponsored by American Association of Clinical Endocrinologists, The Obesity Society, and American Society for Metabolic & Bariatric Surgery. Obesity (Silver Spring) 2013;21(Suppl 1):S1–27; and American Academy of Pediatrics and the American College of Obstetricians and Gynecologists. Guidelines for perinatal care. 7th edition. Washington, DC: American Academy of Pediatrics; American College of Obstetricians and Gynecologists; 2012.

Vegetarians

There are varying types of vegetarian diets, including ovolactovegetarian (includes dairy and egg products), ovovegetarian (includes eggs), lactovegetarian (includes dairy products), and vegan (excludes eggs, dairy, and any other animal products). Alternative protein sources for these women include beans, peas, soy, nuts, nut butter, and milk and egg products. Minerals that may be deficient in their diets include iron, calcium, zinc, and vitamin B_{12}. Laboratory testing for these specific nutrients may be indicated.

Common Exposures

Historically, pregnant women were advised to abstain from caffeine. However, those earlier studies that demonstrated an increased risk of adverse obstetric outcomes such as miscarriage, poor fetal growth, and stillbirth were subject to substantial bias.[59] Additionally, the risk of those outcomes occurring generally increased with fairly substantive doses of caffeine, such as greater than 4 cups of coffee a day.[60,61] Most current research suggests that smaller amounts of caffeine intake, less than 200 to 300 mg daily, are not associated with increased risk of adverse obstetric outcomes.

It is particularly important that general food safety precautions, such as ensuring meat and dairy-containing foods are appropriately refrigerated, are followed during pregnancy because pregnant women are more susceptible to the effects of infections from certain microorganisms. Ensuring foods are pasteurized and/or appropriately cooked can lower the risk of acquiring infections such as Listeria and toxoplasmosis. Listerial infections are associated with increased risk for pregnancy complications such as preterm delivery and stillbirth.[62] Toxoplasmosis infections can result in ventriculomegaly and other fetal-neonatal complications.[63] Wearing gloves when gardening may also reduce the risk of exposure to toxoplasmosis.[64]

Although current recommendations from professional organizations do not recommend universal screening for lead exposure, risk assessment should be performed at the first prenatal visit and testing of lead levels performed if any risk factors are identified. High lead levels have been associated with a greater risk of obstetric complications such as miscarriage, poor fetal growth, and neurodevelopmental impairment.[65]

LACTATION
Physiology and Production

Breastfeeding and breast milk are the global standard for infant feeding. The World Health Organization, the US Surgeon General, the American Academy of Pediatrics, the American Congress of Obstetricians and Gynecologists, the American Academy of Family Practice, and the Academy of Breastfeeding Medicine all support this statement. The American Academy of Pediatrics further recommends exclusive breastfeeding for the first 6 months and breastfeeding at least through the first year of life.[66] Similar to pregnancy, energy and nutritional requirements also differ during lactation and breastfeeding.

Women who breastfeed require approximately 500 kcal more per day than is recommended for nonpregnant women.[67] The estimate is derived from the mean volume of breast milk produced per day (mean 780 mL, range 450–1200 mL) and the energy content of milk (67 kcal/100 mL).[68] During pregnancy, most women store an extra 2 to 5 kg (19,000–48,000 kcal) in tissue, mainly as fat, in physiologic preparation for lactation. If women do not consume the extra calories, then body stores are used to maintain lactation. It is not unusual for lactating women to lose 0.5 to 1.0 kg per month after the first postpartum month.[69]

There are even fewer evidence-based recommendations for nutrient intake during breastfeeding compared with pregnancy. Lactation is considered successful when the breast-fed infant is gaining an appropriate amount of weight. The recommended daily allowance for protein during lactation is an additional 25 g per day. Requirements of many micronutrients increase compared with pregnancy, with the exception of vitamins D and K, calcium, fluoride, magnesium, and phosphorus. As such, it is recommended that women continue to take a prenatal vitamin daily while they are breastfeeding (see **Tables 2** and **3**). Weight loss during lactation does not usually impact the quantity or quality of breast milk, but maternal deficiencies in magnesium, vitamin B_6, folate, calcium, and zinc have been described during lactation.[68,70] Both fat (vitamins A, D, K) and water-soluble vitamins (vitamins C, B_1, B_6, B_{12}, and folate) are secreted into breast milk and their levels are reduced in breast milk when there is a maternal vitamin deficiency.[71–73] Fortunately, these vitamin deficiencies in breast milk respond to maternal supplementation. On the other hand, calcium, phosphorus, and magnesium levels in breast milk are independent of maternal serum levels and diet.[74] Maternal factors such as stress, anxiety, and smoking can decrease milk production, but the quantitative and caloric value of breast milk does not change with dieting and exercise.[75–82] Moreover, a woman's weight, BMI, body fat percentage, and weight gain during pregnancy do not influence milk production.[83–85]

Special Considerations

Multiple gestations
Approximately 40% to 90% of mothers of twins initiate breastfeeding.[86] The production of milk is primarily determined by infant demand rather than the maternal capacity to lactate. As such, for women attempting to breastfeed twins and triplets, the supply will meet the demand. Continuation of micronutrient supplementations given antenatally in the form of a prenatal vitamin is appropriate for women who are breastfeeding twins. Twins can breastfeed either simultaneously or separately.

Obesity
Several studies have demonstrated that women with obesity have decreased rates of initiating breastfeeding and breastfeed for shorter durations compared with normal weight women.[87] Biological (ie, delayed lactation), psychological (ie, embarrassment related to body size and difficulty in breastfeeding discreetly), mechanical (ie, larger breasts and nipples that create difficulties with latching), and medical (ie, cesarean deliveries, diabetes, thyroid dysfunction) factors have been theorized to explain these findings, but the exact cause is likely a combination of factors. To combat this trend and increase the likelihood that women with obesity attain their breastfeeding goals, they need additional support and encouragement to breastfeed, including assistance with appropriate latching techniques and demonstration of appropriate infant positions, to aid with initiation and continuation of lactation.

Bariatric surgery
Women who have had bariatric surgery are also advised to follow the recommendation of breastfeeding for at least 6 months. Laboratory evaluation of micronutrient levels, as described in **Table 7** for pregnant women, is also recommended for breastfeeding women after bariatric surgery, with one group suggesting they be tested as frequently as every 3 months.[88] The infant's provider also should be aware of the mother's history of bariatric surgery, as well as any of her specific dietary restrictions or identified nutrient deficiencies. For women who have a gastric banding procedure, a recommendation is to keep the band deflated until the successful establishment of breastfeeding.[89] Though few studies have evaluated the nutritional content of breast milk

produced by lactating women after bariatric surgery, it is likely similar to other women. Although infants who are born to women with obesity have a higher rate of early childhood obesity, this may be offset by the reduced risk of early childhood obesity in infants who are predominantly breastfed.[90–92]

Vegetarians

Recommended dietary guidelines for vegetarians during lactation are lacking. Vitamin D supplements are recommended for women who do not drink milk or other food fortified with vitamin D. A vitamin B_{12} supplement (2.6 µg/d) is also recommended for women who consume ovolactovegetarian and vegan diets.[93] Another recommendation is to consume 1200 to 1500 mg per day of calcium because of the possible decreased intake and absorption from a plant-based diet.[94] The FDA recommends similar precautions regarding avoiding higher mercury-content fish during lactation. Adverse neonatal effects have not been demonstrated with ordinary maternal fish consumption during breastfeeding.

ONLINE RESOURCES FOR CLINICIANS

www.phenxtoolkit.org Screening questions to identify nutritional issues or deficiencies in patients.

http://resources.iom.edu/Pregnancy/WhatToGain.html?_ga=1.247807815.195235449.1445895119 BMI calculator

http://fnic.nal.usda.gov/interactiveDRL. Calculators for daily energy needs and interactive dietary reference intakes for health care professionals

http://www.choosemyplate.gov/supertracker-tools/daily-food-plans/moms.html Allows health care professionals to estimate energy and nutrient requirements during pregnancy and lactation

www.marchofdimes.com/pregnancy/nutrition_indepth.html Resource for general prenatal dietary guidelines from the March of Dimes

http://iom.nationalacademies.org/Activities/Children/PregnancyWeightDissemination/2013-SEP-09/~/media/Files/About%20the%20IOM/Pregnancy-Weight/Providers Bro-Final.pdf?_ga=1.148168439.195235449.1445895119 Review on how to implement the IOM gestational weight gain guidelines

http://iom.nationalacademies.org/Activities/Children/PregnancyWeightDissemination/2013-SEP-09/ToolKit.aspx Webinar that reviews a toolkit on implementing the IOM gestational weight gain guidelines.

http://iom.nationalacademies.org/Activities/Children/PregnancyWeightDissemination/2013-SEP-09/~/media/Files/About%20the%20IOM/Pregnancy-Weight/IOM PregnancyMythsFactsEnglish.pdf Myths for providers to dispel during the course of prenatal care

http://www.foodsafety.gov/risk/pregnant/chklist_pregnancy.html Checklist of foods to avoid during pregnancy

http://www.fda.gov/food/foodborneillnesscontaminants/metals/ucm393070.htm Resource from the FDA on fish consumption during pregnancy

https://www.breastfeeding.asn.au/bf-info/common-concerns%E2%80%93mum/diet Breastfeeding information and nutrition

SUMMARY AND FUTURE CONSIDERATIONS

Nutrition counseling is a cornerstone of prenatal care for all women during pregnancy and it also extends to lactation. Clinicians should be aware of the physiologic adaptations that occur during pregnancy and lactation, as well as how these changes influence the nutritional needs of pregnant and lactating women. One area of research that would assist providers and women in meeting their nutritional requirements and gestational weight gain goals is the measurement of diet and physical activity that is specific to pregnancy. Effective interventions that target health behaviors are also needed to improve a woman's nutritional status and assist her in meeting the gestational weight gain goals.

REFERENCES

1. Forsum E, Lof M. Energy metabolism during human pregnancy. Annu Rev Nutr 2007;27:277–92.
2. Trumbo P, Schlicker S, Yates AA, et al. Food and Nutrition Board, Institute of Medicine: dietary reference intakes for energy, carbohydrate, fiber, fat, fatty acids, cholesterol, protein, and amino acids. Washington, DC: National Academies Press; 2002.
3. Hytten F, Chamberlain G. Clinical physiology in obstetrics. Oxford (United Kingdom): Blackwell Scientific Publications; 1991.
4. Pitkin RM. Folate and neural tube defects. Am J Clin Nutr 2007;85(1):285S–8S.
5. Otten JJ, Hellwig JP, Meyers LD. Dietary reference intakes. The essential guide to nutrient requirements. Washington, DC: National Academies Press; 2006.
6. Lassi ZS, Salam RA, Haider BA, et al. Folic acid supplementation during pregnancy for maternal health and pregnancy outcomes. Cochrane Database Syst Rev 2013;(3):CD006896.
7. Siega-Riz AM, Mehta U. Clinical updates in Women's Health Care. In: Artal R, editor. Nutrition, vol. 13. Washington, DC: American College of Obstetricians and Gynecologists; 2014. p. 1–93.
8. ACOG Committee on Obstetric Practice. ACOG Committee opinion no. 495: vitamin D: screening and supplementation during pregnancy. Obstet Gynecol 2011;118(1):197–8.
9. Humphrey JH, West KP Jr, Sommer A. Vitamin A deficiency and attributable mortality among under-5-year-olds. Bull World Health Organ 1992;70(2):225–32.
10. Wenstrom KD. The FDA's new advice on fish: it's complicated. Am J Obstet Gynecol 2014;211(5):475–8.e1.
11. Myers GJ, Davidson PW, Cox C, et al. Prenatal methylmercury exposure from ocean fish consumption in the Seychelles child development study. Lancet 2003;361(9370):1686–92.
12. Hibbeln JR, Davis JM, Steer C, et al. Maternal seafood consumption in pregnancy and neurodevelopmental outcomes in childhood (ALSPAC study): an observational cohort study. Lancet 2007;369(9561):578–85.
13. Genuis SJ, Schwalfenberg GK. Time for an oil check: the role of essential omega-3 fatty acids in maternal and pediatric health. J Perinatol 2006;26(6):359–65.
14. Grandjean P, Weihe P, White RF, et al. Cognitive deficit in 7-year-old children with prenatal exposure to methylmercury. Neurotoxicol Teratol 1997;19(6):417–28.
15. Administration USFaD. Fish: what pregnant women and parents should know. 2014. Available at: http://www.fda.gov/Food/FoodborneIllnessContaminants/Metals/ucm393070.htm. Accessed October 15, 2015.
16. Makrides M, Gibson RA, McPhee AJ, et al. Effect of DHA supplementation during pregnancy on maternal depression and neurodevelopment of young children: a randomized controlled trial. JAMA 2010;304(15):1675–83.
17. Felig P. Maternal and fetal fuel homeostasis in human pregnancy. Am J Clin Nutr 1973;26(9):998–1005.

18. Freinkel N. Banting Lecture 1980. Of pregnancy and progeny. Diabetes 1980; 29(12):1023–35.
19. Stehbens JA, Baker GL, Kitchell M. Outcome at ages 1, 3, and 5 years of children born to diabetic women. Am J Obstet Gynecol 1977;127(4):408–13.
20. Rizzo T, Metzger BE, Burns WJ, et al. Correlations between antepartum maternal metabolism and child intelligence. N Engl J Med 1991;325(13):911–6.
21. Silverman BL, Rizzo T, Green OC, et al. Long-term prospective evaluation of offspring of diabetic mothers. Diabetes 1991;40(Suppl 2):121–5.
22. Institute of Medicine. Weight gain during pregnancy: reexamining the guidelines. Washington, DC: National Academic Press; 2009.
23. Institute of medicine. Nutrition during pregnancy. Washington, DC: National Academic Press; 1990.
24. Deputy NP, Sharma AJ, Kim SY. Gestational weight gain - United States, 2012 and 2013. MMWR Morb Mortal Wkly Rep 2015;64(43):1215–20.
25. Johnson J, Clifton RG, Roberts JM, et al. Pregnancy outcomes with weight gain above or below the 2009 Institute of Medicine guidelines. Obstet Gynecol 2013; 121(5):969–75.
26. Casele HL, Dooley SL, Metzger BE. Metabolic response to meal eating and extended overnight fast in twin gestation. Am J Obstet Gynecol 1996; 175(4 Pt 1):917–21.
27. Rosello-Soberon ME, Fuentes-Chaparro L, Casanueva E. Twin pregnancies: eating for three? Maternal nutrition update. Nutr Rev 2005;63(9):295–302.
28. Goodnight W, Newman R. Society of Maternal-Fetal M. Optimal nutrition for improved twin pregnancy outcome. Obstet Gynecol 2009;114(5):1121–34.
29. Luke B. Nutrition in multiple gestations. Clin Perinatol 2005;32(2):403–29, vii.
30. Young BC, Wylie BJ. Effects of twin gestation on maternal morbidity. Semin Perinatol 2012;36(3):162–8.
31. Luke B, Gillespie B, Min SJ, et al. Critical periods of maternal weight gain: effect on twin birth weight. Am J Obstet Gynecol 1997;177(5):1055–62.
32. Luke B, Minogue J, Witter FR, et al. The ideal twin pregnancy: patterns of weight gain, discordancy, and length of gestation. Am J Obstet Gynecol 1993;169(3): 588–97.
33. National institute of health. The practical guide: identification, evaluation, and treatment of overweight and obesity in adults. NIH Publication 2000. No. 98–4083.
34. Obesity: preventing and managing the global epidemic. Report of a WHO consultation. World Health Organ Tech Rep Ser 2000;894:i–xii, 1–253.
35. Ogden CL, Carroll MD, Kit BK, et al. Prevalence of childhood and adult obesity in the United States, 2011-2012. JAMA 2014;311(8):806–14.
36. Hauger MS, Gibbons L, Vik T, et al. Prepregnancy weight status and the risk of adverse pregnancy outcome. Acta Obstet Gynecol Scand 2008;87(9):953–9.
37. Cnattingius S, Bergstrom R, Lipworth L, et al. Prepregnancy weight and the risk of adverse pregnancy outcomes. N Engl J Med 1998;338(3):147–52.
38. ACOG Practice Bulletin No 156: obesity in pregnancy. Obstet Gynecol 2015; 126(6):e112–26.
39. Walsh JM, McGowan CA, Mahony R, et al. Low glycaemic index diet in pregnancy to prevent macrosomia (ROLO study): randomised control trial. BMJ 2012;345:e5605.
40. Dodd JM, Grivell RM, Crowther CA, et al. Antenatal interventions for overweight or obese pregnant women: a systematic review of randomised trials. BJOG 2010; 117:1316–26.

41. Campbell F, Johnson M, Messina J, et al. Behavioural interventions for weight management in pregnancy: a systematic review of quantitative and qualitative data. BMC Public Health 2011;11:491.
42. Tanentsapf I, Heitmann BL, Adegboye AR. Systematic review of clinical trials on dietary interventions to prevent excessive weight gain during pregnancy among normal weight, overweight and obese women. BMC Pregnancy Childbirth 2011; 11:81.
43. Oteng-Ntim E, Varma R, Croker H, et al. Lifestyle interventions for overweight and obese pregnant women to improve pregnancy outcome: systematic review and meta-analysis. BMC Med 2012;10:47.
44. Thangaratinam S, Rogozinska E, Jolly K, et al. Effects of interventions in pregnancy on maternal weight and obstetric outcomes: meta-analysis of randomised evidence. BMJ 2012;344:e2088.
45. Barker DJ, Osmond C, Kajantie E, et al. Growth and chronic disease: findings in the Helsinki Birth Cohort. Ann Hum Biol 2009;36(5):445–58.
46. Barker DJ. The developmental origins of adult disease. Eur J Epidemiol 2003; 18(8):733–6.
47. Paulen ME, Zapata LB, Cansino C, et al. Contraceptive use among women with a history of bariatric surgery: a systematic review. Contraception 2010;82(1):86–94.
48. Teitelman M, Grotegut CA, Williams NN, et al. The impact of bariatric surgery on menstrual patterns. Obes Surg 2006;16(11):1457–63.
49. Gosman GG, King WC, Schrope B, et al. Reproductive health of women electing bariatric surgery. Fertil Steril 2010;94(4):1426–31.
50. Shankar P, Boylan M, Sriram K. Micronutrient deficiencies after bariatric surgery. Nutrition 2010;26(11–12):1031–7.
51. Mechanick JI, Youdim A, Jones DB, et al. Clinical practice guidelines for the perioperative nutritional, metabolic, and nonsurgical support of the bariatric surgery patient—2013 update: cosponsored by American Association of Clinical Endocrinologists, The Obesity Society, and American Society for Metabolic & Bariatric Surgery. Obesity (Silver Spring) 2013;21(Suppl 1):S1–27.
52. Gudzune KA, Huizinga MM, Chang HY, et al. Screening and diagnosis of micronutrient deficiencies before and after bariatric surgery. Obes Surg 2013;23(10): 1581–9.
53. American College of Obstetricians and Gynecologists. ACOG Practice Bulletin no. 105: Bariatric surgery and pregnancy. Obstet Gynecol 2009;113(6):1405–13.
54. Simon SR, Zemel R, Betancourt S, et al. Hematologic complications of gastric bypass for morbid obesity. South Med J 1989;82(9):1108–10.
55. Heber D, Greenway FL, Kaplan LM, et al. Endocrine and nutritional management of the post-bariatric surgery patient: an Endocrine Society Clinical Practice Guideline. J Clin Endocrinol Metab 2010;95(11):4823–43.
56. Alvarez-Cordero R, Aragon-Viruette E. Post-operative complications in a series of gastric bypass patients. Obes Surg 1992;2(1):87–9.
57. Halverson JD. Micronutrient deficiencies after gastric bypass for morbid obesity. Am Surg 1986;52(11):594–8.
58. American Psychiatric Association. Treatment of patients with eating disorders, third edition. American Psychiatric Association. Am J Psychiatry 2006;163(7 Suppl): 4–54.
59. Bracken MB. Potential confounding still clouds the possible association of maternal caffeine intake and low birth weight. Evid Based Med 2015;20(1):37.
60. CARE Study Group. Maternal caffeine intake during pregnancy and risk of fetal growth restriction: a large prospective observational study. BMJ 2008;337:a2332.

61. Bech BH, Nohr EA, Vaeth M, et al. Coffee and fetal death: a cohort study with prospective data. Am J Epidemiol 2005;162(10):983–90.

62. Committee on Obstetric Practice, American College of Obstetricians and Gynecologists. Committee opinion no. 614: management of pregnant women with presumptive exposure to Listeria monocytogenes. Obstet Gynecol 2014;124(6): 1241–4.

63. Neu N, Duchon J, Zachariah P. TORCH infections. Clin Perinatol 2015;42(1): 77–103, viii.

64. Prevention CfDCa. Parasites - toxoplasmosis. 2013. Available at: http://www.cdc. gov/parasites/toxoplasmosis/prevent.html. Accessed October 15, 2015.

65. Committee on Obstetric Practice. Committee opinion No. 533: lead screening during pregnancy and lactation. Obstet Gynecol 2012;120(2 Pt 1):416–20.

66. Section on Breastfeeding. Breastfeeding and the use of human milk. Pediatrics 2012;129(3):e827–41.

67. Guidelines for perinatal care. 7th edition. Washington, DC: American Academy of Pediatrics; American College of Obstetricians and Gynecologists; 2012.

68. Nutrition during lactation. Washington, DC: Institute of Medicine; National Academy Press; 1991.

69. Weekly SJ. Diets and eating disorders: implications for the breastfeeding mother. NAACOGS Clin Issu Perinat Womens Health Nurs 1992;3(4):695–700.

70. Gartner LM, Greer FR, Section on Breastfeeding and Committee on Nutrition, et al. Prevention of rickets and vitamin D deficiency: new guidelines for vitamin D intake. Pediatrics 2003;111(4 Pt 1):908–10.

71. Butte NF, Calloway DH. Evaluation of lactational performance of Navajo women. Am J Clin Nutr 1981;34(10):2210–5.

72. Hollis B, Lambert PW, Horst RL. Factors affecting the antirachitic sterol content of native milk. In: Holick MF, Gray K, Anast CS, editors. Perinatal calcium and phosphorous metabolism. Amsterdam (NY): Elsevier Science Publishers BV; 1983. p. 157.

73. von Kries R, Shearer M, McCarthy PT, et al. Vitamin K1 content of maternal milk: influence of the stage of lactation, lipid composition, and vitamin K1 supplements given to the mother. Pediatr Res 1987;22(5):513–7.

74. Prentice A. Calcium supplementation during breast-feeding. N Engl J Med 1997; 337(8):558–9.

75. Schanler RJ, Hurst NM. Human milk for the hospitalized preterm infant. Semin Perinatol 1994;18(6):476–84.

76. Hopkinson JM, Schanler RJ, Fraley JK, et al. Milk production by mothers of premature infants: influence of cigarette smoking. Pediatrics 1992;90(6):934–8.

77. Vio F, Salazar G, Infante C. Smoking during pregnancy and lactation and its effects on breast-milk volume. Am J Clin Nutr 1991;54(6):1011–6.

78. Andersen AN, Lund-Andersen C, Larsen JF, et al. Suppressed prolactin but normal neurophysin levels in cigarette smoking breast-feeding women. Clin Endocrinol (Oxf) 1982;17(4):363–8.

79. Dewey KG. Effects of maternal caloric restriction and exercise during lactation. J Nutr 1998;128(2 Suppl):386S–9S.

80. Dewey KG, Lovelady CA, Nommsen-Rivers LA, et al. A randomized study of the effects of aerobic exercise by lactating women on breast-milk volume and composition. N Engl J Med 1994;330(7):449–53.

81. Dusdieker LB, Hemingway DL, Stumbo PJ. Is milk production impaired by dieting during lactation? Am J Clin Nutr 1994;59(4):833–40.

82. McCrory MA, Nommsen-Rivers LA, Mole PA, et al. Randomized trial of the short-term effects of dieting compared with dieting plus aerobic exercise on lactation performance. Am J Clin Nutr 1999;69(5):959–67.
83. Dewey KG, Heinig MJ, Nommsen LA, et al. Maternal versus infant factors related to breast milk intake and residual milk volume: the DARLING study. Pediatrics 1991;87(6):829–37.
84. Butte NF, Garza C, Stuff JE, et al. Effect of maternal diet and body composition on lactational performance. Am J Clin Nutr 1984;39(2):296–306.
85. Michaelsen KF. Nutrition and growth during infancy. The Copenhagen Cohort Study. Acta Paediatr Suppl 1997;420:1–36.
86. Flidel-Rimon O, Shinwell ES. Breast feeding twins and high multiples. Arch Dis Child Fetal Neonatal Ed 2006;91(5):F377–80.
87. Wojcicki JM. Maternal prepregnancy body mass index and initiation and duration of breastfeeding: a review of the literature. J Womens Health (Larchmt) 2011; 20(3):341–7.
88. Kaska L, Kobiela J, Abacjew-Chmylko A, et al. Nutrition and pregnancy after bariatric surgery. ISRN Obes 2013;2013:6.
89. Dixon JB, Dixon ME, O'Brien PE. Pregnancy after lap-band surgery: management of the band to achieve healthy weight outcomes. Obes Surg 2001;11(1):59–65.
90. Arenz S, Ruckerl R, Koletzko B, et al. Breast-feeding and childhood obesity–a systematic review. Int J Obes Relat Metab Disord 2004;28(10):1247–56.
91. Owen CG, Martin RM, Whincup PH, et al. Effect of infant feeding on the risk of obesity across the life course: a quantitative review of published evidence. Pediatrics 2005;115(5):1367–77.
92. Ip S, Chung M, Raman G, et al. Breastfeeding and maternal and infant health outcomes in developed countries. Evid Rep Technol Assess (Full Rep) 2007;(153): 1–186.
93. Picciano MF. Pregnancy and lactation: physiological adjustments, nutritional requirements and the role of dietary supplements. J Nutr 2003;133(6):1997S–2002S.
94. Venti CA, Johnston CS. Modified food guide pyramid for lactovegetarians and vegans. J Nutr 2002;132(5):1050–4.

Nutrition in Children and Adolescents

Mark R. Corkins, MD, CNSC, SPR[a], Stephen R. Daniels, MD, PhD[b],*,
Sarah D. de Ferranti, MD, MPH[c], Neville H. Golden, MD[d], Jae H. Kim, MD, PhD[e],
Sheela N. Magge, MD, MSCE[f], Sarah Jane Schwarzenberg, MD[g]

KEYWORDS

• Nutrition • Infants • Children • Adolescents • Breastfeeding • Formula • Diet

KEY POINTS

- The healthiest and most appropriate feeding at birth for a newborn infant begins with their own mother's breastfeeding.
- Parents control the home food environment and should ensure preferential access to healthful foods, allowing children to choose among these options.
- Parents should also be alert to foods that present a choking hazard. Children do not learn to chew with a grinding motion until age 4.
- Existing data demonstrate that children generally do not meet recommended targets for a healthy diet.
- Chronic illnesses can have their onset during adolescence. These diseases may be further complicated by nutritional deficiencies.

[a] Pediatric Gastroenterology, University of Tennessee Health Sciences Center, 49 North Dunlap Street, Memphis, TN 38105, USA; [b] Department of Pediatrics, Children's Hospital Colorado, University of Colorado School of Medicine, 13123 East 16th Avenue, B065, Aurora, CO 80045, USA; [c] Preventive Cardiology Clinic, Department of Cardiology, Children's Hospital Boston, Harvard University Medical School, 300 Longwood Avenue, Boston, MA 02115, USA; [d] Division of Adolescent Medicine, Department of Pediatrics, Lucile Packard Children's Hospital Stanford, Stanford University School of Medicine, 770 Welch Road, Palo Alto, CA 94304, USA; [e] Neonatal-Perinatal Medicine Fellowship, Supporting Premature Infant Nutrition Program, Rady Children's Hospital of San Diego, University of California San Diego Health, 3020 Children's Way, San Diego, CA 92123, USA; [f] Division of Endocrinology and Diabetes, Center for Translational Science, Patient and Clinical Interactions (formerly CRC), CTSI, Children's National Health System, The George Washington University School of Medicine and Health Sciences, 111 Michigan Ave NW, Washington, DC 20010, USA; [g] Pediatric Gastroenterology, Hepatology and Nutrition, Masonic Children's Hospital, University of Minnesota, 2450 Riverside Avenue, Pediatric Ambulatory Services East Building, Minneapolis, MN 55454, USA
* Corresponding author.
E-mail address: Stephen.Daniels@childrenscolorado.org

Med Clin N Am 100 (2016) 1217–1235
http://dx.doi.org/10.1016/j.mcna.2016.06.005
0025-7125/16/$ – see front matter © 2016 Elsevier Inc. All rights reserved.
medical.theclinics.com

INTRODUCTION

In some aspects, pediatric nutrition is easier than adult nutrition, in that children have a ready "marker" for nutrition status: growth. Although an approximation, appropriate growth implies adequate intake of the basic nutrients. Thus, one of the best initial tools to assess nutritional status in pediatric patients is the standardized growth curves. There are curves for length (age <3 years), height (for >3 years), head circumference (age <3 years), and weight (both under and over 3 years). Children under 2 years of age are plotted on the World Health Organization (WHO) growth curves and those 2 years of age and older on the Centers for Disease Control and Prevention (CDC) curves.[1,2]

In other aspects, however, pediatric nutrition is more difficult. The caloric needs vary by age, as does the need for various nutrients. In gross terms, the most rapid growth occurs during infancy and the number of calories needed per kilogram body weight is the greatest. The growth then slows and the number of calories per kilogram body weight decreases. But because the child is constantly growing, the total number of calories needed is always increasing. For other nutrients such as calcium the needs vary by age with an increased need during puberty. The requirements of the various nutrients over the years have been published.[3]

Children who fall below the standard growth curves may have malnutrition. There is recognition that malnutrition in the developed world often occurs in the presence of a disease process. These processes are often accompanied by the presence of inflammation, which has profound effects on nutrition and growth. Pediatric malnutrition is now etiology based with a statement of the underlying disease process, whether or not inflammation is present, and then the supportive anthropometric measurements (**Table 1**).[4] Chronic malnutrition leads to growth stunting and the loss of potential functional capacity.

This article describes nutritional needs for children and adolescents through developmental stages, and then reviews the influence of nutrition on early brain development, risk for food allergies, and cardiometabolic risks, including obesity, hypertension, and hyperlipidemia.

BIRTH TO 1 YEAR

The healthiest and most appropriate feeding at birth for a newborn infant begins with their own mother's breastfeeding. The American Academy of Pediatrics (AAP) and the WHO recommend that exclusive breastfeeding should be maintained for at least

Table 1
Primary anthropometric indicators

	Mild Malnutrition	Moderate Malnutrition	Severe Malnutrition
Weight for height (z score)[a]	−1 to −1.9	−2 to −2.9	−3 or greater
BMI for age (z score)	−1 to − 1.9	−2 to −2.9	−3 or greater
Length/height (z score)	No data	No data	−3
Mid-upper arm circumference (z score)	Greater than or equal to −1 to −1.9	Greater than or equal to −2 to −2.9	Greater than or equal to −3

[a] The z score is a statistical measurement based on the mean and standard deviation of the distance of a score from the mean in a group of scores.

Data from USDA Center for Nutrition Policy and Promotion. Estimated calorie needs per day by age, gender, and physical activity level. Available at: http://www.cnpp.usda.gov/sites/default/files/usda_food_patterns/EstimatedCalorieNeedsPerDayTable.pdf. Accessed June 9, 2016; and Institute of Medicine. Dietary reference intakes for energy, carbohydrate, fiber, fat, fatty acids, cholesterol, protein, and amino acids. Washington (DC): The National Academies Press; 2002.

6 months to ensure optimal growth, development, and health.[5] This period is followed by concurrent breastfeeding with the introduction of complementary foods until at least 12 months of age, and continuation of breastfeeding for as long as mutually desired by mother and baby.

The first produced breast milk is called colostrum, a dense, concentrated milk that confers immunologic protection to the newborn.[6] Colostrum functions to provide an initial rich concentration of nutrients, but also confers passive immunity with antibodies as well as immunologically active factors such as lysozymes, lactoferrin, complement, and interleukins. Aiding the establishment of breastfeeding of colostrum is early skin-to-skin care that involves the immediate attachment of a newborn onto their mother's upper body.[7]

Within the first week, colostrum transitions to a more mature milk that is comparatively less dense in protein and bioactive compounds, but more dense in fat and carbohydrates, resulting in slightly higher energy density (colostrum 19 vs mature 20 kcal/oz.).

There is wide variability in the nutrient content of breast milk between feedings from the same mother, over the lactation period, and between mothers.[8,9] Despite this, infants are able to consume an appropriate amount of milk to satisfy their hunger and growth needs because they can compensate for lower calories by drinking greater volumes each day.

Despite a wide range of maternal diets, breast milk generally provides an adequate calorie density and macronutrient content for most infants to grow. Changes in maternal diet do not greatly alter breast milk content, with a few exceptions such as severe malnutrition. Maternal dietary intake of specific fatty acids alters the fatty acid profile but not the amount of fat of their breast milk.[10] For instance, a mother ingesting large amounts of fish oil produces breast milk that has a high fraction of omega 3 fatty acids in her milk.

The benefits of breastfeeding have been documented extensively.[11] The clearest benefits relate to protection against infection, such as upper respiratory infection, pneumonia, otitis media, urinary tract infection, sepsis, and meningitis. Breastfeeding also significantly reduces the incidence of sudden infant death syndrome, allergy, asthma, type 1 diabetes, celiac disease, and obesity. There are several efforts to increase exclusive breastfeeding globally (WHO, CDC, Healthy 2020; available: www.healthypeople. gov). Breastfeeding prevalence in the United States (2014) has been increasing steadily for the past decade with 79.2% having any breastfeeding and 49% doing any breastfeeding at 6 months. Exclusive breastfeeding prevalence is lower at 40.7% by 3 months, decreasing to 18% by 6 months. The Baby Friendly Initiatives (available: www.bfhi.org) have been highly successful in increasing breastfeeding rates with their 10-step program that promotes best practices for breastfeeding for healthy term newborns along with restrictions in promotion of pacifiers and infant formula.

Breast milk would be a complete nutrition for infants with the exception of inadequate vitamin D content owing to societal reduction in sunlight exposure from clothing, increased use of sunscreen, and migrating to places further away from the equator (2015).[12] Recently, mothers have been shown to provide adequate vitamin D in their milk when supplemented with 6400 IU of vitamin D during lactation, although this practice has not been adopted widely.[13] The recommendation for breastfed infants continues to be a daily liquid supplement of 400 IU of vitamin D[14] (Institute of Medicine dietary reference intakes for calcium and vitamin D). This can be as vitamin D alone or in combination with other vitamins.

Infant formulas are modern formulations of cow's milk-based protein and carbohydrate with plant-based lipids along with other additives to provide a complete nutritional source for infants. There are now numerous and complex infant formula options available in North America that act primarily as nutritional substitutes for breast milk in the first year of life.[15] It is worth noting that there have been limited attempts to mimic most of the biologically active functions of the hundreds of different bioactive compounds in breast milk. Infant formulas have been able to include nucleotides, luteins, prebiotic oligosaccharides, and probiotics that can confer some of the bioactive benefits of breast milk.[16]

Weaning refers to the time when infants transition from breast milk to solid foods. *Complementary feeding* is the process starting when breast milk alone is no longer sufficient to meet the nutritional requirements of infants, and therefore other foods and liquids are needed, along with breast milk (WHO definition). The AAP and WHO recommend complementary foods to begin after 6 months of age.[15] Weaning from breastfeeding is quite variable and can generally take place over the first 2 years. This weaning period is a highly vulnerable time for infant nutrition deficiencies to occur. It is advised to avoid including excess amounts of fruit juices and keep to unsweetened 100% fruit juices. It is helpful to avoid excess salty and sweet additives to their solid foods.

With formula feeding, earlier introduction may occur after 4 months. Very early introduction of solids presents a risk for food allergies or celiac disease with early exposure of gluten-containing foods in those with susceptible HLA markers known to be associated with celiac disease.[17] Interestingly, later introduction of gluten-containing foods beyond 7 months of age also increases the risk of celiac disease. Concurrent introduction of gluten with breast milk is also beneficial.

There have been past concerns that several food proteins that pose high allergic risk need to be avoided within the first year, but more recent evidence suggests the opposite, that lack of exposure to some food proteins such as peanuts, egg, and fish protein actually increase one's risk of developing food allergies to those proteins.[18] The introduction of food proteins concurrently with breastfeeding is the best method of introduction.[11]

Meeting the iron needs of most infants during the first year of life remains a worldwide challenge. Infants may be at greater risk of iron deficiency after 6 months of age owing to reduced iron stores and limited iron content in breast milk.[19] The AAP recommends breast milk or iron-fortified infant formula and avoiding whole cow's milk until 1 year of age.[20] Therefore, complementary foods that are high or enriched in iron such as iron-fortified cereals and meat products are favored.

AGE 1 TO 4 YEARS

As the infant becomes a toddler, many changes are occurring, including major changes in diet. At around 1 year of age, the growth in height and weight starts to slow down. This is when many parents notice a substantial decline in the child's appetite. This transition is often difficult for parents as their "healthy eater" becomes a "picky eater," but it is a normal shift, reflecting a change in energy balance.

This age range is one in which adultlike eating patterns are established over time. However, parents should expect this to be a process, not a quick transition. For example, children may develop very narrow preferences for certain foods for periods during this age range. Parents may try to introduce new foods but can be met with resistance.

If there is a concern about a toddler's diet, there are several things to consider. First, it is important to assess whether the child is growing and developing appropriately. Second, it may help to do a nutritional assessment. Often, the child is getting adequate calories, macronutrients, and micronutrients, despite the limited choices. Third, it should be recognized that children may need to experience new foods and new tastes multiple times before accepting them. This may take as many as 10 to 12 attempts over time.[21] Parents should be careful how they interpret their child's response to food. A frown or grimace may be more owing to it being new than to not liking the food. Remember that this is an age range for toddlers where virtually everything they experience is new. Sometimes, limiting their likes and dislikes in the food arena is a way of controlling their environment. It is important that parents not turn eating into a confrontational experience.

Parents control the home food environment. They should ensure preferential access to healthful foods, including fruits, vegetables, whole grains, and low-fat dairy, and allow children to choose among these options. Similarly, parents should limit foods and beverages, beginning with those high in added sugar and in saturated fat. An approach to appropriate serving sizes is presented in **Table 2**.

This age range is also a time where parents can establish routines around meal times. The toddler should eat with the rest of the family. There should be no television or other media to distract from the meal. This family approach to meals has been associated with lower risk of obesity for children and adolescents.[22]

It is important to recognize that energy requirements are modest in this age range. A general estimate is that a child needs approximately 40 calories per day for each inch of height. So a toddler at 30 inches would require about 1200 calories a day to sustain appropriate growth. This suggests that the serving size for a young child should be about one-quarter the size that would be appropriate for an adult.

Parents should also be alert to foods that present a choking hazard. Children do not learn to chew with a grinding motion until age 4. This leaves them vulnerable to aspiration of some foods. Such foods include hot dogs and other meats (unless cut into small, nonround pieces), nuts, whole grapes, raw carrots, and popcorn.

Finally, because the dietary approach provided will give the toddler adequate calories, vitamins, and minerals, children do not need nutritional supplements during this age range. The toddler, who gets foods from the various food groups, even with a relatively small portion sizes compared with adults, will have appropriate nutrition without adding supplements.

Table 2
Appropriate diet for children age 2 years

Food Group	Approximate Percent of Calories per Day[a]	Serving Size
Whole grains (6 servings)	20	Bread ¼-½ slice Cereal ¼ cup (dry)
Vegetables (2–3 servings)	6	Cooked 1 tablespoon per year of age
Fruits (2–3 servings)	6	Fresh fruit ½ piece
Dairy (2–3 servings)	33	Milk ½ cup Cheese ½ ounce
Meat, fish, poultry (2 servings)	20	1 ounce (2 tablespoons ground meat)

[a] Based on 1200 total calories per day. This leaves approximately 10% to 15% of calories to be distributed among these categories or to come from other categories, such as legumes.

FEEDING THE 4- TO 12-YEAR-OLD CHILD

The ages of 4 to 12 years span years of continued growth and also transition. There is continued somatic growth, although at a rate less dramatic than the periods that preceded it (infancy and toddlerhood), and the age to follow (adolescence). During these years, children begin to spend time away from home, eating without supervision by their parents. By this time children have generally mastered the physical tasks of feeding themselves (using a cup, a spoon and fork), and can now begin to learn about eating a balanced and diverse diet. Although food continues to be provided by adults, and meals are still quite supervised during the early years, by the end of this period children can be more independent about their food and beverage choices. This age is a key opportunity for parents and other involved adults to teach children healthy eating habits and to promote self-regulation based on appetite, before the struggle for autonomy, so characteristic of adolescence, fully manifests itself.

Dietary recommendations for children ages 4 to 12 years are similar to those for other periods of childhood and include promoting the intake of fruits and vegetables, fiber and seafood, and lean proteins. Calcium remains a priority for bone growth. It is recommended that children consume minimal amounts of sugary beverages, desserts, fast foods, and foods high in salt. The main difference from other ages is caloric intake necessary for optimal growth, which increases gradually from age 4 to 6 (1200–1800 kcal/d) to age 12 (1400–2000 kcal/d) and should be adjusted to account for physical activity. Portion sizes should increase over these years; for example, from 4 to 6 tablespoons of vegetables per serving at age 4 to one-half cup per serving for a 12 year old.[23,24] Recommended portion sizes and total daily portions by age and by daily calorie targets can be found at http://health.gov in the Dietary Guidelines for America.

Existing data demonstrate that children generally do not meet recommended targets for a healthy diet. When dietary recalls from the National Health and Nutrition Examination Survey[25] are used to calculate healthy eating index scores, most children do not achieve scores in the optimal level and many are much lower than recommended, with younger children having better diets than older children.[26] The most important deficits are in vegetable intake, whole grains, legumes, and seafood. The most concerning areas of excess are desserts and sugary beverages, which supply as much as 40% of daily energy consumption.[27] Not only are these foods high in calories and low in nutrients, but they also tend to crowd out more beneficial foods containing vitamins and other micronutrients.[25]

A number of strategies can be used at the individual level and at the level of the family unit to improve dietary habits and quality, including meal timing and frequency, mindful eating, using environmental strategies to stack the deck in favor of a healthy diet, getting kids involved in the process, including everyone in the family in healthy eating, and making better choices when eating out (**Table 3**). Parental modeling is an important factor for children in this age range. Having soda and fruit drinks in the home was associated with a worse healthy eating index score.[28] There are also interventions in place at the national, state, and local levels aimed at promoting healthier diets in 4- to 12-year-olds, with school lunch and breakfast programs being the cornerstone programs for this age group. In fact, school lunch and breakfast programs have been shown to protect families from food insufficiency.[29] Available evidence suggests that prior school lunch and breakfast programs did not meet the recommendations set by the Dietary Guidelines for Americans.[30] There is optimism, and some early evidence, that new school food standards are improving dietary quality.[31,32]

Table 3
Approaches to promote healthy eating behaviors in 4- to 12-year-olds

Concepts	Eating Behaviors
Meal timing and frequency	No meal skipping Eat breakfast. Do not go longer than 5 hours without eating.
Mindful eating	Before you reach for more food or drink, be aware of what your body is telling you. Consider whether you are truly hungry, or you are eating for other reasons (fatigue, stress, boredom, etc). Minimize eating in front of a screen.
Stack the deck	Create a food safe environment – put more healthy foods in the house and keep unhealthy foods out. Serve vegetables first.
Get kids involved in the process	Ask children to come up with ideas of healthy foods they like to eat. Take children to the grocery store to find new and healthy foods. Get children cooking in the kitchen.
Eat healthy as a family	Encourage parents to model healthy eating. Do not provide different meals for different family members.
Healthier eating out	Order extra vegetables if they are not included in your meal. Know your food - investigate your favorite take-out and choose a healthier option from the menu. Plan ahead to bring healthier options.

ADOLESCENTS, AGES 13 TO 18

Outside of the first year of life, adolescence is the period of greatest growth and development across the lifespan. Longitudinal height increases 20%, body weight doubles, 40% to 60% of peak bone mass is accrued, muscle mass increases, blood volume expands, and the heart, brain, lungs, liver, and kidney all increase in size. As a result, nutritional requirements increase dramatically and may exceed those of adulthood. During adolescence, differences in body size and composition between boys and girls become accentuated and affect nutritional requirements.

Adolescence is a time of increasing autonomy with reduced parental supervision of meals and snacks. Peer pressure replaces parental authority and poor dietary habits may often be established during the adolescent years. Skipping of meals (especially breakfast) becomes more common and there is increased consumption of snacks, fast foods, sweetened beverages, and foods high in sodium and saturated fats, with reduced intake of fruits, vegetables, dairy products, whole grains, lean meats, and fish. Data from the National Health and Nutrition Examination Survey reveal that in 2011 to 2012, 34.5% of 12- to 19-year-olds were overweight or obese.[33] Adolescence is also the usual time of onset of eating disorders, when young people become preoccupied with body shape and weight and voluntarily embark on self-restrictive diets to achieve their perceived "thin ideal" weight. Finally, a number of chronic illnesses such as type 1 diabetes, inflammatory bowel disease, and celiac disease can have their onset during adolescence. These diseases, because of a combination of dietary limitations and increased metabolic requirements associated with chronic inflammation, together with increased requirements for growth and development, may be further complicated by nutritional deficiencies.

ADOLESCENT GROWTH AND DEVELOPMENT

In contrast with other age groups, nutritional requirements during adolescence depend more on sexual maturity rating (Tanner staging) than on chronologic age. The stages of sexual maturity rating for girls and boys are shown in **Table 4**. In girls, onset of puberty is 9 to 11 years of age and peak height velocity occurs early in puberty, usually between Tanner stages 2 and 3 of breast development. Menarche occurs late, usually between Tanner stage 4 and 5 of breast development and 2 to 3 years after onset of breast development. The median age of menarche in the United States is 12.4 years and occurs earlier in African Americans (12.06 years) than Hispanics (12.25) or Caucasians (12.55).[34] Longitudinal growth is usually complete 1 year after menarche.

In contrast with girls, the onset of puberty in boys is 10 to 13 years and peak height velocity occurs later in puberty, usually between Tanner genital stages 4 and 5. As a result, boys grow on average for 2 years longer than girls. Increased muscle mass development occurs during Tanner genital stages 4 and 5, secondary to increasing androgen levels. In both boys and girls, peak bone mass acquisition occurs

Table 4 Sexual maturity rating for boys and girls		
Girls Stage	**Breast Development**	**Pubic Hair Development**
SMR 1[a]	Prepubertal; nipple elevation only.	Prepubertal, no pubic hair.
SMR 2	Small, raised breast bud.	Sparse growth of downy hair along labia.
SMR 3	Enlargement of breast extending beyond areola.	Increased amount of hair. Hair darker, coarser and more curled.
SMR 4	Further enlargement of the breast. Areola and nipple form a secondary mound above the level of the breast.	Hair resembles adult type, but does not extend to thighs.
SMR 5	Mature, adult contour, with areola in same contour as breast, and only nipple projecting.	Adult type and quantity, extends to thighs.
Boys Stage	**Genital Development**	**Pubic Hair Development**
SMR 1	Prepubertal; no change in size of testes, scrotum, or penis.	Prepubertal; no pubic hair.
SMR 2	Enlargement of scrotum and testes; reddening and change in texture in skin of scrotum; little or no penis enlargement.	Sparse growth of downy hair at base of penis.
SMR 3	Increase in size of penis, mainly in length; continued growth of testes and scrotum.	Hair is darker, more coarse and more curled; increase in amount.
SMR 4	Enlargement of penis with growth in breadth in addition to length; further growth of testes and scrotum, darkening of scrotal skin.	Hair resembles adult type, but not spread to medial aspect of thighs.
SMR 5	Adult size and shape genitalia.	Adult type and quantity, spread to highs.

[a] SMR Sexual maturity rating.

approximately 6 to 12 months after peak height velocity. In girls, puberty is accompanied by increased accumulation of body fat, whereas in boys there is an increase in the proportion of lean body mass.

The onset and tempo of puberty is variable and adolescents do not necessarily follow the CDC or WHO growth curves, which were derived from cross-sectional population-based data. Early maturing adolescents may be taller than their peers during early puberty but may end up as shorter adults. Similarly, late maturing adolescents continue to grow after their peers have stopped growing, and may cross percentiles for height, weight and body mass index (BMI). Assessment of Tanner staging can inform the provider about nutritional requirements for that particular adolescent. Chronic energy deprivation during a period of growth and development can lead to growth stunting, pubertal delay, menstrual abnormalities in girls, and interference with peak bone mass accrual.

NUTRITIONAL REQUIREMENTS DURING ADOLESCENCE

The estimated caloric requirements to maintain energy balance are shown in **Table 5**. Adolescents are prone to imbalances in energy and dietary deficiencies of protein, calcium, iron, folic acid, and vitamins A, D, E, and B_6.

Energy requirements depend on activity level and are higher than those for adults. A moderately active adolescent girl requires approximately 2300 kcal/d and a moderately active boy, 2700 kcal/d.[35] Energy imbalance can lead to both obesity and eating disorders. Female athletes who do not consume sufficient calories for their sport may develop the "female athlete triad," a clinical triad characterized by low energy availability (ie, an energy deficit), menstrual dysfunction (amenorrhea and oligomenorrhea), and reduced bone mineral density.[36] The energy deficit may be intentional in those trying to drop weight or unintentional in those who are not meeting their energy requirements because of lack of knowledge or poor advice from their coach. Girls with the triad are at increased risk for stress fractures.

Protein requirements increase during adolescence to support increased muscle mass. Calcium and vitamin D are necessary for bone accretion and achievement of optimal peak bone mass and dietary deficiencies of calcium and vitamin D are prevalent in teens. The major source of calcium is milk products. Milk consumption in adolescents has declined at the same time that soda consumption has increased. Between 17% and 47% of adolescents are vitamin D deficient and the prevalence of deficiency is higher in teens than in younger children.[37] Iron requirements increase during adolescence to support increased muscle mass and higher hemoglobin levels in both boys and girls, and to offset menstrual losses in menstruating girls.

EATING DISORDERS

More than 90% of patients with eating disorders are diagnosed before the age of 25 years. The mean age of onset for anorexia nervosa is early to mid adolescence and for bulimia nervosa late adolescence. Eating disorders occur in all racial and ethnic groups with a 9:1 female predominance. However, increased prevalence in males and in younger children has been noted in recent years. Even though the diagnostic criteria for anorexia nervosa and bulimia nervosa are more inclusive with the publication of the fifth edition of the *Diagnostic and Statistical Manual of Mental Disorders* (DSM-5),[38] the prevalence of disordered eating and subclinical eating disorders far exceeds that of fully diagnosed cases. The key features of anorexia nervosa are significant weight loss leading to a low weight for age, distortion of body image, and preoccupation with shape and weight. Medical complications include

Table 5
Estimated calorie needs per day by age, gender, and physical activity level

	Male			Female[c]		
Activity level[b]	Sedentary	Moderately Active	Active	Sedentary	Moderately Active	Active
Age (y)						
2	1000	1000	1000	1000	1000	1000
3	1200	1400	1400	1000	1200	1400
4	1200	1400	1600	1200	1400	1400
5	1200	1400	1600	1200	1400	1600
6	1400	1600	1800	1200	1400	1600
7	1400	1600	1800	1200	1600	1800
8	1400	1600	2000	1400	1600	1800
9	1600	1800	2000	1400	1600	1800
10	1600	1800	2200	1400	1800	2000
11	1800	2000	2200	1600	1800	2000
12	1800	2200	2400	1600	2000	2200
13	2000	2200	2600	1600	2000	2200
14	2000	2400	2800	1800	2000	2400
15	2200	2600	3000	1800	2000	2400
16	2400	2800	3200	1800	2000	2400
17	2400	2800	3200	1800	2000	2400
18	2400	2800	3200	1800	2000	2400
19–20	2600	2800	3000	2000	2200	2400
21–25	2400	2800	3000	2000	2200	2400
26–30	2400	2600	3000	1800	2000	2400
31–35	2400	2600	3000	1800	2000	2200
36–40	2400	2600	2800	1800	2000	2200
41–45	2200	2600	2800	1800	2000	2200
46–50	2200	2400	2800	1800	2000	2200
51–55	2200	2400	2800	1600	1800	2200
56–60	2200	2400	2600	1600	1800	2200
61–65	2000	2400	2600	1600	1800	2000
66–70	2000	2200	2600	1600	1800	2000
71–75	2000	2200	2600	1600	1800	2000
76+	2000	2200	2400	1600	1800	2000

Estimated amounts of calories[a] needed to maintain calorie balance for various gender and age groups at 3 different levels of physical activity. The estimates are rounded to the nearest 200 calories for assignment to a USDA Food Pattern. An individual's calorie needs may be higher or lower than these average estimates.

[a] Based on Estimated Energy Requirements (EER) equations, using reference heights (average) and reference weights (healthy) for each age-gender group. For children and adolescents, reference height and weight vary. For adults, the reference man is 5 feet 10 inches tall and weighs 154 pounds. The reference woman is 5 feet 4 inches tall and weighs 126 pounds. EER equations are from the Institute of Medicine.

[b] Sedentary means a lifestyle that includes only the light physical activity associated with typical day-to-day life. Moderately active means a lifestyle that includes physical activity equivalent to walking about 1.5 to 3 miles per day at 3 to 4 miles per hour, in addition to the light physical activity associated with typical day-to-day life. Active means a lifestyle that includes physical activity equivalent to walking more than 3 miles per day at 3 to 4 miles per hour, in addition to the light physical activity associated with typical day-to-day life.

[c] Estimates for females do not include women who are pregnant or breastfeeding.

From USDA – Center for Nutrition Policy and Promotion. Available at: http://www.cnpp.usda.gov/sites/default/files/usda_food_patterns/EstimatedCalorieNeedsPerDayTable.pdf. Accessed June 9, 2016; and Dietary reference intakes for energy, carbohydrate, fiber, fat, fatty acids, cholesterol, protein, and amino acids. Washington (DC): The National Academies Press; 2002.

bradycardia, cardiac arrhythmias, vital sign instability, electrolyte disturbances, nutritional anemia, increased transaminases, growth retardation, pubertal delay, amenorrhea in girls, and reduced bone mass in both boys and girls. Key features of bulimia nervosa are recurrent episodes of bingeing with inappropriate compensatory behaviors that include purging, excessive exercise, periods of starvation, and use of diet pills, laxatives, and/or diuretics. In contrast with anorexia nervosa, where weight is low, patients with bulimia nervosa are usually of normal weight. Avoidant restrictive food intake disorder, a new diagnostic category in DSM-5, describes those patients who avoid certain foods because of color, texture, or fear of choking or vomiting. There is no distortion in body weight and no fear of gaining weight, but the eating behaviors interfere with normal growth and development. The medical provider plays an important role in the diagnosis and management of eating disorders, usually as part of a multidisciplinary team.[39]

INFLUENCE OF NUTRITION ON EARLY BRAIN DEVELOPMENT

Healthy, normal neurodevelopment is a complex process involving cellular and structural changes in the brain that proceed in a specified sequence.[40,41] Timing is crucial; once a particular developmental sequence fails, it may be possible to retrieve some lost function, but not all of it. Healthy development requires that all necessary factors be present at their biologically defined time points and that no inhibitory factors be present.

The period from conception to age 2 years (the "first 1000 days") is a time of tremendous opportunity for neurodevelopment, and a time of tremendous vulnerability.[40] In the presence of a supportive environment, an attached primary provider, and a healthy diet, the brain will thrive. In the presence of toxic stress, emotional deprivation, and a deficient diet, the child is unlikely to have optimal brain development. Both adequate overall nutrition (ie, absence of malnutrition) and provision of adequate amounts of key micronutrients at critical periods in development are necessary for normal brain development.

Macronutrient sufficiency is necessary for normal brain development. Early malnutrition is associated with lower IQ scores, reduced school success, and more behavioral dysregulation.[42] Availability of increased resources, as in higher socioeconomic conditions, may mitigate some or all of the effects of early malnutrition.[43] However, the classic study of early malnutrition, the Dutch Famine study, is instructive in this regard. Pregnant women in Holland, along with the rest of the country, experienced severe food restrictions for several months after World War II. Children born to these women generally experienced adequate food intake after birth, and did not exhibit IQ deficits into adulthood. However, as adults they had increased psychiatric disease (eg, schizophrenia) and increased risk of addiction. Thus, the impact of severe malnutrition in early childhood can be reduced by subsequent environmental enrichment, but not completely normalized.[41]

In addition to generalized malnutrition, deficiencies of individual nutrients may have substantial impact on neurodevelopment. Prenatal and early infancy iron deficiency is associated with long-term neurobehavioral damage that may not be reversible, even with later iron supplementation. Maternal iron deficiency, limited availability of maternal iron (eg, cigarette smoking or maternal hypertension), or conditions that increase fetal iron demand (such as maternal diabetes), may lead to newborn iron deficiency and associated long-term cognitive deficits.[44] Adolescent iron deficiency is also associated with neurocognitive impairment, but is reversible with iron treatment.[44] Iodine is essential for synthesis of thyroid hormone, which is crucial in neurodevelopment. Deficiency of iodine in pregnant women leads to cretinism in the child, with attendant severe irreversible developmental delays. Postnatal mild to moderate chronic iodine deficiency is associated with reduced performance on IQ tests.[41] Women living in iodine-deficient areas of the world require attention to supplementation during pregnancy.[45] Long-chain polyunsaturated fatty acids, which include docosahexaenoic acid and arachidonic acid are important for normal development of vision and may also impact neurocognitive development.[45] Traditions in complementary feeding, or restricted diets owing to poverty, may reduce infant intake of many key factors in normal neurodevelopment, including zinc, protein, and iron.[45]

Nutrition plays a critical role in neurodevelopment. Nutrient deficiencies during fetal life and early childhood may have long-lasting impact on cognitive development, behavior, and emotional well-being. Insuring adequate nutrition during these periods and screening for deficits, when appropriate, is critical.

FOOD ALLERGIES

An allergy is an immune reaction to a protein. Published studies indicate that 4% to 8% of children in the United States have a food allergy.[46] There are many adverse reactions to foods that are not based on an immune reaction. The non–immune-based processes are usually called intolerances and may be caused by maldigestion, or toxic or pharmacologic reactions to foods. The allergic reactions by the immune system can be with antibody-based responses, or mixed or cellular responses.

The antibody-based reactions are the more acute and severe; these reactions range anywhere from anaphylaxis to urticaria. Normally these are IgE mediated. A sensitized individual when exposed to the triggering food protein has IgE binding that results in the release of a variety of immune mediators. The end result depends on the mediators released and can cause symptoms in the skin, gastrointestinal tract, respiratory tract, and cardiovascular system. The IgE reactions have the potential to become life threatening.

T lymphocytes can also react to food proteins and result primarily in gastrointestinal symptoms, typically enteropathy or enterocolitis. Clinically, patients present with vomiting or diarrhea. There is also a set of disorders that are a mixture of IgE and non-IgE reactions. These disorders result in an infiltration of the gastrointestinal mucosa by eosinophils. The location involved within the gastrointestinal tract varies. Therefore, symptoms can vary from vomiting, abdominal pain, to weight loss or poor weight gain.

Many times, the diagnosis of food allergies is made by history because there is minimal testing available. For IgE-mediated reactions, skin prick testing can be done. A positive test means that an IgE antibody is present but not necessarily clinical disease. The same is true of the blood radioallergosorbent test (RAST) and these tests require correlation with clinical history. Using these tests as a general screen for nonspecific symptoms leads to a high number of positive tests that may not be relevant clinically. The best test to diagnosis food allergies is the oral food challenge. This is done under medical observation with the best test being when the family and observer are all blinded to whether the food protein is present or not. The eosinophilic disorders are diagnosed based on biopsies from the gastrointestinal mucosa. The histology suggests the allergic process but does not identify the causative agent.

The most common foods that are causative for allergic reactions in the United States are milk, soy, egg, wheat, peanut, tree nuts, fish, and shellfish.[47] The primary therapy for food allergies is strict avoidance of the food resulting in the allergy. For those with anaphylaxis-type reactions, the prescription of an epinephrine injector is necessary. Some patients have multiple food allergies and this can lead to concerns about nutritional deficiencies. The allergic process in the esophagus, eosinophilic esophagitis, has been treated successfully with a topical steroid approach.

The course of childhood food allergies depends on the food to which the child is sensitive. The great majority of children allergic to milk, soy, eggs, and wheat will lose the response by 5 years of age. This is in contrast with the peanut, tree nuts, and seafood allergic reactions, which are commonly lifelong.[46]

FOOD SAFETY

Infants and children are particularly susceptible to infections or toxic contaminants in food. Food products and contaminants that are generally harmless or cause minimal harm in healthy adults may represent both immediate- and long-term risk when ingested by infants and children. In general, the younger the child and the higher the dose ingested, the more serious the potential effects.

Infant botulism is an example. Exposure of infants to spores of *Clostridium botulinum* occurs through ingestion of infected soil or honey. In the gastrointestinal, tract the spores germinate, colonize the tract, and the bacteria produce botulinum toxins A and B.[48] Infantile botulism is characterized by progressive weakness, frequently requiring prolonged ventilator support. About 94 cases per year of infant botulism are reported to the CDC, but many cases may go unrecognized. A history of honey consumption is seen in 15% of cases, and 25% of honey products contain spores. Although the amount of spores in honey is harmless to older children, children under the age of 1 year should not be given honey or products containing honey.[49]

Other foods unsafe for infants and children include raw milk and products made with raw milk, meat, poultry, eggs, fish, and products made with them.[50,51] These products can carry bacterial, viral, or parasitic contamination that can lead to illness in any person. However, infants and children are at increased risk because of their less mature immune systems and more rapid rate of dehydration. Contaminated food may lead to classic gastrointestinal symptoms, including vomiting, diarrhea, and abdominal cramps, but some agents cause more serious illness. *Escherichia coli* 0157:H7 is associated with hemolytic–anemia syndrome, for example, which may lead to renal failure.

Toxins present in food may also pose a risk for infants and children. Pesticide residue, agents added during food processing, and naturally occurring toxins may pose risks to the developing child's brain when present in high levels. Mercury is a known contaminant in the food chain (eg, swordfish, mackerel). Blood concentrations of methylmercury may be increased in children born to mothers ingesting mercury contaminated fish. Infants are at especially high risk with exposure to this neurodevelopmental toxin.[52]

The CDC, the AAP, and other agencies provide guidance for providers and families that can reduce risk of infectious and toxic food contamination or limit risk of ingesting contaminants if present. Use of these resources will ultimately reduce risk to children.

NUTRITION FOR OBESITY, DYSLIPIDEMIA, AND HYPERTENSION

The pediatric obesity epidemic has led to the need for widespread nutritional intervention during childhood. Overweight in children is defined as a BMI at the 85th percentile or greater for age and sex, and obesity is defined as a BMI at the 95th percentile or greater for age and sex.[53,54] The prevalence of obesity in 2- to 19-year-old US children is 16.9%,[33] with increasing risks of comorbidities such as dyslipidemia and hypertension associated with excess adiposity.

Efforts to stem the tide of obesity have progressively turned scientists' attention to earlier childhood, and the fetal environment. In the 1990s, Barker[55] introduced the concept of the fetal origins of adult disease, underscoring the importance of maternal nutrition and fetal growth during pregnancy. He proposed that undernutrition of the fetus in utero leads to metabolic changes and fetal programming, later resulting in increased risk for adult diseases such as coronary artery disease, diabetes, and hypertension.[55] The "thrifty phenotype hypothesis" suggests that malnutrition in the intrauterine environment leads to permanent adaptive metabolic changes in the fetus, which may be mismatched to an extrauterine environment with excess nutrition and a sedentary lifestyle.[56,57] One of the mechanisms suggested for these adaptive changes is epigenetic, the phenomenon of the environment interacting with the human genome, causing methylation changes in DNA and posttranslational histone modifications. These changes are heritable, and thought to contribute to fetal programming of later disease risk.[58,59] Thus, an infant born with intrauterine growth retardation may undergo changes in utero causing later insulin resistance and cardiometabolic disease.

Obesity is often not only a state of overnutrition, but of poor nutrition, with an excess of nonnutritive, energy-dense foods. If an overweight or obese child is young enough, they may be able to work toward weight maintenance, allowing statural growth "into" his or her weight. However, if the child already carries significant excess weight by adult standards, weight loss may be indicated. This can often be done through lifestyle modification involving both increased physical activity and improved nutrition.[54] In the United States, common sources of nonnutritive calories include soft drinks, energy drinks, and fast food. Elimination or limitation of these foods and drinks improves nutritional status and can result in weight loss. An energy deficit of approximately 300 to 400 kcal/d should result in a weight loss of approximately 1 pound per week.[54] Physical activity producing energy expenditure is an important part of health promotion. It is recommended that children do at least 60 minutes of moderate to vigorous activity daily. Sedentary activities such as television, computer use not related to school, handheld electronics, video games, and cell phones should be kept to less than 2 hours per day.[54]

Nutritional changes can be made in consultation with a pediatric nutritionist, by setting short-term goals and tracking progress, with frequent follow-up and rewards for successful accomplishment of goals. Nutritional changes should not be portrayed as punitive to the child, and in general should be made by the family as whole, with an emphasis on healthy eating for a lifetime. Children should be encouraged to eat at least 5 servings of fruits and vegetables daily, and to increase fiber intake. They should not skip meals, and portion sizes should be limited. Short-term fad diets are not recommended, and in some cases can be dangerous for children, who still need appropriate amounts of vitamins and minerals for growth. Multiple free nutritional resources are available for families, including www.choosemyplate.gov and www.healthychildren.org (accessed April 4, 2016). The AAP "Healthy Active Living for Families" page at www.healthychildren.org (accessed April 4, 2016) advocates the "5-2-1-0" campaign—5 servings of fruits and vegetables per day, no more than 2 hours of screen time per day, 1 hour of physical activity per day, and 0 sugar-sweetened beverages. Some have added 8 to this, representing 8 hours of sleep per night. This is a straightforward message for childhood healthy living that has been advocated broadly.

Lifestyle change can be difficult, and childhood obesity can lead to multiple complications, such as dyslipidemia. Dyslipidemia can occur as a consequence of obesity or in hereditary forms. The current prevalence of 1 or more abnormal lipids in US children 6 to 19 years of age is approximately 20%,[60–62] with evidence of some decrease in prevalence between 1999 to 2000 and 2011 to 2012.[62] Autopsy studies have shown that atherosclerosis begins in youth, indicating that prevention and treatment during childhood is preferable. For confirmed hyperlipidemia, the recommended population diet includes an average intake of less than 10% of total calories from saturated fatty acids, 20% to 30% of calories from total fat, and less than 300 mg/d of cholesterol. Polyunsaturated fatty acids should be up to 10% and monounsaturated fatty acids 10% to 15% of total calories. The diet should consist of approximately 55% of total calories from carbohydrates (optimally replacing simple with complex carbohydrates such as whole grains) and 15% from protein.[54,63] It is also recommended to limit trans fatty acids to less than 1% of total calories or, if possible, to eliminate trans fats completely from the diet. For children at high cardiovascular risk, further restriction of saturated fat to less than 7% and total cholesterol to less than 200 mg/d are recommended.[64]

Another potential complication of obesity is hypertension. In youth, blood pressure is categorized by percentile for age, sex, and height.[65] In 3- to 11-year-olds, blood pressure at the 90th percentile or greater but less than the 95th percentile is categorized as prehypertension, 95th percentile or greater but less than the 99th percentile + 5 mm Hg is considered stage 1 hypertension, and 99th percentile or greater + 5 mm Hg is considered stage 2 hypertension. Among 12- to 17-year-olds, the same categories apply except that prehypertension also includes blood pressure of 120/80 mm Hg or greater but less than the 95th percentile.[24] Using the National Health and Nutrition Examination Survey data in 8- to 17-year-olds, the prevalence of "high" blood pressure (blood pressure at or above the 95th percentile) has decreased from 3% in 1999 to 2000 to 1.6% in 2011 to 2012. The prevalence of "borderline high" ($\geq$90th percentile but <95th percentile, or $\geq$120/80 mm Hg but <95th percentile) and "high or borderline high" have remained approximately the same, with a prevalence of 9.4% and 11%, respectively, in the 2011 to 2012 survey.[62] Elevated blood pressure is associated with increased BMI and weight loss of 5% to 10% of initial body weight has been associated with a decrease in blood pressure.[24]

The Cardiovascular Health Integrated Lifestyle Diet (CHILD-1) is the first stage in dietary modification for children felt to be at increased cardiovascular risk.[24] It is important that appropriate calories and nutrients are provided for growth and development. A diet plan associated with some weight loss and with significantly decreased blood pressure is the Dietary Approach to Stop Hypertension (DASH diet), which was developed initially for adults.[66] This diet is low in saturated fat, sugar, and sodium, and high in potassium in composition.[67,68] More specific restriction of sodium, initially started at 2-3 g/d, may be helpful as well, especially in salt-sensitive individuals.

SUMMARY

Nutrition is a critical factor for appropriate child and adolescent development. Because individuals in the pediatric age group are growing and developing, appropriate nutrition changes according to age. It is also clear that nutrition is an important element for prevention of disease development, especially for chronic diseases such as obesity, diabetes, hypertension, and dyslipidemia.

Many children and adolescents live in home, school, and other environments that do not promote optimum nutrition. This is in part what leads to increased consumption of calorie-dense, but nutrient-poor foods and beverages, including sugar-sweetened beverages. Thus, families must work to provide improved food environments to encourage optimum nutrition. The stakes are high in that early primordial prevention of risk factors for chronic disease, such as cardiovascular disease, is important, and dietary habits established early may be carried through adult life.

REFERENCES

1. World Health Organization (WHO). The WHO child growth standards. Available at: http://www.who.int/childgrowth/en. Accessed July 12, 2016.
2. Centers for Disease Control and Prevention (CDC), National Center for Health Statistics. Growth charts. Available at: http://www.cdc.gov/growthcharts. Accessed July 12, 2016.
3. American Academy of Pediatrics Committee on Nutrition. Appendix E. In: Kleinman RE, Greer FR, editors. Pediatric nutrition. 7th edition. Elk Grove (IL): American Academy of Pediatrics; 2014. p. 1355.
4. Becker P, Corkins MR, Carney LN, et al, Academy of Nutrition and Dietetics and the American Society for Parenteral and Enteral Nutrition. Consensus Statement of the Academy of Nutrition and Dietetics/American Society for Parenteral and Enteral Nutrition: Indicators Recommended for the Identification and Documentation of Pediatric Malnutrition (Undernutrition). Nutr Clin Pract 2015;30(1):147–61.
5. Kramer MS, Kakuma R. Optimal duration of exclusive breastfeeding. Cochrane Database Syst Rev 2012;(8):CD003517.
6. Ballard O, Morrow AL. Human milk composition: nutrients and bioactive factors. Pediatr Clin North Am 2013;60(1):49–74.
7. Moore ER, Anderson GC, Bergman N, et al. Early skin-to-skin contact for mothers and their healthy newborn infants. Cochrane Database Syst Rev 2012;(5):CD003519.
8. Cooper AR, Barnett D, Gentles E, et al. Macronutrient content of donor human breast milk. Arch Dis Child Fetal Neonatal Ed 2013;98(6):F539–41.
9. De Halleux V, Rigo J. Variability in human milk composition: benefit of individualized fortification in very-low-birth-weight infants. Am J Clin Nutr 2013;98(2): 529S–35S.
10. Innis SM. Impact of maternal diet on human milk composition and neurological development of infants. Am J Clin Nutr 2014;99(3):734S–41S.
11. Hoyt AE, Medico T, Commins SP. Breast milk and food allergy: connections and current recommendations. Pediatr Clin North Am 2015;62(6):1493–507.
12. McGuire E. Vitamin D and breastfeeding: an update. Breastfeed Rev 2015;23(2): 26–32.
13. Hollis BW, Wagner CL, Howard CR, et al. Maternal versus infant vitamin D supplementation during lactation: a randomized controlled trial. Pediatrics 2015;136(4): 625–34.
14. Wagner CL, Greer FR, American Academy of Pediatrics Section on Breastfeeding, American Academy of Pediatrics Committee on Nutrition. Prevention of rickets and vitamin D deficiency in infants, children, and adolescents. Pediatrics 2008;122(5):1142–52.
15. Kleinman RE, Greer F. Pediatric nutrition handbook. 7th edition. Elk Grove Village (IL): American Academy of Pediatrics; 2012.
16. Capeding R, Gepanayao CP, Calimon N, et al. Lutein-fortified infant formula fed to healthy term infants: evaluation of growth effects and safety. Nutr J 2010;9–22. http://dx.doi.org/10.1186/1475-2891-9-22.
17. Pinto-Sanchez MI, Verdu EF, Liu E, et al. Gluten introduction to infant feeding and risk of celiac disease: systematic review and meta-analysis. J Pediatr 2016;168: 132–43.e3.

18. Fleischer DM, Sicherer S, Greenhawt M, et al. Consensus communication on early peanut introduction and the prevention of peanut allergy in high-risk infants. Ann Allergy Asthma Immunol 2015;115(2):87–90.
19. Qasem W, Fenton T, Friel J. Age of introduction of first complementary feeding for infants: a systematic review. BMC Pediatr 2015;15:107.
20. Baker RD, Greer FR. Committee on Nutrition of the American Academy of Pediatrics. Diagnosis and prevention of iron deficiency and iron-deficiency anemia in infants and young children (0-3 years of age). Pediatrics 2010;126(5):1040–50.
21. Anzman-Frasca S, Savage JS, Marini ME, et al. Repeated exposure and associate conditioning promote preschool children's liking of vegetables. Appetite 2012;58:543–53.
22. Berge JM, Wall M, Hsueh TF, et al. The protective role of family meals for youth obesity: 10-year longitudinal associations. J Pediatr 2015;166:296–301.
23. Kleinman RE, Greer FR. Pediatric Nutrition. 7th Edition. Chicago (IL): American Academy of Pediatrics; 2014.
24. Expert Panel on Integrated Guidelines for Cardiovascular Health and Risk Reduction in Children and Adolescents, National Heart, Lung, and Blood Institute. Expert panel on integrated guidelines for cardiovascular health and risk reduction in children and adolescents: summary report. Pediatrics 2011;128(Suppl 5): S213–56.
25. Marriott BP, Olsho L, Hadden L, et al. Intake of added sugars and selected nutrients in the United States, National Health and Nutrition Examination Survey (NHANES) 2003-2006. Crit Rev Food Sci Nutr 2010;50(3):228–58.
26. Banfield EC, Liu Y, Davis JS, et al. Poor adherence to US Dietary Guidelines for Children and Adolescents in the National Health and Nutrition Examination Survey Population. J Acad Nutr Diet 2016;116(1):21–7.
27. Reedy J, Krebs-Smith SM. Dietary sources of energy, solid fats, and added sugars among children and adolescents in the United States. J Am Diet Assoc 2010;110(10):1477–84.
28. Santiago-Torres M, Adams AK, Carrel AL, et al. Home food availability, parental dietary intake, and familial eating habits influence the diet quality of urban Hispanic children. Child Obes 2014;10(5):408–15.
29. Huang J, Barnidge E. Low-income Children's participation in the National School Lunch Program and household food insufficiency. Soc Sci Med 2015;150:8–14.
30. Hopkins LC, Gunther C. A historical review of changes in nutrition standards of USDA child meal programs relative to research findings on the nutritional adequacy of program meals and the diet and nutritional health of participants: implications for future research and the summer food service program. Nutrients 2015;7(12):10145–67.
31. Schwartz MB, Henderson KE, Read M, et al. New school meal regulations increase fruit consumption and do not increase total plate waste. Child Obes 2015;11(3):242–7.
32. Merlo C, Brener N, Kann L, et al. School-level practices to increase availability of fruits, vegetables, and whole grains, and reduce sodium in school meals - United States, 2000, 2006, and 2014. MMWR Morb Mortal Wkly Rep 2015;64(33):905–8.
33. Ogden CL, Carroll MD, Kit BK, et al. Prevalence of childhood and adult obesity in the United States, 2011-2012. JAMA 2014;311(8):806–14.
34. American Academy of Pediatrics Committee on Adolescence, American College of Obstetricians and Gynecologists Committee on Adolescent Health Care, Diaz A. Menstruation in girls and adolescents: using the menstrual cycle as a vital sign. Pediatrics 2006;118(5):2245–50.

35. American Academy of Pediatrics Committee on Nutrition. Pediatric nutrition 7th edition: adolescent nutrition. Elk Grove Village (IL): American Academy of Pediatrics; 2014.

36. Nattiv A, Loucks AB, Manore MM, et al. American College of Sports Medicine position stand. The female athlete triad. Med Sci Sports Exerc 2007;39(10): 1867–82.

37. Golden NH, Abrams SA, Committee on Nutrition. Optimizing bone health in children and adolescents. Pediatrics 2014;134(4):e1229–43.

38. American Psychiatric Association. Diagnostic and statistical manual of mental disorders. 5th edition. Washington, DC: American Psychiatric Association; 2013.

39. Golden NH, Katzman DK, Sawyer SM, et al. Update on the medical management of eating disorders in adolescents. J Adolesc Health 2015;56(4):370–5.

40. Wachs TD, Georgieff M, Cusick S, et al. Issues in the timing of integrated early interventions: contributions from nutrition, neuroscience and psychological research. Ann N Y Acad Sci 2014;1308:89–106.

41. Prado EL, Dewey KG. Nutrition and brain development in early life. Nutr Rev 2014;72:267–84.

42. Grantham-McGregor S. A review of studies of the effect of severe malnutrition on mental development. J Nutr 1995;125:2233S–8S.

43. Troche F, Echevarria G. The effect of birthweight on childhood cognitive development in a middle-income country. Int J Epidemiol 2011;40:1008–18.

44. Georgieff MK. Long-term brain and behavioral consequences of early iron deficiency. Nutr Rev 2011;69(Suppl 1):S43–8.

45. Monk C, Georgieff MK, Osterholm EA. Research review: maternal prenatal distress and poor nutrition—mutually influencing risk factors affecting infant neurocognitive development. J Child Psychol Psychiatry 2013;54:115–30.

46. American Academy of Pediatrics Committee on Nutrition. Food allergy. In: Kleinman RE, Greer FR, editors. Pediatric nutrition. 7th edition. Elk Grove (IL): American Academy of Pediatrics; 2014. p. 845.

47. Walla CLS, Feuling MB, Glimenez LM, et al. Food allergies. In: Corkins MR, editor. The A.S.P.E.N. Pediatric nutrition support core curriculum. 2nd edition. Silver Spring (MD): American Society for Parenteral and Enteral Nutrition; 2015. p. 289.

48. Centers for Disease Control and Prevention (CDC). Botulism. Available at: http://www.cdc.gov/nczved/divisions/dfbmd/diseases/botulism/. Accessed December 3, 2015.

49. Cox N, Hinkle R. Infant botulism. Am Fam Physician 2002;65:1388–92.

50. American Academy of Pediatrics Committee on Nutrition. Food safety: infectious disease. In: Kleinman RE, Greer FR, editors. Pediatric nutrition. 7th edition. Elk Grove Village (IL): American Academy of Pediatrics; 2014. p. 1225–49.

51. Committee on Infectious diseases, Committee on Nutrition, American Academy of Pediatrics. Consumption of raw or unpasteurized milk and milk products by pregnant women and children. Pediatrics 2014;133:175–9.

52. American Academy of Pediatrics Committee on Nutrition. Food Safety: pesticides, industrial chemicals, toxins, antimicrobial preservatives, irradiation, and food contact substances. In: Kleinman RE, Greer FR, editors. Pediatric nutrition. 7th edition. Elk Grove Village (IL): American Academy of Pediatrics; 2014. p. 1252–84.

53. American Academy of Pediatrics Committee on Nutrition. Pediatric obesity. In: Kleinman RE, Greer FR, editors. Pediatric nutrition. 7th edition. Elk Grove (IL): American Academy of Pediatrics; 2014. p. 1355.

54. Barlow SE. Expert committee recommendations regarding the prevention, assessment, and treatment of child and adolescent overweight and obesity: summary report. Pediatrics 2007;120:S164.
55. Barker DJ. The fetal and infant origins of disease. Eur J Clin Invest 1995;25(7): 457–63.
56. Hales CN, Barker DJ. The thrifty phenotype hypothesis. Br Med Bull 2001;60: 5–20.
57. Calkins K, Devaskar SU. Fetal origins of adult disease. Curr Probl Pediatr Adolesc Health Care 2011;41(6):158–76.
58. Raychaudhuri N, Raychaudhuri S, Thamotharan M, et al. Histone code modifications repress glucose transporter 4 expression in the intrauterine growth-restricted offspring. J Biol Chem 2008;283(20):13611–26.
59. Simmons RA. Developmental origins of beta-cell failure in type 2 diabetes: the role of epigenetic mechanisms. Pediatr Res 2007;61(5 Pt 2):64R–7R.
60. Dai S, Yang Q, Yuan K, et al. Non-high-density lipoprotein cholesterol: distribution and prevalence of high serum levels in children and adolescents: United States National Health and Nutrition Examination Surveys, 2005-2010. J Pediatr 2014; 164(2):247–53.
61. Kit BK, Carroll MD, Lacher DA, et al. Trends in serum lipids among US youths aged 6 to 19 years, 1988-2010. JAMA 2012;308(6):591–600.
62. Kit BK, Kuklina E, Carroll MD, et al. Prevalence of and trends in dyslipidemia and blood pressure among US children and adolescents, 1999-2012. JAMA Pediatr 2015;169(3):272–9.
63. American Academy of Pediatrics. National Cholesterol Education Program: report of the expert panel on blood cholesterol levels in children and adolescents. Pediatrics 1992;89(3 pt 2):525–84.
64. US Department of Agriculture, US Department of Health and Human Services. Dietary guidelines for Americans, 2012. 7th edition. Washington, DC: US Government Printing Office; 2010.
65. National High Blood Pressure Education Program Working Group on High Blood Pressure in Children and Adolescents. The fourth report on the diagnosis, evaluation, and treatment of high blood pressure in children and adolescents. Pediatrics 2004;114(2 Suppl 4th Report):555–76.
66. Gidding SS, Dennison BA, Birch LL, et al, American Heart Association, American Academy of Pediatrics. Dietary recommendations for children and adolescents: a guide for practitioners: consensus statement from the American Heart Association. Circulation 2005;112(13):2061–75.
67. Mertens IL, Van Gaal LF. Overweight, obesity, and blood pressure: the effects of modest weight reduction. Obes Res 2000;8(3):270–8.
68. Couch SC, Saelens BE, Levin L, et al. The efficacy of a clinic-based behavioral nutrition intervention emphasizing a dash-type diet for adolescents with elevated blood pressure. J Pediatr 2008;152(4):494–501.

Nutrition Recommendations in Elderly and Aging

Hope Barkoukis, PhD, RDN, LD

KEYWORDS

- Aging • Physiologic changes of aging • Nutrition screening tools for older adults
- Nutrition recommendations for older adults • Geriatric giants, nutrition and aging

KEY POINTS

- Optimal nutritional status is a cornerstone for healthy aging. Early identification of older adults who are at risk of insufficient caloric and nutrient adequacy, defined as nutritional risk, is paramount to maintaining health, independence, quality of life, and longevity.
- Maintaining optimal health and well-being in the older adult requires an understanding of how physiologic changes influence nutritional status.
- Familiarity with available validated nutrition screening and assessment tools for the older adult is critical to providing evidence based practice.

INTRODUCTION

Aging is defined as the collective series of physiologic changes that occur in an organism over time, resulting in progressive deterioration of functioning, increased vulnerability to disease, and reduced viability.[1] Primary aging, or senescence, refers to the intrinsic age-related changes independent of disease processes or the environment. Secondary aging includes the interaction of senescence with disease processes and environmental influences. Considerable heterogeneity in health trajectory, health status, and quality of life exist at any given age.[2] According to the Administration on Aging, 14.1% of the US population are categorized as older adults (age ≥65); by 2040, this figure is expected to reach 21.7%.

Optimal nutritional status is a cornerstone for healthy aging. Aging increases the prevalence of malnutrition due to numerous factors, including physiologic changes, social and environmental influences, decreased physical functioning, cognitive decline, and multimorbidities.[3] Early identification of older adults who are at risk of insufficient caloric and nutrient adequacy, defined as nutritional risk, is paramount to maintaining health, independence, quality of life, and longevity.

Department of Nutrition, School of Medicine, Case Western Reserve University, 10900 Euclid Avenue, Cleveland, OH 44106, USA
E-mail address: Hope.Barkoukis@case.edu

Med Clin N Am 100 (2016) 1237–1250
http://dx.doi.org/10.1016/j.mcna.2016.06.006
0025-7125/16/$ – see front matter © 2016 Elsevier Inc. All rights reserved.

medical.theclinics.com

This article reviews the following: (1) physiologic and pathophysiologic changes of aging, (2) nutrition screening and assessment tools for older adults, (3) specific nutrition recommendations for older adults and how they differ from younger persons, and (4) important disorders and risk factors that predispose older adults to increased morbidity and functional decline, including "geriatric giants" along with nutrition recommendations to address these issues.

PHYSIOLOGIC AND PATHOPHYSIOLOGIC CHANGES OF AGING
Dysphagia

The changes in swallowing physiology from primary and secondary aging translates to a conservative dysphagia prevalence estimate of approximately 8% of older adults worldwide, 15% of community-dwelling older adults in the United States, 68% of nursing home residents, approximately 64% of patients with stroke, and 45% of those with dementia in the United States.[4] Nutritional status is at risk because the presence of dysphagia generally leads to reduced or altered oral food and liquid intake, thus increasing malnutrition risk and negatively impacting functional capacity.

Primary age-related changes influencing swallowing include reduced muscle mass; loss of connective tissue elasticity that impacts the flow of ingested foods through the upper digestive tract; and decreases in saliva production, taste sensitivity, and olfaction.[4] These collective changes generally are subtle but progress to slow the collective swallowing processes, increase risk of swallowed foods penetrating into the upper airway, and increase post-swallow residue accumulation during meals.[5]

Best practice dysphagia management is a team approach including the physician, speech language pathologist, and the registered dietitian nutritionist. A "one-size-fits-all" strategy is not recommended. Universally the goals are to optimize oral nutrition and hydration intake and nutritional status, and prevent related morbidities, such as risk of aspiration and pneumonia. The main concepts of dietary modification are to thicken liquids to slow swallowing transit time, alter food texture and size to improve swallowing safety, maintain nutritional and hydration intake, and reduce the risk of aspiration.[4] Plans are currently under way to create universal descriptors and best practice guidelines for international dysphagia management[5]; in the United States there is a National Dysphagia Diet, published in 2002 by the American Dietetic Association, providing clear guidelines defining diet level categories, clarification of viscosity levels, and evidence-based best nutritional practices.[6]

Gastroesophageal Reflux Disease

Gastroesophageal reflux disease or GERD is defined as symptoms and mucosal damage that develops secondary to the reflux of gastric contents into the esophagus.[7] In the United States, the most commonly reported upper gastrointestinal disorder in older adults is GERD with approximately 10% to 20% reporting symptoms at least once weekly and 15% to 40% experiencing symptoms at least once monthly.[7] The etiology of GERD includes reduced salivary production, delayed gastric emptying, and an altered antireflux barrier. The reduced salivary production decreases salivary bicarbonate response to the presence of acid in the esophagus, thus impairing esophageal acid clearance.[7] During aging, the lower esophageal sphincter (LES) has transient relaxations, not accompanied by swallowing, thereby promoting acid reflux and altering its intended function as an antireflux barrier.[7] Commonly used medications for hypertension, cardiovascular disease, and depression also decrease LES pressure.

Evaluation of GERD in the older adult is critical, and the main treatment goals would include alleviation of symptoms, healing the esophagitis, and preventing complications. Lifestyle modification techniques would be a cornerstone of most initial therapy, and these include weight loss; increased physical activity; decreasing meal volume, dietary fat; avoiding dietary irritants, such as alcohol, tomatoes, coffee, and onions; elevating the head of the bed when sleeping; and avoiding ingestion of foods before bedtime.[7]

Gastrointestinal Motility

The rate of gastric emptying influences nutrient absorption as well as rate of appearance into plasma.[8,9] Numerous factors impact gastric-emptying rates, including liquid versus solid meals, meal volume, the ratio between liquid versus solid in one meal, the amount and type of dietary fibers present in the meal, the specific kinetics of nutrient absorption, and the type of carbohydrate and protein in the meal.[8,9] Given the plethora of etiologic factors and the heterogeneity of study designs, conflicting data have been reported on the impact of primary aging on gastric-emptying rates. In the context of these noted limitations, generally speaking, slower gastric-emptying rates for large meals have been repeatedly demonstrated in older versus younger adults, whereas studies using liquid or small meals have not universally observed this delayed gastric response.[10]

Other changes associated with primary and secondary aging are impaired esophageal peristalsis, decreased transpyloric flows, decreased gastric contractile force, and post meal peristalsis, but no evidence of altered small intestine transit times.[10] The transit times and motility patterns in the small intestine seem to be maintained with aging, but very limited data are available.[8] The effect of primary aging on colonic transit time has been challenging due to the impact of confounding factors.[8,10]

Constipation

Chronic constipation not associated with irritable bowel syndrome is defined as infrequent stools (defined as <2 per week), and/or difficulty in passage of stools such that there is a sense of incomplete stool evacuation, straining, hard or lumpy stools, a prolonged time to evacuate stool, or the need for assistance via manual techniques to induce stool passage for a 3-month period of time within the prior year.[11] This condition is one of the most frequently diagnosed gastrointestinal problems in the older adult. Self-reported constipation has been reported at 26% in women and 16% in men 65 years or older in a free-living environment. Chronic constipation in long-term care facilities has a documented prevalence of approximately 57% in women and 64% in men.

Both primary and secondary aging factors are associated with the etiology of chronic constipation. Primary factors include alterations in colonic motility and physiology, including reduced neuron number in the myenteric plexus, reduced response to direct stimulation, increased collagen deposition in the colon, reduced colonic segmental motor coordination, decreased sphincter pressure (both resting and maximally stimulated), decreased squeeze pressure, and diminished rectal wall elasticity.[11] Secondary aging contributory factors include insufficient total calorie and fluid intake; diets low in dietary fiber; high-fat diets; hyperglycemic and hypokalemic conditions; impaired and/or limited mobility; cognitive and neurologic disorders; increased dependence (nursing home residence vs community dwelling); a variety of medications, including the use of anticholinergic agents, opioid analgesics, calcium supplements, calcium channel blockers, and nonsteroidal anti-inflammatory drugs; autoimmune disorders; diabetes mellitus; psychological disorders; and travel.

Clinical evaluation includes a physical examination, including anal examination, a detailed history, and assessment of the primary and secondary etiology. Identification of high risk factors, such as involuntary weight loss, family history of colorectal cancer or inflammatory bowel disease, positive fecal occult blood testing, iron deficiency anemia, acute onset of symptoms, sudden change in bowel habits, or hematochezia, would warrant a thorough diagnostic evaluation of the colon.[11]

When the physician determines that a nonpharmacologic approach to management can be initiated, it is of value to include the dietitian and/or nurse educator to discuss dietary factors, increases in physical activity as medically appropriate, and toilet training. The referral to a registered dietitian nutritionist can help the patient to review current food and fluid ingestion to assess customary intake of how these factors are influencing the constipation. Specifically, determination of dietary fiber quantity and sources are of value to create a plan for increasing fluid and fiber to meet recommended amounts. Slowly increasing total daily dietary fiber from food sources is recommended as the initial treatment step for chronic constipation with no identified secondary etiology and at a mild-to-moderate severity level because stool bulk will increase and colonic transit time will decrease with increased total daily dietary fiber.

Dietary Reference Intakes (DRI) dietary fiber recommendations in the older adult age categories are 21 g per day for women and 30 g daily for men.[12] Dietary fiber intake of older adults has consistently been observed to be significantly lower than these recommended levels.[13] Dietary fiber should be slowly added to the diet at increments of approximately 3-g to 5-g increases twice weekly until the goal is met to minimize bloating and gas secondary to the increased fiber levels. Fiber-rich foods, such as whole fruits, vegetables, whole-grains, bran, and prune juice, can be incorporated as tolerated. Wheat bran has been observed to be a very effective laxative resulting in a dose-response increase in stool size.[14] Care should be taken to modify dietary fiber levels in congruence with an understanding of a full evaluation for adequate total daily caloric and fluid intake. Older adults with poor appetite or anorexia must be carefully monitored to avoid excess satiety from the addition of dietary fiber. Hydration adequacy should also be determined, with increased amounts of fluid recommended as dietary fiber ingestion increases.[13]

Chronic constipation should be monitored under physician guidance because individuals with constipation secondary to refractory slow transit issues or pelvic floor dyssynergia may respond poorly to increased dietary fiber and instead may need to avoid fiber increases to instead focus on use of pharmacologic agents.[14] Current pharmacologic agents include bulking agents, stool softeners, stimulant laxatives, and osmotic agents.[14]

Gastrointestinal Absorption

Universal malabsorption of nutrients is not a primary consequence of healthy aging. Animal models do not support the observation of global changes in villus height, crypt depth, or changes in total surface area for absorption with primary aging.[8] Currently available data do not indicate malabsorption of dietary protein or fat. It is, however, not known if brush border peptidases, amino acid or peptide transporters are affected by primary aging. Similarly, it is not known whether absorption of essential fatty acids, specifically linoleic and α-linolenic acid is altered with aging.[8] Limited evidence of modest carbohydrate malabsorption is complicated by use of breath test data, which are influenced by intestinal bacteria.[10]

The best data for micronutrient malabsorption associated with primary aging includes calcium, vitamin B_{12}, and magnesium.[10,13] There is a long latency period for B_{12} deficiency: as long as 2 to 5 years, even in the case of complete loss of absorption and enterohepatic reabsorption.[15] DRI recommendations for magnesium are not altered for adults aged 51 to 70 or older than age 70; however, with increasing age, dietary magnesium absorption declines, urinary magnesium losses increase, and ingestion of food sources with magnesium decreases, all of which may predispose to magnesium deficiency. The precise extent of the altered absorption secondary to primary aging is not known.[12]

Calcium homeostasis is critical to numerous physiologic processes, and intestinal calcium absorption is a key component of maintaining calcium balance.[16] Absorption occurs via a passive nonsaturable absorption route called the paracellular pathway and the metabolically driven transport pathway called transcellular.[8,16] The paracellular pathway involves passive transport throughout most of the intestine that is highly influenced by the luminal concentration of $Ca2+$. The effect of primary aging on paracellular absorption is unknown.[8,16] By contrast, transcellular pathway is an active, saturable process regulated by nutritional and physiologic factors, predominantly active in the duodenum and jejunum. The main proteins involved with the transcellular pathway are all reduced with aging.[8,16]

Total intestinal calcium absorption depends on several factors, including the total quantity of calcium consumed, transit time spent in the various components of the small and large intestines, and the percentage of soluble calcium available for absorption, as determined by the intestinal pH. In healthy adults, the average pH of the small intestine is 7.3, whereas the duodenum is generally at a pH of 6.0 and the large intestine 6.6. Optimal calcium solubility occurs with a pH of approximately 6.0 and as pH increases, solubility decreases.

Enhanced intestinal absorption of calcium across the intestine is controlled by the active form of vitamin D, 1, 25 (OH)2D3. Intestinal calcium absorption is also influenced by the physiologic state of the individual. Absorption efficiency increases during periods of increased need and/or low dietary calcium in infancy, children, adolescence, and adulthood, but this adaptation has not been observed in older adults.[10] A reduced absorption of calcium in aging has been well documented, with numerous etiologic factors reported, including decreased levels of vitamin D, and atropic gastritis, which negatively impacts the transformation of calcium into soluble forms. Clear elucidation of all the mechanisms impacting absorption in aging is still being actively investigated.[16]

NUTRITION SCREENING AND ASSESSMENT TOOLS FOR THE OLDER ADULT

Although numerous nutritional assessment and screening tools exist, most were developed for heterogeneous population groups. The following diagnostic tools **(Table 1)** have been developed and validated specifically for use in older adults.[17]

- DETERMINE Checklist: The Nutrition Screening Initiative (NSI, 2005), created and validated this simple, self-administered set of 10 questions to identify older adults in community settings who are at "nutritional risk." Included in the NSI are Level 1 and Level 2 in-depth assessment components validated to assess malnutrition.[18]
- Mini Nutrition Assessment (MNA) is one of the most extensively validated tools to assess malnutrition in free-living, hospitalized, or nursing home residents age 65 and older. The 18-question assessment is conducted and then scored (www.mna-elderly.com).[19]
- MNA short form (MNA-SF) and revised MNA-SF are validated against the original tool but only include 6 questions. The revised MNA-SF has exchanged the inclusion of body mass index (BMI) for calf circumference. This tool can be incorporated into electronic medical records, and is available via online interactive tools

Table 1
Nutrition screening and assessment tools

Tool Name	Format	Validated Population	Includes
DETERMINE Checklist	10 questions self-administered	Elderly in: Community Settings	Checklist is only a screening tool. Levels I and II Assessment tools are available as part of this toolkit
Mini Nutrition Assessment (MNA) (www.mna-elderly.com)	18 questions administered by professional	Elderly in: Community settings, Hospital, Nursing homes	Assessment and screening
Mini Nutrition (MNA) Assessment-Short Form	6 questions administered by professional or self-administered	Elderly in: Community, Hospital, Nursing homes	Assessment and screening
Geriatric Nutrition Risk Index (GNR)	6 questions administered by professional	Elderly in: Hospital	Assessment

in many languages (www.mna-elderly.com). Most recently, a validated, self-administered version is available at that same Web site.[19]

- The Geriatric Nutrition Risk Index (GNRI) classifies hospitalized elderly patients based on a nutrition-related risk index. It has been validated as a prognostic indicator of morbidity and mortality in this population.[20]

NUTRITION SCREENING, THE OLDER ADULT AND BODY MASS INDEX

A BMI between 18.5 and 24.9 kg/m^2 has been adopted by numerous health organizations, including the World Health Organization (WHO), as an inexpensive, easy-to-use method of defining a normal, healthy body weight range for adults based on reduced risk of mortality. A BMI of $\leq$18.5 kg/m^2 is classified as underweight, the overweight range is 25.0 to 29.9 kg/m^2, class 1 obesity is 30.0 to 34.9 kg/m^2, class 2 obesity is 35.0 to 39.9 kg/m^2 and class 3 obesity is $\geq$40.0 kg/m^2.[21] BMI is often used as a core component of nutritional screenings for older adults.[22] Recently the validity of using BMI in the older adult population as a singular screening tool is being questioned because of some key concerns, including the following:

- BMI does not capture changes in body weight or body composition and these considerations are very significant in risk determination for loss of skeletal muscle mass and functional status, nutrient deficiencies, and increased hospital admission.[23] Unintended weight loss of $\geq$5% in the prior 1 to 6 months is considered high nutritional risk.[24]
- Current BMI threshold values are too restrictive for use in older adults because they do not account for the considerable variability in functional and metabolic alterations associated with aging.[25]
- Screening limited to one parameter, such as BMI or body weight, using the current lower threshold of 18.5 kg/m^2, results in undernutrition being insufficiently identified or determined too late to reverse a state of vulnerability that can cascade into an inability to maintain optimal nutritional status. Earlier intervention

could result using a higher value for the lower threshold cutoff for the older population.[22,24]

- The trigger value recommended for nutrition interventions in long-term care facilities is a minimum BMI of 21 kg/m^2 rather than the current cutoff of 18.5 because malnutrition in institutionalized elderly leads to an increased rate of morbidity and mortality.[22] Being underweight reflects a chronic energy insufficiency in older adults that translates to higher functional and lean body mass loss, and nutritional insufficiencies that persist after discharge.[22,24]

BODY MASS INDEX AND RISK OF MORTALITY IN OLDER ADULTS

Evidence is also emerging that the normal weight range and overweight BMI threshold may have different associations with mortality risk in older versus younger adults. The association between BMI and all-cause mortality for adults age 65 and older has been observed to be a U-shaped curve with the nadir of the curve between 24.0 and 30.9 kg/m^2. A lower mortality risk has been seen in several systematic reviews with community-dwelling older adults in the overweight BMI range, heterogeneous effects in morbidity at the class 1 and class 2 obesity levels, and a higher risk at the lower normal range values.[25,26] Therefore, current data questions whether the WHO BMI weight classification ranges are also suitable for mortality risk assessment in an older adult population and if unilateral weight loss interventions in the overweight classification should be advised in the older adult population.[26]

These data from meta-analyses and cohort studies of community-dwelling older adults have been challenged on the basis of insufficient factor adjustments, inadequate attention to preexisting conditions, and selective survival. Nonetheless, these U-shaped curves have been reported in several studies, including 5 years of follow-up and statistical analyses that accounted for these factors.[22,25,26]

NUTRITION RECOMMENDATIONS FOR OLDER ADULTS: DIETARY REFERENCE INTAKES

Nutrient reference guidelines, called DRIs,[12] have been established by the Institute of Medicine for healthy individuals from infancy through age 70. Dietary recommendations for total daily calories, essential nutrients, and important food components, such as dietary fiber for older adults, are designated in the age categories of 51 to 70 and ≥70. Tables of these quantitative DRI values and the evidence to support these recommendations are available online at http://www.iom.edu/dri. Limited evidence is available for healthy older adults, consequently recommendations for older adults remain the same as for adults ages 19 to 50, with the exception of Vitamins D, B_6, B_{12}, iron, and calcium. **Table 2** identifies DRI nutrient recommendations specific to older adults, including the key evidence to support these recommendations.

ASSESSING MICRONUTRIENT STATUS

Screening for micronutrient status in all older adults is not generally recommended, unless there is suspicion of deficiency. Nutrients at highest risk for insufficiency include vitamin D, vitamin B_{12}, and calcium.

Vitamin D[12,27]:

- Functions: maintenance of calcium and phosphate balance, proper bone mineralization.
- Risk factors for deficiency: limited sun exposure, dark skin pigmentation, adults 65 years or older with a history of falls and nontraumatic fractures, BMI ≥30 kg/m^2, renal or hepatic disease, malabsorptive syndromes.

Table 2
Nutrient recommendations for older adults from the Dietary reference intakes (DRIs)

Nutrient	DRI Recommendations Specific for Adults Ages ≥51–70 y	Evidence Supporting DRI Recommendations
Vitamin D	Age ≥70: Men and women: recommendation increases to 800 IU	Age-related absorption changes; insufficient dietary intake.
Vitamin B_6	Age ≥51 increased recommendations: Men: 1.7 mg/d; women: 1.5 mg/d	Limited data in older adults, but increased intake needed to maintain plasma 5 pyridoxal phosphate of 20 nmol/L. Plasma levels reflects tissue stores.
Vitamin B_{12}	Quantity recommendations identical throughout adulthood, but crystalline sources recommended for both genders of adults ≥50 y	Naturally occurring food sources of B_{12} are not as readily absorbed as crystalline formulations of the vitamin. Recommended that adults older than 50 ingest foods fortified with the vitamin or vitamin B_{12} supplements.
Calcium	Age ≥51–70: Women: recommendation increases to 1200 mg/d; Age ≥70: Women and men: recommendation increases to 1200 mg/d.	Age-related absorption changes; insufficient dietary intake.
Iron	Age ≥51: Women: recommendation lowered to 5 mg/d; Ages 19–70: Men: recommendations remain the same.	Postmenopausal women menses monthly losses stop. No mechanism to excrete iron in adults.

- Signs/symptoms of deficiency include bone pain and muscle weakness. Vitamin D deficiency is defined by the Institute of Medicine as serum levels of 25-hydroxyvitamin D less than 20 ng/mL (50 nmol/L) and insufficiency as 20 to 30 ng/mL (50–70 nmol/L).
- Therapy: Treat deficiency or insufficiency with oral cholecalciferol (vitamin D3) 50,000 IU per week for 8 weeks, and then reassess 25-hydroxyvitamin; maintenance dosage from dietary and supplemental sources is 600 to 800 IU daily.
- The US Preventive Services Task Force currently recommends screening those at high risk for deficiency or the presence of osteoporosis, but does not have sufficient evidence to recommend for or against general screening.

Vitamin B_{12} (cobalamin)[12,28–32]:
- Functions: Necessary for DNA synthesis and red blood cell production.
- Risk factors for deficiency: physiologic or pathophysiologic changes of aging, particularly those associated with gastrointestinal absorption, decreased intrinsic factor, presence of atrophic gastritis. Prolonged use of medications, such as metformin, proton pump inhibitors, and histamine H2 blockers, interfere with vitamin absorption. Inadequate intake risk could be a concern for vegans, or those abusing alcohol, although most deficiency presentations are not because of a primary dietary deficiency.
- Signs/symptoms of deficiency: Vitamin deficiency results in classic hematologic manifestations of megaloblastic, macrocytic anemia (macrocytic anemia is characterized by tachycardia, palpitations, generalized weakness, and fatigue and

pallor). Common neurologic manifestations include cognitive impairment, paresthesias, peripheral neuropathies, sensory and neurologic abnormalities, decreased muscle strength, functional disability, abnormalities of gait, and behavioral changes.

- Risks of nontreatment: Untreated deficiency of this vitamin results in irreversible neurologic damage necessitating early screening and diagnosis.
- No guidelines exist regarding frequency of screening asymptomatic adults for the vitamin deficiency. Measurements of serum B_{12} are not sufficiently sensitive to independently screen for deficiency, as levels will be maintained at the expense of tissue depletion and no gold standard for deficiency exists. For this reason, various indicators being used to indicate a deficiency include holotranscobalamin (holoTC) as an early marker of depletion, serum B_{12} <258 pmol/L and serum homocysteine (Hcy) >10 μmol/L, serum B_{12} <258 pmol/L and serum methylmalonic acid (MMA) >0.2 μmol/L.
- Elevated Hcy or MMA are functional metabolites used to screen for the vitamin deficiency concomitant to serum vitamin levels, as these will accumulate at later stages of the vitamin's deficiency. Hcy elevations can be secondary to either B_{12} or folate deficiencies, whereas MMA is specific to a B_{12} deficiency. The sensitivity of both markers will be impaired with impaired renal status or diabetes.
- Therapy recommendations: Regardless of etiology, intramuscular administration or oral doses (1–2 mg daily) given for 8 weeks are equally effective to correct the deficiency followed by monthly maintenance doses of 1 mg.
- Lowering elevated plasma homocysteine levels via B_{12} administration has had no observed effect on cognitive domains, global cognitive functioning, cognitive decline in mild to moderate Alzheimer disease, or cardiovascular outcomes in older adults.

Calcium[12,16,33]:

- Older adults should be preferentially encouraged to consume dietary sources of calcium, such as milk, yogurt, and cheeses, and nondairy, such as dark green vegetables, including kale and broccoli, and fortified foods.
- Older adults are often lactose intolerant and hence tend to avoid dairy products. Encourage lactose-free milk consumption or low lactose dairy products, such as aged cheeses (cheddar and Swiss) and yogurt. Small quantities of lactose consumed (less than 12 g), especially if ingested with other foods, generally have been reported to result in minimal or no symptoms.
- When calcium supplementation is advised, the 2 available forms include calcium carbonate, which requires an acidic environment for absorption, so this should be taken with food, and calcium citrate, which does not rely on an acidity for absorption, allowing for ingestion to occur either with or without food. This form is advisable for those with gastrointestinal alterations, such as achlorhydria, a condition commonly reported in older adults.
- The efficiency of absorption decreases with supplemental doses greater than 500 mg. Accordingly, advice should be given to not exceed this level of supplementation at any one time.

"GERIATRIC GIANTS" AND THE ROLE OF NUTRITION

"Geriatric giants" is the term coined for risk factors that predispose to functional decline.[34] These disorders have nutrition components and/or can be affected by nutritional status. The clinician must recognize the status of current nutrition recommendations for these risk factors. The remainder of this article focuses on nutrition aspects of these disorders.

ANOREXIA OF AGING AND ENERGY HOMEOSTASIS

Primary aging has been associated with anorexia secondary to a multiplicity of nonphysiologic and physiologic causes, as well as progressive decrease in caloric intake.[35,36] Reduced appetite, lowered energy intake, and reduced energy expenditure contribute to decreased resting metabolic rate (RMR) of approximately 1% to 2% per decade between the ages of 20 and 70.[13] Collectively, these factors increase the risk for sarcopenia and osteopenia, with unintended weight loss (or weight stability if increased fat mass concomitantly occurs).[37] A validated rapid screening tool for anorexia is the Simplified Nutrition Assessment Scale, SNAQ.[34,36]

Maintaining weight or increasing weight gain secondary to unintentional weight loss in nursing home residents has identified a variety of mealtime changes, including providing adequate individual feeding assistance, changing the mealtime routine, altering the dining environment, and staff training.[38] A systematic review of 36 studies evaluated a range of interventions for their impact on improving food/caloric intake and body weight/weight status.[38] Direct interventions related to food assistance, increasing staff knowledge, providing real food snacks and flavor enhancers, and improving the dining environment resulted in positive outcomes. Commercial oral energy dense supplements have demonstrated small (1.2-kg averages) but consistent positive effect on weight gain, but compliance in clinical settings ranges from 14% to 97%, depending on flavor, texture, dysphagia, and comorbidity.[39] The European Society for Clinical Nutrition and Metabolism has recommended oral nutrition supplements to maintain or improve the nutritional status of frail older adults.[40–42] Treatments should identify the core underlying causes and use a multidisciplinary team including dietitians, speech or occupational therapists, and social service.

Appetite stimulant medications, such as megestrol, have insufficient data to establish optimal dose or determine efficacy in reducing mortality.[35] Other appetite-inducing agents, such as mirtazapine, are frequently used but have insufficient data to support efficacy for this purpose.[35]

Frailty

Adults older than 70 and any individual with unintended weight loss of ≥5% should be screened for frailty.[34] Physical frailty is defined as a "medical syndrome with multiple causes and contributors characterized by diminished strength, endurance, and reduced physiologic function that increases an individual's vulnerability for developing increased dependency and/or death."[34,36] Validated tools are available to assess frailty, such as the FRAIL scale.[36]

Nutritional status in frail older adults should be assessed using one of the tools described previously and a registered dietitian nutritionist should be included in the treatment team to identify medical nutrition concerns, such as calorie and protein needs, micronutrient insufficiencies, and the need for feeding assistance. Randomized clinical trials have demonstrated that daily protein supplementation, including 30 g of high-quality protein and 6 months of resistance-type exercise training, improved strength and physical performance capacity in frail older adults.[43,44]

Sarcopenia

Sarcopenia, an unintended loss of muscle mass, results in loss of muscle function and strength, reduced independent mobility, and increased risk for falls, fractures, disability, and hospital and long-term care admissions.[45,46] In 2009, the European Working Group on Sarcopenia in Older Adults identified a consensus definition including anthropometric (appendicular muscle mass $\leq$7.23 kg/m^2 for men and $\leq$5.67 kg/m^2 for women, assessed by dual-energy x-ray absorptiometry) and functional (gait speed <1 m/s or hand grip strength $\leq$30 kg for men and $\leq$20 kg for women) criteria.[47] The SARC-F (strength, assistance, rise, climb, falls) consists of 5 questions and is a validated and rapid screen with high specificity for sarcopenia diagnosis.[36,48]

The etiology and progression of sarcopenia is multifactorial, but modifiable factors regarding progression rate and risk reduction include prolonged resistance exercise training programs designed by exercise physiologists or physical therapists,[49] adequacy of total caloric intake, provision of 1.1 to 1.2 g/kg per day of high-quality protein, and satisfactory vitamin D status.[46]

More recently, data on healthy older adults have observed a blunted sensitivity of muscle anabolism, or anabolic resistance, to meal or exercise stimuli. This anabolic resistance necessitates the provision of approximately 30 g of high-quality dietary protein per meal (assuming 3 meals daily), with no less than 2.2 g and no greater than 3.0 g of leucine in that dietary protein per meal for optimal postprandial muscle mass synthesis.[50] Stated differently, anabolic resistance means that lower quantities of meal protein do not appear to maximally stimulate muscle protein synthesis in older adults, as occurs in younger adults.[50] These recommendations are not "high-protein" diets, but provide approximately 1.1 to 1.2 g of protein per kilogram of body weight. This is slightly above the current adult DRI protein recommendations of 0.8 g per kilogram of body weight. The European Union Geriatric Medicine Society appointed an international study group to review current studies on protein needs with aging, and their recommendations were 1.0 to 1.2 g protein per kilogram of body weight daily.[46]

Upper levels for protein or amino acids have not been established by the Institute of Medicine.[12] No evidence of negative effects in the renal function of healthy adults has been observed, but the International Society for Renal Nutrition and Health does recommend protein restriction for those with existing renal disease.[37,50]

MILD COGNITIVE IMPAIRMENT AND DEPRESSION

According to the US Preventive Services Task Force, the prevalence of mild cognitive impairment ranges from 3% to 42% in adults 65 years or older, with widely documented racial and ethnic disparities, including a prevalence of 15.91% in black individuals, 11.55% in Hispanic individuals, and approximately 2.98% in whites.[51] Consistent evidence demonstrating that nutritional supplementation of any type slows cognitive decline or improves cognitive function in either healthy or cognitively impaired older adults is lacking.[52] The role of folate deficiency needs additional study, but may be a contributing factor for onset and progression of neuropsychiatric diseases and depression in older adults.[52] B vitamin and omega-3 supplementations appear to confer no benefit in modulating Alzheimer disease.[53] Epidemiologic studies have shown no consistent benefit with multivitamins, despite the observation from multiple studies that patients with Alzheimer disease were deficient in vitamins B, C, K, E, selenium, and iron.[53] Current investigations are focused on the role of a Mediterranean-type diet and cognitive functioning. Mediterranean diets vary, but include olive oil, wine, an abundance of vegetables and fruits, moderate amounts of dairy products, low to moderate amounts of poultry and red meats, and an abundance of breads, cereals, beans, and nuts.[53,54]

REFERENCES

1. Masoro EJ. The physiology of aging. In: Boron WF, Boulpaep EL, editors. Medical physiology: a cellular and molecular approach. 2nd edition. Philadelphia: Saunders Elsevier; 2012. p. 1281–92.
2. Lowsky DJ, Olshansky SJ, Bhattacharya J, et al. Heterogeneity in healthy aging. J Gerontol A Biol Sci Med Sci 2014;69(6):640–9.
3. Morley JE. Undernutrition in older adults. Fam Pract 2012;29(Suppl 1):i89–93.
4. Sura L, Madhaven A, Carnaby G, et al. Dysphagia in elderly: management and nutritional considerations. Clin Interv Aging 2012;7:287–98.
5. Cichero J, Steele C, Duivestein J, et al. Need for international terminology and definitions for texture modified foods and thickened liquids used in dysphagia management: global initiative. Curr Phys Med Rehabil Rep 2013;1:280–91.
6. National Dysphagia Diet Task Force. National dysphagia diet: standardization for optimal care. Chicago: American Dietetic Association; 2002.
7. Chait M. Gastroesophageal reflux disease: important considerations in elderly. World J Gastrointest Endosc 2010;2(12):388–96.
8. Remond D, Shahar DR, Gille D, et al. Understanding the gastrointestinal tract of the elderly to develop dietary solutions that prevent malnutrition. Oncotarget 2015;6(16):13858–98.
9. O'Mahony D, Leary P, Wuigley E. Aging and intestinal motility: a review of factors that affect intestinal motility in the aged. Drugs Aging 2002;19(7):515–27.
10. Bhutto A, Morley JE. The clinical significance of gastrointestinal changes with aging. Curr Opin Clin Nutr Metab Care 2008;11:651–60.
11. Mounsey A, Raleigh M, Wilson A. Management of constipation in older adults. Am Fam Physician 2015;92(6):500–4.
12. Institute of Medicine, Food and Nutrition Board. Dietary reference intakes for energy, carbohydrate, fiber, fatty acids, cholesterol, protein and amino acids. Washington, DC: National Academies Press; 2002.
13. Bernstein M. Position of the Academy of Nutrition and Dietetics: food and nutrition for older adults: promoting health and wellness. J Acad Nutr Diet 2012;112(8): 1255–77.
14. Gallegos-Orozco J, Foxx-Orenstein A, Sterler S, et al. Chronic constipation in the elderly. Am J Gastroenterol 2012;107:18–25.
15. Carmel R. Cobalamin (vitamin B12). In: Ross AC, Caballero B, Cousins RJ, et al, editors. Modern nutrition in health and disease. 11th edition. Baltimore (MD): Lippincott Williams & Wilkins; 2014. p. 369–89.
16. Weaver C, Heaney R. Calcium. In: Ross AC, Caballero B, Cousins RJ, et al, editors. Modern nutrition in health and disease. 11th edition. Baltimore (MD): Lippincott Williams & Wilkins; 2014. p. 133–50.
17. Van Bokhorst-de van Schueren MA, Guaitoli PR, Jansma EP, et al. A systemic review of malnutrition screening tools for the nursing home setting. J Am Med Dir Assoc 2014;15:171–84.
18. Posner B, Jette A, Smith K, et al. Nutrition and health risks in elderly, the nutrition screening initiative. Am J Public Health 1993;83(7):972–8.
19. MNA® Mini Nutritional Assessment [Internet]. Nestle Nutrition Institute. 2013. [cited 2016 Apr 4]. Available at: http://www.mna-elderly.com/. Accessed April 4, 2016.
20. Bouillanne O, Morineau G, Dupont C, et al. Geriatric nutrition risk index: a new index for evaluating at risk elderly medical patients. Am J Clin Nutr 2005;82(4): 777–82.

21. Centers for Disease Control and Prevention (CDC). Division of Nutrition, Physical Activity and Obesity. Washington, DC. Available at: http://www.cdc.gov/healthyweight/assessments/bmi/adult_bmi/. Accessed April 4, 2016.
22. Cereda E, Pedrolli C, Zagami A, et al. Body mass index and mortality in institutionalized elderly. J Am Med Dir Assoc 2011;12(3):174–8.
23. de Boer A, Ter Horst GJ, Lorist MM. Physiological age-related changes associate with reduced food intake in older persons. Ageing Res Rev 2013;12:316–28.
24. Beck AM. At which body mass index and degree of weight loss should hospitalized elderly patients be considered at nutritional risk? Clin Nutr 1998;17(5):195–8.
25. Winter JE, MacInnis RJ, Wattanapenpaiboon N, et al. BMI and all-cause mortality in older adults: a meta-analysis. Am J Clin Nutr 2014;99(4):875–90.
26. Wu CY, Chou YC, Huang N, et al. Association of body mass index with all-cause and cardiovascular disease mortality in the elderly. PLoS One 2014;9(7):e102589.
27. Bordelon P, Ghetu MV, Langan R. Recognition and management of vitamin D deficiency. Am Fam Physician 2009;80(8):841–6.
28. Obeid R, Jung J, Falk J, et al. Serum vitamin B12 status in patients with type 2 diabetes. Biochimie 2013;95:1056–61.
29. Oberlin BS, Tangney CC, Gustashaw KA, et al. Vitamin B12 deficiency in relation to functional disabilities. Nutrients 2013;5(11):4462–75.
30. Berg RL, Shaw GR. Laboratory evaluation for vitamin B12 deficiency: the case for cascade testing. Clin Med Res 2013;11(1):7–15.
31. Langan RC, Zawistoski KJ. Update on vitamin B12 deficiency. Am Fam Physician 2011;83(12):1425–30.
32. Clarke R, Bennett D, Parish S, et al. Effects of homocysteine lowering with B vitamins on cognitive aging: meta-analysis of 11 trials with cognitive data on 22,000 individuals. Am J Clin Nutr 2014;100(2):657–66.
33. Hertzler SR, Savaiano DA. Colonic adaptation to daily lactose feeding in lactose maldigesters reduces lactose intolerance. Am J Clin Nutr 1996;64(2):232–6.
34. Morley JE. Anorexia, weight loss, and frailty. J Am Med Dir Assoc 2010;11(4):225–8.
35. Gaddey HL, Holder K. Unintentional weight loss in older adults. Am Fam Physician 2014;89(9):718–22.
36. Morley JE. Aging successfully: the key to aging in place. J Am Med Dir Assoc 2015;16(12):1005–7.
37. Phillips SM, Fulgoni VL III, Heaney RP, et al. Commonly consumed protein foods contribute to nutrient intake, diet quality, and nutrient adequacy. Am J Clin Nutr 2015;101:346S–1352S.
38. Abbott RA, Whear R, Thompson-Coon J, et al. Effectiveness of mealtime interventions on nutritional outcomes for the elderly living in residential care: a systemic review and meta-analysis. Ageing Res Rev 2013;12:967–81.
39. Lombard K, van SJ, Schuur T, et al. Compliance of energy-dense, small volume oral nutritional supplements in the daily clinical practice on a geriatric ward–an observational study. J Nutr Health Aging 2014;18:649–53.
40. Abizanda P, López MD, García VP, et al. Effects of an oral nutritional supplementation plus physical exercise intervention on the physical function, nutritional status, and quality of life in frail institutionalized older adults: the ACTIVNES Study. J Am Med Dir Assoc 2015;16(5):439.e9-e16.
41. Abizanda P, Sinclair A, Barcons N, et al. Costs of malnutrition in institutionalized and community-dwelling older adults: a systemic review. J Am Med Dir Assoc 2016;17(1):17–23.

42. Volkert D, Berner Y, Berry E, et al. ESPEN guidelines in enteral nutrition: geriatrics. Clin Nutr 2006;25(2):330–60.
43. Tieland M, Dirks ML, van der Zwaluw N, et al. Protein supplementation increases muscle mass gain during prolonged resistance-type exercise training in frail elderly people: a randomized, double-blind, placebo-controlled trial. J Am Med Dir Assoc 2012;13:713–9.
44. Churchward-Venne TΛ, Tieeland M, Verdijk LB, et al. There are no nonresponders to resistance-type exercise training in older men and women. J Am Med Dir Assoc 2015;16:400–11.
45. Bauer JM, Verlaan S, Bautmans I, et al. Effects of a vitamin D and leucine-enriched whey protein nutritional supplement on measures of sarcopenia in older adults, the PROVIDE study: a randomized, double-blind, placebo-controlled trial. J Am Med Dir Assoc 2015;16:740–7.
46. Bauer J, Biolo G, Cederholm T, et al. Evidence-based recommendations for optimal dietary protein intake in older people: a position paper from the PROT-AGE study group. J Am Med Dir Assoc 2013;14:542–59.
47. Cruz-Jentoft AJ, Landi F, Schneider SM, et al. Prevalence of and interventions for sarcopenia in aging adults: a systematic review. Report of the international sarcopenia initiative (EWGSOP and IWGS). Age Ageing 2014;43(6):748–59.
48. Woo J, Leung J, Morley JE. Validating the SARC-F: a suitable community screening tool for sarcopenia? J Am Med Dir Assoc 2014;15:630–4.
49. Morley JE. Exercise: the ultimate medicine. J Am Med Dir Assoc 2015;16:351–3.
50. Layman DK, Anthony TG, Rasmussen BB, et al. Defining meal requirements for protein to optimize metabolic roles of amino acids. Am J Clin Nutr 2015; 101(Suppl):1330S–8S.
51. Lin JS, O'Connor E, Rossom RC, et al. Screening for cognitive impairment in older adults: a systematic review for the U.S. Preventive Services Task Force. Ann Intern Med 2013;159(9):601–12.
52. Araújo JR, Martel F, Borges N, et al. Folates and aging: role in mild cognitive impairment, dementia and depression. Ageing Res Rev 2015;22:9–19.
53. Shah R. The role of nutrition and diet in Alzheimer disease: a systemic review. J Am Med Dir Assoc 2013;14:398–402.
54. Yannakoulia M, Kontogianni M, Scarmeas N. Cognitive health and Mediterranean diet: just diet or lifestyle pattern. Ageing Res Rev 2015;20:74–8.

Nutrition Interventions for Cardiovascular Disease

Janet M. de Jesus, MS, RD[a],*, Scott Kahan, MD, MPH[b], Robert H. Eckel, MD[c]

KEYWORDS

- Physician counseling • Nutrition therapy • Cardiovascular disease • Risk factor
- Treatment • Prevention • Blood pressure • Lipids

KEY POINTS

- Physicians are encouraged to play an active role in nutrition counseling to reduce cardio-vascular disease (CVD) risk.
- Mediterranean (Med)-style and Dietary Approaches to Stop Hypertension (DASH)-style dietary patterns that emphasize vegetables, fruits, and whole grains; include low-fat dairy products, lean protein and fish, and healthy sources of fats improve blood pressure (BP) and lipid management. The dietary pattern should be calorie controlled for weight loss or maintenance.
- Adults who would benefit from low-density lipoprotein cholesterol (LDL-C) lowering should be encouraged to substitute foods sources higher in healthy fats (vegetable oils, nuts, and fish) for foods higher in saturated fats and trans fats. And sodium reduction is encouraged for BP reduction.
- Physicians could inform adults that moderate alcohol intake may reduce CVD risk but adults who abstain from alcohol are not encouraged to begin.
- Physicians should also counsel patients on weight control/loss and the importance of regular physical activity.

INTRODUCTION

CVD is the number one cause of death in the United States despite a 40% reduction from 2001 to 2011.[1] Advances in CVD risk factor screening and detection, pharmacologic treatment, and decreased tobacco use have contributed to the significant

Disclosures: The authors have nothing to disclose.
[a] Center for Translation Research and Implementation Science (CTRIS), National Heart, Lung, and Blood Institute, National Institutes of Health, Rockledge 1 Building, Room 6189, MSC 7960, Bethesda, MD 20817, USA; [b] George Washington University, The School of Medicine and Health Sciences, Department of Health Policy, 1020 19th Street NW, Suite 450, Washington, DC, 20036, USA; [c] Division of Endocrinology, Metabolism, and Diabetes, University of Colorado Denver Anschutz Medical Campus, Research Complex 1 South, 12801 East 17th Avenue room 7107 8106, Aurora, CO 80045, USA
* Corresponding author.
E-mail address: dejesusjm@mail.nih.gov

Med Clin N Am 100 (2016) 1251–1264
http://dx.doi.org/10.1016/j.mcna.2016.06.007
0025-7125/16/Published by Elsevier Inc.

medical.theclinics.com

reduction, but CVD continues to be a major source of morbidity and mortality. The cause of CVD includes several modifiable risk factors, including an unhealthy diet and sedentary lifestyle, high LDL-C, high BP, overweight and obesity, diabetes, and smoking. Approximately one-third of Americans have high levels of LDL-C or high BP[1,2]; 9% of the US population has diabetes[3] and there continues to be a staggering burden of overweight and obesity in America as more than one-third of US adults are have obesity.[4] Racial and ethnic disparities are highly prevalent in CVD with communities of color and lower socioeconomic status having a disproportionally higher prevalence of CVD risk factors and CVD-related mortality.[5–9] A strong body of evidence exists on the lifestyle interventions for CVD risk reduction.[10] Nutrition and physical activity behaviors are key modifiable factors and physicians should play an active role in counseling patients on lifestyle change and referring them to more intense interventions when appropriate.[11]

This article describes the nutrition interventions for preventing and treating CVD and its associated risk factors. Although several nutrition intervention areas have shown effectiveness for CVD, the most promising of these are measures to control BP and lipids, which is the focus of this article. Nutrition interventions for diabetes and overweight and obesity are covered in other articles in this issue, and interventions for tobacco cessation, physical activity, and pharmacotherapy, which are additionally effective at lowering CVD risk, are beyond the scope of this article. This article focuses on dietary pattern interventions, including the Med-style and the DASH-style patterns. Additionally, evidence for the role of specific nutrients, including dietary fats, sodium, and alcohol intake, on CVD risk reduction is discussed.

DIETARY PATTERN INTERVENTIONS

There is increasing research on the effect of dietary patterns on BP and lipid management and CVD risk. Nutrition research on CVD risk factors includes a long history on the study of individual dietary components, such as dietary fats and sodium. In the past decade there has been an increased emphasis on the study of dietary patterns rather than individual nutrients. Dietary patterns in research can be defined by the amount and type of food groups and/or based strictly on target nutrients. A variety of dietary patterns have been studied looking at the effect on CVD risk factors and outcomes, notably the Mediterranean and DASH diets. Other popular diet patterns have not been consistently shown to improve CVD risk and therefore are not discussed. It is commonly believed that vegetarian diets improve CVD risk factors; however, evidence for the benefits of vegetarian dietary patterns and CVD risk factors is not well established. Despite the inconsistent evidence, physicians should support patients who are interested in consuming a vegetarian diet for religious, environmental, ethical, or other reasons and should recommend that all patients increase intake of fruits and vegetables.

Mediterranean-Style Dietary Pattern

A Med-style dietary pattern has been studied in numerous trials, yet the pattern is not consistently defined in research studies.[12] Common characteristics of this dietary pattern[13] include increased fruits and vegetable, whole grain, and fatty fish intake; decreased red meat (while emphasizing lean meat) intake; including nuts; and consuming oils and margarine blended with rapeseed or flaxseed oils instead of butter or other fats. The dietary pattern is also generally moderate in fat (32%–35% of total calories), lower in saturated fat (9%–10% of calories), and higher in fiber compared with the typical American diet.[10]

Randomized clinical trials (RCTs) and cohort studies have examined the effects of the Med-style diet on BP, lipids, and CVD events. This dietary pattern has been recommended in the American Heart Association (AHA)/American College of Cardiology (ACC) guideline for CVD prevention. A notable Spanish study, Prevención con Dieta Mediterránea (PREDIMED), compared an intervention group given advice to consume a Med-style diet (either supplemented with olive oil or nuts) versus a control diet given advice to consume a low-fat intake on CVD risk factors and events among high-risk individuals. After 3 months, there was a reduction in systolic and diastolic BP in the Med diet group but no difference in lipids.[14] After 4 years, BP improved in both groups, which is suspected to be due to the dietary counseling and interaction in either group.[15] Diastolic BP was lower in the Med-style diet group compared with the control group. A prospective cohort study found that better adherence to the Med-style diet (based on scores) was associated with lower levels of systolic and diastolic BP.[16] After 4.8 years, there was a reduction in major cardiovascular events in the Med-style diet groups compared with the control group.[17] An important strength of this study was the monitoring of dietary compliance using random and periodic measures of urinary hydroxytyrosol (olive oil) and plasma alpha-linolenic acid (nuts). In summary, the Med-style dietary pattern, especially when supplemented with olive oil and nuts, has been shown to reduce incidence of CVD events and lower BP.

Dietary Approaches to Stop Hypertension Dietary Pattern

Strong evidence exists for the DASH dietary pattern to improve BP, lipids, and CVD risk. The DASH pattern emphasizes intake of vegetables, fruits, and whole grains; includes low-fat dairy products, poultry, fish legumes, nontropical vegetable oils, and nuts; and limits sweets, sugar-sweetened beverages, red meats, and saturated fat. The DASH pattern includes a higher amount of whole grains and lower amount of refined grains compared with the Med-style diet. The food composition of the DASH diet compared with the control diet in the DASH trials is in **Table 1**. Controlled feeding trials have been conducted on the pattern and variations of DASH to study the effect on BP and lipids. The DASH dietary pattern, compared with a typical American diet and a pattern with a higher amount of fruits and vegetables, reduced BP in the entire study population by an average of 5.5 mm Hg/3.0 mm Hg and was most

Table 1
Food composition of Dietary Approaches to Stop Hypertension diet versus control diet

Food	Dietary Approaches to Stop Hypertension diet—Number of Servings/Day	Control Diet—Number of Servings/Day
Fruits	5.2	1.6
Vegetables	4.4	2.0
Low-fat dairy	2.0	0.1
Regular-fat dairy	0.7	0.4
Nuts and beans	0.7	0.0
Red meat	0.5	1.5
Fish	0.5	0.2
Snacks and sweets	0.7	4.1

Data from Eckel RH, Jakicic JM, Ard JD, et al. 2013 AHA/ACC guideline on lifestyle management to reduce cardiovascular risk: a report of the American College of Cardiology/American Heart Association Task Force on Practice Guidelines. J Am Coll Cardiol 2014;63(25 Pt B):2960–84.

effective in lowering BP in African Americans and those with hypertension.[18] Systolic BP was lowered significantly more in African Americans (6.8 mm Hg) than in whites (3.0 mm Hg) and in hypertensive subjects (11.4 mm Hg) than in nonhypertensive subjects (3.4 mm Hg).[19] The BP lowering effect was confirmed in 2 subsequent trials in which sodium[20] and macronutrient levels were varied.[21]

Studies also demonstrated that the DASH dietary pattern leads to some lipid benefits. When compared with the standard American diet, the DASH diet pattern lowered LDL-C by 11 mg/dL but also lowered high-density lipoprotein cholesterol (HDL-C) by 4 mg/dL, whereas triglycerides were unchanged.[18,20] It is thought that the lower level of saturated fat (compared with the control) contributes to the LDL-C lowering whereas the lower saturated fat and higher carbohydrate content contribute to the HDL-C lowering. To address this issue, the Optimal Macronutrient Intake Trial to Prevent Heart Disease (OmniHeart) trial studied macronutrient variations of DASH in which 10% of the carbohydrates were substituted with either monounsaturated fatty acids (MUFAs) or protein. The MUFA substitution resulted in a similar effect on LDL-C and BP but did not lower HDL-C.[21] In summary, the DASH pattern and variations offer a variety of options that are beneficial to BP and lipid parameters.

DIETARY FATS AND CHOLESTEROL
Saturated Fat

In addition to discussing overall dietary patterns with patients, certain nutrients, including saturated fat and sodium, have been shown to be important considerations for CVD prevention. Although the intake of saturated fat has declined in the past few decades, the median intake still remains at approximately 11% of total calories.[22,23] A large body of evidence, including RCTs and epidemiologic studies, is available on the effect of saturated and trans fat on LDL-C and cardiovascular risk.[12] There is clear evidence on the benefit of lowering saturated fat intake and the replacement of saturated fat with other macronutrients in lowering LDL-C. Two meta-analyses of controlled feeding trials illustrated the effect of replacing saturated fatty acids (SFAs) and trans fatty acids (TFAs) with other macronutrients.[24,25] The analyses demonstrated that LDL-C is lowered when SFAs are replaced with unsaturated fat, especially polyunsaturated fatty acids (PUFAs). When SFAs are substituted with carbohydrates, LDL-C is lowered but the replacement leads to lowering HDL-C and increasing triglycerides, and this is considered a positive impact given that LDL-C is the main target of treatment. RCTs testing dietary patterns with different levels of saturated fat also showed the consistency of a lower saturated fat dietary pattern and lower LDL-C.[18,20,26] The dietary patterns in those trials included other nutrient differences and, therefore, it was not possible to isolate the effect of saturated fat; however, the evidence on the effect of saturated fat on levels of LDL-C is strong and consistent. **Table 2** shows the macronutrient composition of the RCTs with varying levels of saturated fat and the effect on lipids. Results of these studies showed that dietary patterns with 5% to 6% of saturated fat reduced LDL-C and HDL-C in comparison to dietary patterns with 14% to 15% saturated fat.[10] The 2013 AHA/ACC Guideline on Lifestyle Management to Reduce Cardiovascular Risk recommends that adults who would benefit from LDL-C lowering aim for a dietary pattern that is 5% to 6% of calories from saturated fat.[10] The 2010 Dietary Guidelines for Americans recommend the general public consume less than 10% of total calories from saturated fat.[27] In summary, RCTs demonstrate that replacing SFAs with unsaturated fatty acids, especially PUFAs and perhaps MUFAs, has a positive impact on lipid profiles by lowering LDL-C. Replacing SFAs with carbohydrate may be less desirable because in addition to

Table 2
Macronutrient composition and lipid effects in Dietary Approaches to Stop Hypertension, Dietary Approaches to Stop Hypertension–sodium, and DELTA

	Total Fat (% kcal)	Saturated Fatty Acid (% kcal)	Carbohydrate (% kcal)	Protein (% kcal)	Baseline Low-Density Lipoprotein Cholesterol of Participants	Effect on Low-Density Lipoprotein Cholesterol (Compared with Control)	Effect on High-Density Lipoprotein Cholesterol and/or Triglycerides (Compared with Control)
DASH	27	6	55	18	<160 mg/dL	−11 mg/dL	HDL-C: −4 mg/dL
DASH: control	36	14	51	14	—	—	—
DASH-na	27	6	58	15	<160 mg/dL	−13 mg/dL	HDL-C: −4 mg/dL Triglycerides: +5 mg/dL
DASH-na: control	38	15	49	13	—	—	—
DELTA[a]: low saturated fat	26	5	59	15	"Healthy"	−11%	HDL-C: −11% Triglycerides: no change
DELTA: step 1	29	9	55	15	—	−7%	HDL-C: −7% Triglycerides: +9%
DELTA: control	34	15	48	15	—	N/A	N/A

[a] Dietary Effects on Lipoproteins and Thrombogenic Activity
Data from Refs. [12,18,20,26]

lowering LDL-C, HDL-C is lowered and triglycerides are increased. That there is a wide variety of grains available and consumption of whole grains and limiting refined grains is a beneficial component of desirable eating patterns.

The observational evidence on SFA and CVD risk has been debated in the literature.[28] Two meta-analyses reviewed the evidence on the relationship of saturated fat and CVD and concluded that replacing SFAs with PUFAs reduces the risk of CVD events and coronary mortality.[29,30] Other meta-analyses in which the replacement for SFAs was generally replaced with carbohydrates did not show a relationship between SFA intake and CVD events or deaths.[31–33] Therefore, it was also concluded that reducing total fat or replacing SFAs with carbohydrates was not shown to reduce CVD risk. Based on this finding, it is not recommended to limit total carbohydrate but instead include whole grains and limit refined grains. Limited evidence suggests that replacing SFAs with MUFAs leads to CVD risk reduction but more evidence is available on the beneficial impact of substitution of plant sources of MUFAs (such as olive oil and nuts) for SFAs.[34]

In summary, health care providers are encouraged to counsel patients on replacing food sources of saturated fat with foods higher in unsaturated fatty acids. Americans should strive to consume desirable dietary fat instead of reducing total fat. Patients should be encouraged to choose vegetable oils that are higher in unsaturated fats and low in SFAs, such as soybean, corn, olive, and canola oils, instead of animal fats and tropical oils that are high in SFAs.

Trans Fat

Strong evidence demonstrates the effect of TFAs on LDL-C and cardiovascular risk. It is widely accepted that consumption of trans fat should be limited in the diet.[35] TFA can be produced by a process called hydrogenation in which hydrogen is added to vegetable oil to make it more solid and shelf-stable, producing partially hydrogenated oils (PHOs).[36] PHOs are included in some processed foods, such as baked goods, frozen foods, and margarine. A minimal amount of TFA occurs naturally in some animal products and milk. The US intake of trans fat has decreased in the past decade as a result of policy and product reformulation.[37] Numerous efforts have led to the decreases in trans fat intake, including the US Food and Drug Administration establishment of product-labeling and menu-labeling regulation, the US Department of Agriculture nutrition standards in schools, and local policy discouraging the use of PHOs.[37–41] The Food and Drug Administration recently determined that PHOs, the primary dietary source of industrially produced trans fat, are not generally recognized as safe for use in human food.[42] In summary, significant progress has been made to decrease industrially produced trans fat in the food supply but physicians should continue to counsel patients who would benefit from LDL-C lowering to limit trans fat intake.

Omega-3 Fatty Acids

The evidence on the benefit of omega-3 (n-3) fatty acids on CVD risk is inconsistent.[43] Polyunsaturated omega-3 fatty acids (eicosapentaenoic acid [EPA] and docosahexaenoic acid [DHA]) are present in many types of fish. Limited observational evidence suggests that consumption of EPA and DHA omega-3 fatty acids may reduce the risk of coronary heart disease in individuals at high risk for CVD.[43] One methods issue is that most of the research is on fish oil supplements as opposed to intake of naturally occurring omega-3 fatty acids in fish and seafood. Research is still under way to determine the health effects of omega-3 fatty acids. A large RCT, the Vitamin D and Omega-3 Trial (VITAL), is currently testing the effect of EPA and DHA and vitamin D supplements in the primary prevention of heart disease, stroke, and cancer among 20,000 healthy participants in the United States.[44] These results will be available in the next few years and will inform the scientific community about the effects of omega-3 fatty acids on CVD risk. Despite the inconsistent evidence on the benefit of omega-3 fatty acids on CVD, fish and seafood are good sources of protein that are important components of heart healthy dietary patterns and should be recommended by physicians.

Dietary Cholesterol

Historically, federal and nongovernment organizations have recommended limiting dietary cholesterol intake to 200 mg to 300 mg per day due to the effect on blood lipids.[27,45,46] Methods for reviewing the scientific literature for developing clinical guidelines have become more rigorous than guidelines developed in the past. The AHA/ACC Guideline on Lifestyle Management to Reduce Cardiovascular Risk concluded that there was not enough evidence to make a recommendation to reduce intake of dietary cholesterol for the reduction of LDL-C.[10] The guideline was based on a systematic review of the evidence on meta-analyses and systematic reviews published from 1990 to 2009.[12] Most of the studies did not examine the effects of dietary cholesterol independent of other components of the diet that affect blood cholesterol levels, such as saturated fats and trans fats. Several recent analyses were unable to form a conclusion on the relationship between dietary cholesterol or egg intake and CVD due to heterogeneous studies and methodologic flaws and, therefore, it was recommended that further research is needed.[47–50] The 2015 to 2020 Dietary Guidelines for Americans report states that adequate evidence is not available for a quantitative limit for dietary cholesterol specific to the Dietary Guidelines. The report suggested that research is needed on the dose-response relationship between dietary cholesterol and blood cholesterol levels.[51] It is important for physicians to emphasize that saturated fat and trans fat are the most important nutrients that have an effect on LDL-C and they should be substituted with healthy fats (discussed previously).

GLYCEMIC INDEX

The glycemic index indicates a food's effect on blood glucose compared with the same amount of pure glucose. The preponderance of evidence on glycemic index–varied diets does not show benefits for CVD risk factors in populations without diabetes. A recent modified version of the DASH dietary pattern, the OmniCARB, was used to examine the impact of glycemic index in the setting of high versus low CHO diets on lipids and glycemia.[52] The following interventions were tested: (1) a high-glycemic index (65% on the glucose scale), high-carbohydrate diet (58% energy); (2) a low-glycemic index (40%), high-carbohydrate diet; (3) a high-glycemic index, low-carbohydrate diet (40% energy); and (4) a low-glycemic index, low-carbohydrate diet. Results showed that diets with low glycemic index of carbohydrate compared with a high glycemic index did not improve insulin sensitivity, lipid levels, or systolic BP. It was concluded that in the context of the DASH diet that varying the glycemic index may not improve CVD risk factors or insulin resistance. Similar results, concluding no benefit of a low glycemic index diet, were reported in an RCT comparing low and high glycemic index diets in overweight men.[53] In addition, 2 reviews of RCTs studying the role of glycemic index and glycemic load on CVD risk factors reported inconsistent effects of the glycemic index of the diet on CVD risk factors.[54,55] In summary, modifying the glycemic index of diets is not beneficial to patients without diabetes. Physicians are not recommended to discuss the glycemic index with patients without diabetes to modify CVD risk factors.

In patients with diabetes, glycemic index has had inconsistent effects on glycemic control. In 1 study, subjects with type 2 diabetes randomized to a low glycemic index diet had reductions in postprandial glucose and transient decreases in total cholesterol/HDL-C; however, there was no effect on hemoglobin A_{1c}.[56] In the most recent (2016) Standard of Medical Care in Diabetes, the American Diabetes Association concluded, "The literature concerning glycemic index and glycemic load in individuals with diabetes is complex."[57] They did conclude, however, that "individuals with diabetes should be encouraged to replace refined carbohydrates and added sugars with whole grains, legumes, vegetables, and fruits. The consumption of sugar-sweetened beverages and 'low-fat' or 'nonfat' products with high amounts of refined grains and added sugars should be discouraged."

SODIUM

Strong and consistent evidence is available on the negative effect of sodium on BP. A recent pooled analysis of clinical trials showed that reducing sodium lowers BP in those with and without hypertension.[58] The DASH-sodium (DASH-Na) was a randomized, crossover feeding trial that tested 3 levels of sodium (3300 mg, 2300 mg, and 1500 mg) within the context of the DASH eating and a control diet.[20] The results showed that the lower the sodium level, the lower the BP level in all subgroups. BP was 7/3 mm Hg lower with intake of the 1500 mg sodium diet compared with the diet with 3300 mg of sodium. Other trials have consistently demonstrated the relationship with sodium and BP, showing that sodium reduction leads to BP lowering.[59,60] Results of the DASH-Na trial also showed that the combination of sodium reduction and consumption of the DASH dietary pattern is more effective at BP lowering than single interventions.[20]

High BP is a major risk factor for CVD mortality.[1] Evidence from RCTs and observational studies is available on the relationship of sodium and CVD. Limited yet consistent evidence from RCTs demonstrates a reduction in sodium-reduced CVD events.[61–63] One of the studies included was a 12-year to 15-year follow-up in which participants who received the sodium intervention had a 30% reduction in relative risk for CVD events.[62] Results from observational studies on sodium and CVD risk have been mixed due to limitations in methodology.[64] Limitations include inadequate estimates of sodium intake, reverse causality, inclusion of populations with existing CVD, and inadequate control of confounding variables in analyses. After considering the strengths and limitations of the observational studies, the Lifestyle Workgroup concluded that higher dietary sodium intake is associated with greater risk for fatal and nonfatal stroke and CVD.[12] A recent study showed an association between both low and high intakes of sodium and a higher rate of CVD.[65] This study included the strength of a large sample size yet a major limitation was the method used to assess sodium intake (spot urine vs 24-h sodium collection), which can provide misleading results. In summary, given the strong effect of sodium on BP, it is important for physicians to recommend dietary patterns that are moderate in sodium.

ALCOHOL

Decades of observational evidence consistently support an association between light to moderate alcohol intake and CVD risk reduction.[66] Numerous prospective studies have shown consistent evidence to reinforce the association of light to moderate alcohol consumption with decreased CVD risk.[67–71] Results of a meta-analysis of prospective studies showed that low intake of alcohol was associated with lower risk of stroke whereas heavy intake was associated with increased risk of stroke.[72] Results from a recent large prospective study concluded that light to moderate alcohol intake was associated with decreased risk of heart attack and heart failure.[73,74] A prospective study in twins recently showed that during a 41-year follow-up, a higher (10-g) daily intake of alcohol intake was associated with lower coronary artery disease risk.[75] The observed cardiovascular protective effect of moderate alcohol intake has been mostly attributed to the increases in HDL-C shown in these studies.[76,77] Other possible mechanisms include improved insulin resistance and glucose metabolism, and genetic factors.[78] Moderate alcohol intake has been shown to have a positive effect on glucose metabolism.[79] Evidence from a meta-analysis of prospective observational studies suggested an association between moderate alcohol intake and a reduced risk of type 2 diabetes.[80] Additionally, results of a recent RCT demonstrated that moderate wine intake among those with controlled type 2 diabetes was safe and moderately decreased metabolic syndrome factors.[81]

There is a well-documented association between moderate alcohol intake and CVD risk reduction, yet it remains important to acknowledge that many adverse effects are frequently associated with excess alcohol intake.[82] Providers should use caution when discussing the potential benefit of moderate alcohol and CVD risk. Patients who already drink alcohol could be made aware that moderate consumption is association with reduced CVD risk in some individuals, yet those who abstain from alcohol intake should not be encouraged to begin consuming alcohol for CVD benefit.

SUMMARY

In summary, physicians are a critical component in communicating the importance of a heart healthy diet for CVD risk reduction. For lipid management and BP control, adults should be encouraged to adjust their eating pattern to one that is closer to a dietary pattern that includes vegetables, fruits, whole grains, lean proteins, and low-fat dairy products. Food sources that are high in saturated fats and trans fat, such as high fat meat, dairy, and some baked goods, should be replaced with foods that are higher in healthier fats, such as vegetable oils and nuts. Nutrition modifications effective for BP control include intake of a DASH-style eating pattern in addition to sodium reduction. The evidence on the benefit of using the glycemic index of foods for CVD risk reduction is limited and, therefore, it is not recommended to be used. Additionally, future research is needed to isolate the effect of dietary cholesterol on LDL-C. Moderate alcohol intake is associated with CVD risk reduction and, therefore, can be included in a heart healthy diet. Finally, in addition to nutrition counseling for BP and lipid management, strong evidence supports physical activity and weight control interventions to reduce CVD risk.[83,84]

REFERENCES

1. Mozaffarian D, Benjamin EJ, Go AS, et al. Heart disease and stroke statistics–2015 update: a report from the American Heart Association. Circulation 2015; 131(4):e29–322.
2. Nwankwo T, Yoon SS, Burt V, et al. Hypertension among adults in the US: National Health and Nutrition Examination Survey, 2011-2012. NCHS Data Brief; No. 133. Hyattsville (MD): National Center for Health Statistics; Centers for Disease Control and Prevention; 2013.
3. Centers for Disease Control and Prevention. National diabetes statistics report: estimates of diabetes and its burden in the United States. 2014. Available at: http://www.cdc.gov/diabetes/pubs/statsreport14/national-diabetes-report-web.pdf. Accessed August 18, 2015.

4. Ogden CL, Carroll MD, Kit BK, et al. Prevalence of childhood and adult obesity in the United States, 2011-2012. JAMA 2014;311(8):806–14.

5. Centers for Disease Control and Prevention. CDC health disparities and inequalities report —United States. Morbidity and Mortality Weekly Report; 2013:62(3).

6. Rodriguez CJ, Cai J, Swett K, et al. High cholesterol awareness, treatment, and control among hispanic/latinos: results from the Hispanic Community Health Study/Study of Latinos. J Am Heart Assoc 2015;4(7):1–10.

7. Rodriguez F, Ferdinand KC. Hypertension in minority populations: new guidelines and emerging concepts. Adv Chronic Kidney Dis 2015;22(2):145–53.

8. Singh GK, Siahpush M. Widening rural-urban disparities in all-cause mortality and mortality from major causes of death in the USA, 1969-2009. J Urban Health 2014;91(2):272–92.

9. Satcher D, Fryer GE Jr, McCann J, et al. What if we were equal? A comparison of the black-white mortality gap in 1960 and 2000. Health Aff (Millwood) 2005;24(2):459–64.

10. Eckel RH, Jakicic JM, Ard JD, et al. 2013 AHA/ACC guideline on lifestyle management to reduce cardiovascular risk: a report of the American College of Cardiology/American Heart Association Task Force on Practice Guidelines. J Am Coll Cardiol 2014;63(25 Pt B):2960–84.

11. Eckel RH. Preventive cardiology by lifestyle intervention: opportunity and/or challenge? Presidential address at the 2005 American Heart Association Scientific Sessions. Circulation 2006;113(22):2657–61.

12. National Heart Lung, and Blood Institute. Lifestyle interventions to reduce cardiovascular risk: systematic evidence review from the Lifestyle Work Group. 2013. Available at: https://www.nhlbi.nih.gov/sites/www.nhlbi.nih.gov/files/lifestyle.pdf. Accessed August 19, 2015.

13. Davis C, Bryan J, Hodgson J, et al. Definition of the Mediterranean diet; a literature review. Nutrients 2015;7(11):9139–53.

14. Estruch R, Martinez-Gonzalez MA, Corella D, et al. Effects of a Mediterranean-style diet on cardiovascular risk factors: a randomized trial. Ann Intern Med 2006;145(1):1–11.

15. Toledo E, Hu FB, Estruch R, et al. Effect of the Mediterranean diet on blood pressure in the PREDIMED trial: results from a randomized controlled trial. BMC Med 2013;11:207.

16. Nunez-Cordoba JM, Valencia-Serrano F, Toledo E, et al. The Mediterranean diet and incidence of hypertension: the Seguimiento Universidad de Navarra (SUN) Study. Am J Epidemiol 2009;169(3):339–46.

17. Estruch R, Ros E, Martinez-Gonzalez MA. Mediterranean diet for primary prevention of cardiovascular disease. N Engl J Med 2013;369(7):676–7.

18. Appel LJ, Moore TJ, Obarzanek E, et al. A clinical trial of the effects of dietary patterns on blood pressure. DASH Collaborative Research Group. N Engl J Med 1997;336(16):1117–24.

19. Svetkey LP, Simons-Morton D, Vollmer WM, et al. Effects of dietary patterns on blood pressure: subgroup analysis of the Dietary Approaches to Stop Hypertension (DASH) randomized clinical trial. Arch Intern Med 1999;159(3):285–93.

20. Sacks FM, Svetkey LP, Vollmer WM, et al. Effects on blood pressure of reduced dietary sodium and the Dietary Approaches to Stop Hypertension (DASH) diet. DASH-Sodium Collaborative Research Group. N Engl J Med 2001;344(1):3–10.

21. Appel LJ, Sacks FM, Carey VJ, et al. Effects of protein, monounsaturated fat, and carbohydrate intake on blood pressure and serum lipids: results of the OmniHeart randomized trial. JAMA 2005;294(19):2455–64.

22. Wright JD, Wang CY. Trends in intake of energy and macronutrients in adults from 1999–2000 through 2007–2008. Hyattsville (MD): National Center for Health Statistics; 2010.

23. Kris-Etherton PM, Lefevre M, Mensink RP, et al. Trans fatty acid intakes and food sources in the U.S. population: NHANES 1999-2002. Lipids 2012;47(10):931–40.

24. Mensink RP, Katan MB. Effect of dietary fatty acids on serum lipids and lipoproteins. A meta-analysis of 27 trials. Arterioscler Thromb 1992;12(8):911–9.

25. Mensink RP, Zock PL, Kester AD, et al. Effects of dietary fatty acids and carbohydrates on the ratio of serum total to HDL cholesterol and on serum lipids and apolipoproteins: a meta-analysis of 60 controlled trials. Am J Clin Nutr 2003; 77(5):1146–55.

26. Ginsberg HN, Kris-Etherton P, Dennis B, et al. Effects of reducing dietary saturated fatty acids on plasma lipids and lipoproteins in healthy subjects: the DELTA Study, protocol 1. Arterioscler Thromb Vasc Biol 1998;18(3):441–9.

27. US Department of Agriculture and the US Departmemt of Health and Human Services. Dietary guidelines for Americans. 7th edition. Washington, DC: U.S. Government Printing Office; 2010.

28. McCulloch M. Saturated fat: not so bad or just bad science? Today's Dietitian 2014. Available at: http://www.todaysdietitian.com/newarchives/111114p32. shtml. Accessed on August 19, 2015.

29. Mozaffarian D, Micha R, Wallace S. Effects on coronary heart disease of increasing polyunsaturated fat in place of saturated fat: a systematic review and meta-analysis of randomized controlled trials. PLoS Med 2010;7(3): e1000252.

30. Hooper L, Summerbell CD, Thompson R, et al. Reduced or modified dietary fat for preventing cardiovascular disease. Cochrane Database Syst Rev 2012;(5):CD002137.

31. Skeaff CM, Miller J. Dietary fat and coronary heart disease: summary of evidence from prospective cohort and randomised controlled trials. Ann Nutr Metab 2009; 55(1–3):173–201.

32. Siri-Tarino PW, Sun Q, Hu FB, et al. Meta-analysis of prospective cohort studies evaluating the association of saturated fat with cardiovascular disease. Am J Clin Nutr 2010;91(3):535–46.

33. Chowdhury R, Warnakula S, Kunutsor S, et al. Association of dietary, circulating, and supplement fatty acids with coronary risk: a systematic review and meta-analysis. Ann Intern Med 2014;160(6):398–406.

34. Jakobsen MU, O'Reilly EJ, Heitmann BL, et al. Major types of dietary fat and risk of coronary heart disease: a pooled analysis of 11 cohort studies. Am J Clin Nutr 2009;89(5):1425–32.

35. Mozaffarian D, Aro A, Willett WC. Health effects of trans-fatty acids: experimental and observational evidence. Eur J Clin Nutr 2009;63(Suppl 2):S5–21.

36. Kadhum AA, Shamma MN. Edible lipids modification processes: a review. Crit Rev Food Sci Nutr 2015. [Epub ahead of print].

37. Doell D, Folmer D, Lee H, et al. Updated estimate of trans fat intake by the US population. Food Addit Contam Part A Chem Anal Control Expo Risk Assess 2012;29(6):861–74.

38. Otite FO, Jacobson MF, Dahmubed A, et al. Trends in trans fatty acids reformulations of US supermarket and brand-name foods from 2007 through 2011. Prev Chronic Dis 2013;10:E85.

39. Food and Drug Administration. Food labeling; nutrition labeling of standard menu items in restaurants and similar retail food establishments; calorie labeling of

articles of food in vending machines; final rule. In: Department of Health and Human Services, editor. Federal register. College Park, MD: Government Printing Office; 2014.

40. Food and Drug Administration. Food labeling: trans fatty acids in nutrition labeling, nutrient content claims, and health claims. In: Department of Health and Human Services, editor. Federal register. College Park, MD: U.S. Government Publishing Office; 2003.

41. Food and Nutrition Service. Nutrition standards in the National School Lunch and School Breakfast Programs. In: US Department of Agriculture, editor. Federal register. Alexandria, VA: Government Printing Office; 2012.

42. Food and Drug Administration. Final determination regarding partially hydrogenated oils. In: US Department of Health and Human Services, editor. Federal register. College Park, MD: Government Printing Office; 2015.

43. Khawaja OA, Gaziano JM, Djousse L. N-3 fatty acids for prevention of cardiovascular disease. Curr Atheroscler Rep 2014;16(11):450.

44. Manson JE, Bassuk SS, Lee IM, et al. The VITamin D and OmegA-3 TriaL (VITAL): rationale and design of a large randomized controlled trial of vitamin D and marine omega-3 fatty acid supplements for the primary prevention of cancer and cardiovascular disease. Contemp Clin Trials 2012;33(1):159–71.

45. American Heart Association Nutrition Committee, Lichtenstein AH, Appel LJ, Brands M, et al. Diet and lifestyle recommendations revision 2006: a scientific statement from the American Heart Association Nutrition Committee. Circulation 2006;114(1):82–96.

46. National Cholesterol Education Program (NCEP) Expert Panel on Detection, Evaluation, and Treatment of High Blood Cholesterol in Adults (Adult Treatment Panel III). Third report of the National Cholesterol Education Program (NCEP) expert panel on detection, evaluation, and treatment of high blood cholesterol in adults (Adult Treatment Panel III) final report. Circulation 2002;106(25):3143–421.

47. Fuller NR, Sainsbury A, Caterson ID, et al. Egg consumption and human cardiometabolic health in people with and without diabetes. Nutrients 2015;7(9): 7399–420.

48. Berger S, Raman G, Vishwanathan R, et al. Dietary cholesterol and cardiovascular disease: a systematic review and meta-analysis. Am J Clin Nutr 2015;102(2): 276–94.

49. Tran NL, Barraj LM, Heilman JM, et al. Egg consumption and cardiovascular disease among diabetic individuals: a systematic review of the literature. Diabetes Metab Syndr Obes 2014;7:121–37.

50. Eckel RH. Eggs and beyond: is dietary cholesterol no longer important? Am J Clin Nutr 2015;102(2):235–6.

51. 2015–2020 Dietary Guidelines for Americans. US Department of Health and Human Services, The US Department of Agriculture, editors. 8th edition. 2015. Available at: http://health.gov/dietaryguidelines/2015/guidelines/. Accessed December 15, 2015.

52. Sacks FM, Carey VJ, Anderson CA, et al. Effects of high vs low glycemic index of dietary carbohydrate on cardiovascular disease risk factors and insulin sensitivity: the OmniCarb randomized clinical trial. JAMA 2014;312(23):2531–41.

53. Shikany JM, Phadke RP, Redden DT, et al. Effects of low- and high-glycemic index/glycemic load diets on coronary heart disease risk factors in overweight/obese men. Metabolism 2009;58(12):1793–801.

54. Kristo AS, Matthan NR, Lichtenstein AH. Effect of diets differing in glycemic index and glycemic load on cardiovascular risk factors: review of randomized controlled-feeding trials. Nutrients 2013;5(4):1071–80.

55. Mirrahimi A, Chiavaroli L, Srichaikul K, et al. The role of glycemic index and glycemic load in cardiovascular disease and its risk factors: a review of the recent literature. Curr Atheroscler Rep 2014;16(1):381.

56. Wolever TM, Gibbs AL, Mehling C, et al. The Canadian Trial of Carbohydrates in Diabetes (CCD), a 1-y controlled trial of low-glycemic-index dietary carbohydrate in type 2 diabetes: no effect on glycated hemoglobin but reduction in C-reactive protein. Am J Clin Nutr 2008;87(1):114–25.

57. American Diabetes Association. Standards of medical care in diabetes. Diabetes Care 2016; 39(Suppl 1):S27.

58. Aburto NJ, Ziolkovska A, Hooper L, et al. Effect of lower sodium intake on health: systematic review and meta-analyses. BMJ 2013;346:f1326.

59. He FJ, Li J, Macgregor GA. Effect of longer-term modest salt reduction on blood pressure. Cochrane Database Syst Rev 2013;(4):CD004937.

60. Mozaffarian D, Fahimi S, Singh GM, et al. Global sodium consumption and death from cardiovascular causes. N Engl J Med 2014;371(7):624–34.

61. Appel LJ, Espeland MA, Easter L, et al. Effects of reduced sodium intake on hypertension control in older individuals: results from the Trial of Nonpharmacologic Interventions in the Elderly (TONE). Arch Intern Med 2001;161(5):685–93.

62. Cook NR, Cutler JA, Obarzanek E, et al. Long term effects of dietary sodium reduction on cardiovascular disease outcomes: observational follow-up of the trials of hypertension prevention (TOHP). BMJ 2007;334(7599):885–8.

63. Chang HY, Hu YW, Yue CS, et al. Effect of potassium-enriched salt on cardiovascular mortality and medical expenses of elderly men. Am J Clin Nutr 2006;83(6): 1289–96.

64. Cobb LK, Anderson CA, Elliott P, et al. Methodological issues in cohort studies that relate sodium intake to cardiovascular disease outcomes: a science advisory from the American Heart Association. Circulation 2014;129(10):1173–86.

65. O'Donnell M, Mente A, Rangarajan S, et al. Urinary sodium and potassium excretion, mortality, and cardiovascular events. N Engl J Med 2014;371(7):612–23.

66. Mukamal KJ, Rimm EB. Alcohol's effects on the risk for coronary heart disease. Alcohol Res Health 2001;25(4):255–61.

67. Thun MJ, Peto R, Lopez AD, et al. Alcohol consumption and mortality among middle-aged and elderly U.S. adults. N Engl J Med 1997;337(24):1705–14.

68. Renaud SC, Gueguen R, Schenker J, et al. Alcohol and mortality in middle-aged men from eastern France. Epidemiology 1998;9(2):184–8.

69. Mukamal KJ, Kronmal RA, Mittleman MA, et al. Alcohol consumption and carotid atherosclerosis in older adults: the Cardiovascular Health Study. Arterioscler Thromb Vasc Biol 2003;23(12):2252–9.

70. Waskiewicz A, Sygnowska E, Drygas W. Relationship between alcohol consumption and cardiovascular mortality–the Warsaw Pol-MONICA Project. Kardiol Pol 2004;60(6):552–62 [discussion: 563].

71. Gaziano JM, Gaziano TA, Glynn RJ, et al. Light-to-moderate alcohol consumption and mortality in the Physicians' Health Study enrollment cohort. J Am Coll Cardiol 2000;35(1):96–105.

72. Zhang C, Qin YY, Chen Q, et al. Alcohol intake and risk of stroke: a dose-response meta-analysis of prospective studies. Int J Cardiol 2014;174(3):669–77.

73. Gemes K, Janszky I, Laugsand LE, et al. Alcohol consumption is associated with a lower incidence of acute myocardial infarction: results from a large prospective population-based study in Norway. J Intern Med 2016;279:365–75.

74. Gemes K, Janszky I, Ahnve S, et al. Light-to-moderate drinking and incident heart failure - the Norwegian HUNT study. Int J Cardiol 2015;203:553–60.

75. Dai J, Mukamal KJ, Krasnow RE, et al. Higher usual alcohol consumption was associated with a lower 41-y mortality risk from coronary artery disease in men independent of genetic and common environmental factors: the prospective NHLBI Twin Study. Am J Clin Nutr 2015;102(1):31–9.

76. Brinton EA. Effects of ethanol intake on lipoproteins. Curr Atheroscler Rep 2012; 14(2):108–14.

77. Brien SE, Ronksley PE, Turner BJ, et al. Effect of alcohol consumption on biological markers associated with risk of coronary heart disease: systematic review and meta-analysis of interventional studies. BMJ 2011;342:d636.

78. Matsumoto C, Miedema MD, Ofman P, et al. An expanding knowledge of the mechanisms and effects of alcohol consumption on cardiovascular disease. J Cardiopulm Rehabil Prev 2014;34(3):159–71.

79. Schrieks IC, Heil AL, Hendriks HF, et al. The effect of alcohol consumption on insulin sensitivity and glycemic status: a systematic review and meta-analysis of intervention studies. Diabetes Care 2015;38(4):723–32.

80. Koppes LL, Dekker JM, Hendriks HF, et al. Moderate alcohol consumption lowers the risk of type 2 diabetes: a meta-analysis of prospective observational studies. Diabetes Care 2005;28(3):719–25.

81. Gepner Y, Golan R, Harman-Boehm I, et al. Effects of initiating moderate alcohol intake on cardiometabolic risk in adults with type 2 diabetes: a 2-year randomized, controlled trial. Ann Intern Med 2015;163(8):569–79.

82. Rehm J, Hingson R. Measuring the burden: alcohol's evolving impact on individuals, families, and society. Alcohol Res 2013;35(2):117–8.

83. Jensen MD, Ryan DH, Apovian CM, et al. 2013 AHA/ACC/TOS guideline for the management of overweight and obesity in adults: a report of the American College of Cardiology/American Heart Association Task Force on Practice Guidelines and The Obesity Society. J Am Coll Cardiol 2014;63(25 Pt B):2985–3023.

84. Berra K, Rippe J, Manson JE. Making physical activity counseling a priority in clinical practice: the time for action is now. JAMA 2015;314:2617–8.

Nutrition Interventions in Chronic Kidney Disease

Cheryl A.M. Anderson, PhD, MPH, MS[a],*, Hoang Anh Nguyen, MD, MPH[b],
Dena E. Rifkin, MD, MS[c]

KEYWORDS

- Chronic kidney disease • Nutrition • Interventions

KEY POINTS

- Dietary modification is recommended in the management of chronic kidney disease (CKD).
- Individuals with CKD often have significant comorbid conditions, such as high blood pressure, diabetes, cardiovascular disease, and obesity, for which dietary modification is also recommended.
- Dietary considerations in CKD can be numerous and complicated for both the provider and patients; adherence to recommendations is difficult for patients to achieve.
- Guiding principles of nutritional management include (1) assessment and monitoring of nutritional status throughout all stages of CKD; (2) creation of an individualized yet comprehensive nutrition plan that meets clinical guidelines and will have favorable effects on CKD and associated comorbidities; and (3) recommendation of meal plans that are feasible, sustainable, and suited for the patients' food preferences and needs.
- Given the high prevalence of CKD and the tremendous burden for patients, diet/nutrition is a modifiable factor that could help impact a major clinical and public health issue.

INTRODUCTION

There are numerous reasons to consider nutrition-related interventions in patients with chronic kidney disease (CKD). CKD results in altered metabolism of many nutrients and their end products. Individuals with CKD may also have multiple comorbidities, including a disproportionate burden of hypertension, type 2 diabetes mellitus, and cardiovascular disease (CVD), all of which are amenable to treatment via changes in nutrition. Indeed, many patients with CKD experience fatal cardiovascular events before needing renal replacement therapy. Further, as CKD progresses, medication regimens

[a] Department of Family Medicine and Public Health, UC San Diego School of Medicine, 9500 Gilman Drive, MC 0725, La Jolla, CA 92093-0725, USA; [b] Department of Nephrology and Hypertension, UCSD Medical Center, 200 West Arbor Drive, San Diego, CA 92102, USA; [c] Department of Nephrology and Hypertension, VA San Diego Healthcare System, 3350 La Jolla Drive, San Diego, CA 92161, USA
* Corresponding author.
E-mail address: c1anderson@ucsd.edu

Med Clin N Am 100 (2016) 1265–1283
http://dx.doi.org/10.1016/j.mcna.2016.06.008
0025-7125/16/$ – see front matter © 2016 Elsevier Inc. All rights reserved.

become increasingly complex; nutrition planning plays an important role in slowing down kidney function decline. Therefore, the objectives of nutrition interventions in CKD include addressing the root causes of CKD (diabetes and hypertension); achieving and maintaining optimal nutritional status and nitrogen balance; preventing buildup of toxic metabolic products, thus, minimizing the risk of uremia; and avoiding complications, such as hyperphosphatemia, anemia, hyperkalemia, hypervolemia, and metabolic acidosis. Through these mechanisms, nutrition interventions, for individuals with CKD, should reduce the risk for secondary hyperparathyroidism, malnutrition, muscle wasting, heart failure, hypertension, fatigue, shortness of breath, nausea, and poor quality of life.

The body of research for nutrition interventions in CKD is growing but still quite limited, as even today the current recommendations are primarily based on expert opinion or extrapolated from research on individuals without CKD. The initial clinical practice guidelines for nutrition in CKD were created by the National Kidney Foundation's Kidney Disease Outcome Quality Initiative (K/DOQI) in an effort to provide consensus practice standards based on evidence, opinion, or a combination of both and were developed by expert, multidisciplinary work groups.[1] Guidelines also exist for earlier stages of disease[2] and for those with hypertension.[3] In general, K/DOQI recommends that routine care for patients include dietary advice from a registered dietitian who is experienced in counseling patients with CKD, which is particularly important, as there will likely be a need to address and prioritize management for multiple diagnoses, such as diabetes or hypertension, in addition to CKD. Another source of nutrition guidance is Kidney Disease: Improving Global Outcomes (K/DIGO), which was established in 2003 as a global organization to develop evidence-based guidelines in kidney disease. Recommendations are embedded in clinical practice guidelines for anemia,[4] blood pressure,[5] mineral and bone disorder,[6] and lipids in CKD.[7] Readers are referred to these guidelines for further background information (**Table 1**).

Given the limited availability of data from clinical trials (**Table 2**), nutrition interventions in CKD are largely driven by the clinical judgments of physicians and renal dietitians. Importantly, to the extent possible, patients should play a key role in informing nutritional plans and interventions. The complexities of a renal diet need to be integrated into patients' cultural preferences, financial constraints, and family centered eating patterns. A comprehensive plan for nutrition is one that focuses on

- Establishing overall healthful dietary patterns
- Promoting fluid, electrolyte, and mineral balance
- Preventing dyslipidemia, elevated blood glucose levels, micronutrient deficiencies, and protein-energy malnutrition
- Maintaining appropriate weight and body composition
- And assessing use of supplements, such as phosphorus binders, iron, and bicarbonate

ESTABLISHING HEALTHFUL DIETARY PATTERNS TO PREVENT CARDIOVASCULAR DISEASE IN CHRONIC KIDNEY DISEASE

The most common causes for CKD are hypertension and type 2 diabetes mellitus. Obesity is also a contributing factor. These risk factors for CKD are nutrition related, and healthful dietary patterns have the potential to prevent or mitigate them and, therefore, reduce the risk of CKD. Common elements of healthful dietary patterns include a variety of vegetables; fruits; grains, of which 50% are whole; fat-free or low-fat dairy, which includes milk, yogurt, cheese, and fortified soy; oils; and sources

Table 1
Nutrition recommendations by the National Kidney Foundation's Kidney Disease: improving global outcomes guideline and American Heart Association/American College of Cardiology guidelines

Nutrients	Amount Recommended by NKF K/DIGO Guidelines for Individuals with CKD	Amount Recommended by AHA/ACC Guidelines (Not Specific for Individuals with CKD)
Energy intake	Adults younger than 60 y: 35 kcal/kg/d; adults 60 y or older: 30–35 kcal/kg/d	Match intake of total energy (calories to overall energy needs)
Fat/lipid	For CKD stages I–IV: 25%–35% of total energy intake come from total fat, <10% from saturated fat, and cholesterol intake should be <200 mg/d	Fat free and low fat
Sodium	<90 mmol/d (<2 g/d) corresponding to 5 g of NaCl	<6 g/d
Potassium	Unrestricted unless serum potassium increases to >5 mEq/dL or potassium-sparing medications are being used	No recommendations
Fluid intake	No recommendations	No recommendations
Phosphorous	Reduce phosphorous intake to 800–1000 mg/d if serum phosphorous >4.6 mg/dL	No recommendations
Calcium/vitamin D	No recommendations	
Acid	Serum bicarbonate concentrations <22 mmol/L then consider treatment	No recommendations
Protein	0.60 g/kg/d for GFR ≤25 mL/min Normal adults and CKD stages I–III: 0.75 g/kg/d	No recommendations
Fiber and fiber supplements	No recommendations	≥5 servings of fruits and vegetables per day ≥6 servings of grain products
Supplements	No recommendations	Antioxidants, soy products (needs more research studies)

Abbreviations: ACC, American College of Cardiology; AHA, American Heart Association; NaCl, sodium chloride; NKF, National Kidney Foundation.

of protein, such as legumes, nuts, seeds, soy, eggs, seafood, and lean meats. These patterns are also reduced in saturated fats, added sugars, and sodium. Although there is now a strong body of evidence of the benefit of healthful dietary patterns on health outcomes, these studies included general population samples and exclude individuals with overt proteinuria. Thus, data are lacking regarding optimal dietary patterns in individuals with CKD. The nutritional guidance offered here are extrapolated from general population research samples that aim to reduce CVD risk factors[8,9] and CVD.[10]

Dietary Approaches to Stop Hypertension, OMNIHeart, and Prevencion con Dieta Mediterranea Dietary Patterns and Cardiovascular Disease Risk Reduction

The Dietary Approaches to Stop Hypertension (DASH) trials provide compelling data about the beneficial effects of a healthful dietary pattern on CVD risk factors (ie, blood

Table 2
Randomized controlled trials of nutrient components and their effects on chronic kidney disease

Nutrients	Clinical Manifestations	State of Science	Randomized Controlled Trials
Fluid	Fluid retention exacerbates hypertension leading to peripheral edema, anasarca, or pulmonary edema.	High urine volume and low urine osmolality are independent risk factors for faster decline in eGFR. High fluid intake does not slow renal disease progression.	• No randomized trials • Hebert et al,[18] 2003 (retrospective study): 442 nonpolycystic kidney disease participants
Sodium	High-sodium diet leads to fluid retention and increased blood pressure.	Low sodium intake lowers 24-h blood pressure, fluid volume, and 24-h urinary protein and albumin. High sodium intake increases NT-proBNP, E/I ratio, eGFR, PCR, and ACR.	• Campbell et al,[19] 2014: 20 participants • McMahon et al,[22] 2013: 25 participants
Potassium	High-potassium diet has shown to lower blood pressure in non-CKD patients, but it not recommended for individuals with CKD.	Low potassium intake causes renal sodium retention and elevation of blood pressure. High potassium intake increases kaliuresis and lowers blood pressure.	Riphagen et al,[20] 2016: 35 non-CKD participants
Phosphorous/calcium	There is adynamic bone disease.	A lanthanum- and phosphate-restricted diet decreases FGF23 levels and reduces 24-h urinary phosphate excretion. For calcium carbonate, there is positive calcium balance and it does not affect phosphorous balance; there is only moderate urinary phosphate excretion. High phosphorous intake increases its regulatory hormone and is associated with mortality in CKD.	• Isakova et al,[34] 2011: 16 participants • Isakova et al,[34] 2013: 39 participants • Sigrist et al,[35] 2013: 30 participants • Hill et al,[36] 2013: 8 participants • Di Iorio et al,[37] 2012: 32 participants

(continued on next page)

Table 2 (continued)			
Nutrients	**Clinical Manifestations**	**State of Science**	**Randomized Controlled Trials**
Acid	There is uremic bone disease, protein-energy wasting, impaired glucose homeostasis, and chronic inflammation.	Low serum bicarbonate has been associated with low serum albumin and high mortality across the spectrum of CKD severity. Correcting acidosis is associated with increased serum albumin, reduced protein catabolic rate, and increases in total essential amino acid concentrations.	• Ballmer et al,[72] 1995: 8 male participants • de Bristo-Ashurst et al,[79] 2009: 134 participants
Protein	Signs of inadequate energy intake, signs of malnutrition	In early CKD stages, reduced protein intake slows down CKD progression. Low protein reduces FGF23 levels, serum phosphate, and urinary phosphate.	Di Iorio et al,[37] 2012: 32 participants

Abbreviations: FGF23, fibroblast growth factor 23; NT-proBNP, N-terminal probrain natriuretic peptide; PCR, polymerase chain reaction.

pressure, total cholesterol, and low-density lipoprotein [LDL] cholesterol). The dietary intervention in the DASH trial emphasized fruits, vegetables, and low-fat dairy products; included whole grains, poultry, fish, and nuts; contained only small amounts of red meats, sweets, and sugar-containing beverages; had decreased amounts of total and saturated fat and cholesterol; and had a modest increase in protein. This dietary pattern was fed to participants for 8 weeks and demonstrated substantial reductions in blood pressure in adults with high normal and stage 1 hypertension.[8] Of note, the magnitude of blood pressure reduction in the hypertensive subgroup was similar to that achieved with pharmacotherapy and was achieved at a fixed sodium intake of 3.2 g/d. Although this study did not include individuals with CKD, adoption of this type of diet should have comparably favorable effects on blood pressure and lipids in patients in the early stages of CKD. This diet should not be routinely recommended for patients with later stages of CKD because its protein and phosphorus content is higher than recommended. The potassium content of the DASH diet was 4700 mg/d; as CKD progresses, this may also be of concern because of its emphasis on fruits and vegetables. The DASH trial included 8 to 10 servings of fruits and vegetables per day; approximately twice the average of 4.3 servings per day consumed by US adults.

Additional evidence about the beneficial effects of healthful dietary patterns comes from the OMNIHeart trial.[9] The OMNIHeart capitalized on knowledge learned from the DASH trials and compared the effect of 3 healthful diets with differing macronutrient profiles on blood pressure and serum lipids. The 3 test diets were a carbohydrate-rich diet, similar to the DASH diet (CARB diet); a diet rich in proteins, approximately half from plant sources; and a diet rich in unsaturated fat (UNSAT), predominantly monounsaturated fat. The UNSAT diet not only had all the DASH diet similarities previously described but was also higher in fat (37% vs 27% for DASH), predominantly monounsaturated fat (21%) primarily from olive and canola oils. Diets were all designed to optimize nutrients known to reduce CVD risk but as noted varied in macronutrient distribution. Each diet was reduced in saturated fat and cholesterol and rich in fruit, vegetables, fiber, potassium, and other minerals. Participants were healthy adults with prehypertension or stage 1 hypertension. Each feeding period in the OMNIHeart study lasted 6 weeks, and body weight was held constant. All 3 intervention diets lowered blood pressure and LDL cholesterol from baseline. Systolic blood pressure was reduced between 8.2 mm Hg and 9.5 mm Hg for all diets, with the greatest reduction occurring with consumption of the high-protein diet. LDL cholesterol was reduced from 11.6 mg/dL to 14.2 mg/dL, with the greatest reduction in the high-protein diet.

Comparisons between OMNIHeart diets were notable. The UNSAT diet resulted in a significantly greater reduction in systolic blood pressure (−2.9 mm Hg), increase in high-density lipoprotein cholesterol (1.1 mg/dL), and lower triglycerides (−9.6 mg/dL) compared with reductions of blood pressure and lipids seen with consumption of the CARB diet (similar to the DASH diet). The UNSAT diet, which contained a high monounsaturated fat content, reduced CVD risk factors beyond that achieved with the other healthy diets. Again, as in the DASH study, individuals with CKD were excluded from the OMNIHeart study. However, these results are likely relevant to patients in the early stages of CKD; adoption of carbohydrate intake levels similar to those in this diet should have comparably favorable effects on blood pressure and lipids in this population. In later stages of CKD, DASH-style diets should not be routinely recommended because the content of some nutrients (ie, protein and phosphorus) are higher than recommended.

A substantial body of evidence supports the consumption of a Mediterranean-style diet to reduce the risk of CVD. In the recent Prevencion con Dieta Mediterranea (PRE-DIMED) study, participants were randomized to one of 3 intervention groups: (1) a Mediterranean diet in which participants were provided a supply of extravirgin olive oil; (2) a Mediterranean diet in which participants were provided a supply of mixed nuts; and (3) lowered fat in the diet (control group). There was a reduction in risk of CVD by nearly 30% in the 2 groups that received advice on a Mediterranean diet.[10]

Fiber Intake and Fiber Supplements

Although it has not been tested explicitly in studies of dietary patterns, there is a growing body of intervention studies showing that increasing fiber intake in patients with CKD through the consumption of foods with added fiber may reduce serum creatinine and improve the estimated glomerular filtration rate (eGFR).[11–13] In these studies, many with very small sample sizes (n < 20), it has been hypothesized that diets that are low in plant fiber and symbiotic organisms can alter normal gut microbiome, leading to overgrowth of bacteria that produce uremic toxins, such as cresyl and indoxyl molecules.[14] The translocation of these toxins into the bloodstream promotes systemic inflammation and CKD progression. Additionally, dietary fiber has been found to be associated with free and total p-cresyl sulfate but not indoxyl sulfate. Fiber supplements decrease plasma p-cresol, an inflammatory component, and plasma urea by increasing stool frequency and eliminate urea nitrogen through the gut.

A limitation of the body of evidence on healthful dietary patterns is the lack of studies on the impact on incident CKD or progression of CKD. One of the few, large, randomized controlled trials focusing on dietary intake in CKD was the Modification of Diet in Renal Disease (MDRD) study[15]; much of what is known about reducing protein intake is extrapolated from this study. Currently, the popularity of dietary patterns that have very-high-protein contents warrant that the potential detrimental effect of these diets be reviewed with patients who use them. These diets vary widely and may contain excessive amounts of protein, phosphorus, or potassium. There are no published studies of the long-term metabolic effects of these diets; but they have been found to deliver a marked acid load to the kidney, increase the risk of stone formation, promote negative calcium balance and increase bone loss, and increase GFR.[16] However, given the paucity of data, research is urgently needed to establish the most healthful dietary patterns for individuals with CKD.

PROMOTING FLUID, ELECTROLYTE, AND MINERAL BALANCE

Monitoring salt and water intake is an important part of dietary therapy among individuals with advanced stages of CKD, because as kidney function declines salt and water retention is common. Fluid retention can exacerbate hypertension, and lead to peripheral edema, anasarca, or pulmonary edema. Generally, thirst regulates water balance adequately when sodium balance is well controlled. If a patient with CKD also has diabetes, hyperglycemia may also increase thirst and result in positive water balance. Urine volume may be a good guide to water intake when indicators such as normal blood pressure, absence of edema, and normal serum sodium suggest that total body water is at the desired level. In these cases, it is recommended that daily water intake equals the urine output plus approximately 500 mL to replace insensible losses.

Although conventional wisdom would suggest that drinking more water is healthful, data do not support this idea.[17] For example, a study using the MDRD database to retrospectively examine the relationship between fluid intake and renal disease progression found that sustained high urine volume and low urine osmolality are independent risk factors for faster decline in GFR.[18] Hebert and colleagues[18] concluded that high fluid intake does not slow renal disease progression and that patients should let thirst be their guide.

In a randomized clinical trial, Campbell and colleagues[19] investigated the effects of dietary sodium reduction on fluid volume, kidney function, and adipokines in 20 patients with hypertension and CKD stages III to IV. Study participants were counseled to consume a low-sodium diet (<100 mmol/d). The trial used a crossover design comparing 2 weeks of high-sodium (additional 120 mmol sodium tablets) and low-sodium intake (placebo). Measurements of blood pressure, adipokines (inflammation markers and adiponectin), volume markers (extracellular to intracellular fluid ratio), N-terminal probrain natriuretic peptide (NT-proBNP), kidney function (eGFR), and proteinuria (urine protein-creatinine ratio and albumin-creatinine ratio). It was found that low-sodium intake lowered both systolic and diastolic blood pressure. The high-sodium diet was associated with increased NT-proBNP, extracellular to intracellular fluid ratio, eGFR, and proteinuria. There was no change in inflammatory markers. It was hypothesized that high sodium intake could induce hyperfiltration associated with increased intraglomerular pressure. Therefore, although an increase in eGFR may be considered a reflection of improved kidney function, under these conditions it may actually reflect a state of hyperfiltration leading to further kidney damage and longer-term kidney function decline. The study duration was not long enough to examine this effect.

Sodium retention occurs with CKD and results in extracellular volume expansion. Although the potential consequences of high dietary sodium intake, including higher blood pressure, fluid retention, and CVD risk, are much more common in individuals with CKD,[5] few trials have been conducted in this population. There is evidence of interplay between sodium and potassium that is important in the development of hypertension.[20] At higher levels of potassium intake, the effects of sodium are attenuated. However, potassium levels are generally monitored because, even at typical levels of potassium intake, renal excretion of potassium can be affected in later stages of CKD and predispose individuals to hyperkalemia. There is also a higher risk of hyperkalemia for patients taking angiotensin-converting enzyme inhibitors or potassium-sparing diuretics.

K/DOQI recommends that potassium be unrestricted unless serum potassium level increases to more than 5 mEq/dL or potassium-sparing medications are being used. Other guidelines suggest that when urine output decreases to less than 1 L/d, potassium should be restricted. Nutritional interventions to promote electrolyte balance must consider the degree to which foods are processed, as processing affects potassium content. Highly refined foods, such as white breads, pasta, rice, and certain cereals, contain little potassium. Although fruits and vegetables are a key source of potassium, they can be incorporated into the diet of patients with CKD if they are carefully selected, the portion size is controlled, and the method of preparation is considered. Serum potassium is under tight homeostatic control; but in stages IV to V of CKD, rich sources of potassium should be avoided if serum potassium levels are increasing.

Given limited data from trials, current recommendations on sodium reduction by NKF/KDOQI are based on findings from the DASH and DASH-Sodium trials. In the DASH-Sodium Trial, adoption of the DASH diet lowered blood pressure when the sodium levels in the intervention diets were compared with a diet with sodium levels similar to what many Americans consume (~3400 mg/d).[21] In addition, blood pressure was lowered in both the DASH and typical American diet groups by reducing the sodium intake from 140 mmol/d to 100 mmol/d (2.4 g/d, the currently recommended upper limit); even greater blood pressure reduction was achieved with the consumption of either diet at a lower level of sodium to 65 mmol/d (1.6 g/d). The greatest magnitude of blood pressure reduction occurred with sodium reduction in those consuming the typical American diet. The DASH and DASH-Sodium trials have demonstrated the efficacy and safety of these diets in adults with high normal blood pressure and hypertension.[2] Although these trials did not include individuals with hypertension and kidney disease, most participants were overweight or obese; adoption of these recommendations should have comparable blood pressure–lowering effects in the CKD population. It is important to emphasize that the blood pressure and lipid effects observed in these trials were achieved with isocaloric feeding and no weight loss.

In 2013, a study by McMahon and colleagues[22] provided data from a 2-week randomized double-blind crossover study of high versus low sodium intake in CKD stages III to IV. Participants were placed on a low-sodium diet for a 1-week run-in and then randomized to either (1) a high-sodium arm (accomplished by the addition of a salt tablet on top of the low-sodium diet) or (2) a low-sodium arm (low sodium diet with the addition of a placebo tablet). Participants were treated for 2 weeks in one arm followed by a 1-week washout period before crossing over to the other arm. They showed dramatic reductions in blood pressure (9.7 mm Hg lower on the low-sodium arm compared with the high-sodium arm), proteinuria, fluid status, and body weight and increases in plasma renin and aldosterone with sodium reduction. The level of blood pressure reduction found in the study is substantial and clinically relevant. In addition, 4 participants required dose reductions of antihypertensive medications because of symptomatic hypotension while in the lower-sodium arm, suggesting the effects may have been even greater if the use of antihypertensive medications were held constant. Moreover, proteinuria was decreased by about 50% during the low-sodium intervention, an effect that was statistically independent of blood pressure changes. As expected, body weight and fluid status decreased; plasma renin and aldosterone concentrations markedly increased during the low-sodium intervention. No effect on arterial stiffness was observed. These data suggest that lowering sodium intake has beneficial effects.

The K/DOQI recommendation for sodium intake is less than 2.4 g/d. It is important to communicate to patients that, contrary to common belief, salt added at the table and while cooking is not the major source of sodium in the American diet.[23] The major sources of sodium in the diet are commercially processed foods (cheese, regular breads, cereals, butter or margarine, canned products, and cured meats) and salted sauces.[23,24]

Elegant and persuasive arguments have been made to support both the potential benefit and potential harms of sodium reduction. Regarding harm, it has been suggested that chronic exposure to high plasma renin and aldosterone may promote atherosclerosis,[25] given that sodium reduction increases plasma renin and aldosterone concentrations. Others have argued that, in the setting of diabetes, dietary sodium reduction may increase renal plasma flow and GFR and may contribute to hyperfiltration in the early stages of diabetic nephropathy.[26,27] These studies raise important questions about the effects of dietary sodium reduction in patients with CKD, and it is unknown whether adverse risks may occur if sodium intake is too low or whether recent paradoxic findings are due to methodological limitations within the studies suggesting harm.[28]

Mineral Balance: Phosphorus, Calcium, Parathyroid Hormone, and Fibroblast Growth Factor 23

High dietary phosphorus intake increases its regulatory hormones, parathyroid hormone (PTH) and fibroblast growth factor 23 (FGF23), and has been associated with end-stage renal disease, CVD, and mortality in CKD.[29] The K/DOQI guidelines in stages III to IV CKD recommend reduced phosphorus intake (800–1000 mg/d) if serum phosphorus levels are greater than 4.6 mg/dL.[1] Reducing phosphorus in the early stages of CKD should reduce the net intestinal absorption of phosphorus and minimize the likelihood of positive phosphate balance.

Dietary counseling for phosphorus reduction can be difficult given that phosphorus is found in many high-protein and dairy food products, including milk and milk products, eggs, peanut butter, sardines, and legumes; phosphorus absorption varies by how much of the phosphorus is in the form of phytate. In a small crossover study of 9 patients with CKD, Moe and colleagues[30] compared the effects of vegetarian and meat diets with equivalent nutrients on markers of phosphorus homeostasis. The findings from this study suggest that the source of protein (vegetarian or meat) is important, with 1 week of a vegetarian diet leading to lower serum phosphorus levels and decreased FGF23 levels. In addition to the source of protein, it is imperative that individuals who consume commercially packaged food products read the ingredients list to identify phosphorus additives.

Although the FGF23 level is not currently measured in routine clinical practice, there is clinical research evidence that an elevation of FGF23 is the earliest and most common manifestation of disordered mineral metabolism in patients with CKD. FGF23 levels increase with dietary phosphate loading and decrease when phosphates are reduced.[31,32] Small randomized interventional trials have examined the effects of lanthanum carbonate, calcium carbonate, low-protein diets, and phosphate reduction on FGF23 levels among patients with CKD stages III to IV.[33–37] In one such trial, with patients with normal phosphorus levels and CKD stages III to V, Isakova and colleagues[33] tested whether decreasing phosphorous intake using dietary reduction, phosphorous binders, or a combination of both would decrease FGF23 levels. Patients consuming a diet with 750 mg phosphorus had a greater reduction in 24-hour urinary phosphate excretion when compared with those on a 1500-mg phosphorus diet. Patients taking lanthanum experienced a significant reduction in 24-hour urinary phosphate excretion compared with baseline, but the difference compared with placebo did not reach significance (64% vs 31%). Despite the significant reductions in 24-hour urinary phosphate excretion, no group demonstrated a significant reduction in FGF23 levels; FGF23 levels increased significantly in those on a 1500-mg phosphorus diet, suggesting dietary phosphorus loading.

In another trial, Isakova and colleagues[34] examined the effects of a 3-month phosphate binder intervention alone or in combination with dietary phosphate reduction achieved through outpatient dietary counseling on FGF23 in patients who had normal serum phosphate levels with CKD stages III to V. The study found that, compared with an ad libitum diet, those on a 900-mg phosphate diet or on lanthanum carbonate alone did not significantly reduce FGF23 levels. However, the dual intervention significantly decreased FGF23 levels throughout the study period, resulting in a 35% reduction by study end.

Another small study found that FGF23 levels were higher among the interventional group versus the controls (72 pg/mL vs 30 pg/mL) at baseline. The study used three 7-day dietary interventions: a high phosphate (2000 mg/d), low phosphate (750 mg/d), and low phosphate plus phosphate binder (aluminum hydroxide, 500 mg 3 times daily with meals), with comparable macronutrient content, administered in random sequence. Serum phosphate remained in the normal range throughout the study. The absolute changes of urinary phosphate and calcium for CKD and controls vary according to diet.[35]

The effects of calcium carbonate (a phosphate binder) on calcium and phosphorous balance and calcium kinetics has been examined in patients with CKD stages III to V.[36] Patients on placebo had neutral calcium and phosphorus balance. Calcium carbonate supplementation (1500 mg/d calcium) produced positive calcium balance, did not affect phosphorus balance, and produced only a modest reduction in urine phosphorus excretion compared with placebo. Additionally, fasting blood and urine biochemistries of calcium and phosphate homeostasis were unaffected by calcium carbonate.

Di Iorio and colleagues[37] studied the effects of dietary phosphate reduction on FGF23 among patients with CKD. After 1 week of a very-low-protein diet (0.3 g/kg body weight per day) supplemented with keto-analogues, reductions were seen in FGF23 level, serum phosphate, and urinary phosphate compared with the low-protein diet week.

In summary, the combination of phosphate binders (lanthanum) plus counseling for a phosphate-reduced diet was found to decrease FGF23 levels in patients with CKD stages III to V and normal serum phosphate levels. However, caution should be taken in using calcium carbonate as a phosphate binder given the possibility of resultant positive calcium balance in patients with CKD stages III to IV. There are no specific K/DOQI guidelines[1] for vitamin D or calcium intake; however, supplemental vitamin D in its active form and supplemental calcium can help maintain blood calcium levels and prevent bone disease. Calcium intake is usually maintained at less than 2000 mg/d, including binders and dietary intake. Additional studies are needed to determine the long-term effects of using calcium carbonate as phosphate binders.

MANAGING NUTRITIONAL DEFICIENCIES IN CHRONIC KIDNEY DISEASE
Preventing Dyslipidemia and Minimizing Elevated Blood Glucose Levels

There is evidence that lipid reduction with pharmacologic therapy slows progression of kidney disease, which allows extrapolation to potential benefit from dietary modification therapy. Decreased saturated fats and cholesterol intake has been shown to be associated with decreased total and LDL cholesterol in patients on hemodialysis but not peritoneal dialysis.[38] Clinical trials of diet therapy to reduce lipids and slow progression of predialysis CKD have not been conducted.

To reduce dyslipidemia and to protect against lipid peroxidation and inflammation, the Kidney Health Australia—Caring for Australasians with Renal Impairment's guidelines for early CKD detection, prevention, and management[39] recommend that adults with CKD consume a Mediterranean-style diet. This recommendation is in accordance with the lifestyle guidelines from the American Heart Association/American College of Cardiology developed for CVD risk reduction.[40] In stages I to IV of CKD, K/DOQI recommends that 25% to 35% of total energy intake come from total fat, less than 10% of total energy intake from saturated fat, and cholesterol intake should be less than 200 mg/d.[1] The objective of these guidelines is to control blood lipid levels and minimize elevated blood glucose and triglycerides. Of note, diet modification for the management of dyslipidemia should be recommended and done in conjunction with other CVD risk-factor-reduction goals, including smoking cessation, weight reduction in those who are overweight, moderation of alcohol intake, and regular exercise or physical activity. Because diets for patients with CKD are restricted in protein, sodium, potassium, and water, it may be difficult to provide sufficient energy without resorting to large intake of refined sugars that may increase triglyceride production. Another challenge when addressing fat intake is maintaining recommended macronutrient balance when lowering saturated fat in the diet. When saturated fat is reduced in the diet, it can be replaced with carbohydrates, protein, or unsaturated fat. The optimal means of replacement of saturated fat is not known. Data from dietary intervention trials suggest that a diet low in saturated fat that uses either protein or unsaturated fats to replace carbohydrates can have favorable effects on blood lipids.[9]

Preventing Micronutrient Deficiencies

Micronutrients, such as vitamin K, vitamin K–dependent proteins, and vitamin D, may influence the regulation of bone calcification in CKD. Proteins that regulate mineralization in the arterial wall and bone, such as matrix Gla protein and osteocalcin, are upregulated by vitamin D and depend on vitamin K for their calcium-binding capacity.[41] Higher dietary intakes of vitamin K are associated with overall healthier dietary patterns, and vitamin K status should be monitored.

An inverse association between 25 hydroxyvitamin D (25[OH]D) levels and markers of inflammation, such as high-sensitivity C-reactive protein, has been observed.[42] Additionally, it has been repeatedly observed in patients on dialysis that those taking active vitamin D supplements have significantly better survival than those who did not take supplements.[43–45] These studies may be subject to confounding and bias, and trials are needed to further elucidate this relationship.

Vitamin K and vitamin D (ie, 25[OH]D) insufficiency has been observed in populations with CKD, and studies are needed to evaluate the relationship between vitamin K and D status and clinical outcomes. It may be very difficult to recommend daily intake for vitamin D with food intake alone; therefore, daily oral supplementation for vitamin D is often suggested (individuals aged between 19 and 52 years: 5 µg; those between 51 and 70 years: 10 µg; and those >70 years: 15 µg; 1 µg = 40 IU). Patients on vitamin D therapy should have their calcium, phosphate, PTH, alkaline phosphate, and 25(OH)D levels monitored regularly.[39]

Preventing Protein-Energy Wasting

In general, guidelines and recommendations are in agreement that controlling protein intake should be a goal in the dietary management of CKD. This view is based on the hypothesis that reduced protein intake slows progression of kidney disease. Data from observational studies are suggestive of a beneficial effect; but this has not been clearly demonstrated in trials, such as the MDRD study whereby the benefits of reducing protein intake were modest[15] and not long-term.[46] Additionally, the optimal level of dietary intake to slow the progression of CKD and maintain proper nutritional status is not known.

On a practical level, when diets are very low in protein, it can be difficult to get patients to consume adequate energy/calories; without enough calories, protein will be used for energy. If there is inadequate protein and calorie intake, protein-energy wasting can occur. Declines in energy and protein intake have been attributed to the symptoms of uremic symptoms that include anorexia, nausea, and fatigue in later stages of CKD. Historically, protein-energy wasting has been the major macronutrient challenge for patients with CKD; but more recent data from the US Renal Data System indicate an increased prevalence of overweight and obesity in the dialysis population.[47] Therefore, the contemporary approach to dietary management must address issues of excess energy consumption.

Generally, individuals with early CKD should consume the recommended dietary intake of protein (0.75–1.0 g/kg ideal body weight per day with adequate amounts of energy/calories).[39] As CKD progresses (eGFR <20 mL/min) but individuals are not yet on dialysis, there is relatively strong evidence underlying the American Diabetes Association's recommendation that protein intake be reduced to 0.3 to 0.5 g/kg body weight per day. Keto acid analogues and vitamin supplements should be added, if needed to maintain adequate nutrition status. On hemodialysis, the recommended protein intake for patients who are clinically stable is 1.1 g/kg ideal body weight per day with emphasis on consuming protein of high biological value.[1]

MAINTAINING APPROPRIATE BODY WEIGHT AND BODY COMPOSITION

Observational epidemiologic studies have shown that patients with end-stage renal disease (ESRD) who are overweight and obese have improved survival,[48,49] whereas a normal or low body mass index (BMI) confers higher all-cause and CVD death risks.[50,51] These findings are in contrast to those in the general population whereby overweight and underweight are associated with reduced survival rates.[52] Given the data on improved survival for those who are overweight and obese, some have suggested that obese patients with ESRD should not be counseled to lose weight or those with normal weight should be counseled to gain weight.[53] But, in contrast, other evidence suggests that physical functioning may be impaired by obesity in patients with ESRD.[48]

Although it is recognized that obesity has complex effects in persons with advanced CKD and ESRD, the cause for improved survival in obese patients with CKD remains obscure. The favorable prognosis with higher BMI may reflect reverse causality, a form of bias, seen because CKD can result in intermediate weight loss before death and this obscures the relationship between obesity and mortality. It might also be a result of intrinsic limitations of BMI in differentiating adipose tissue from lean mass in intermediate BMI ranges.[54]

Weight Loss Recommendations in Chronic Kidney Disease

Given the strong body of evidence of association with beneficial health outcomes, weight loss is a sensible therapeutic strategy for individuals with CKD, although the amount of weight loss required to achieve maximal benefit is unknown. Among the documented benefits of losing weight are reduction in proteinuria by about 80% as well as lower blood pressure and improved insulin sensitivity.[55,56] Furthermore, if an individual is expected to progress to ESRD, most transplant programs have cutoff BMI values above which they will not consider a candidate for transplant. The cornerstone of therapy for management of obesity includes nonpharmacologic strategies focused on weight reduction through healthy eating and increased regular physical activity. Prevention and treatment of obesity should be a first-line objective in the therapeutic approach of patients with diabetic and nondiabetic CKD, as high BMI has been categorized as the second leading preventable cause of death, after cigarette smoking.[57] Although studies of intentional weight loss to slow progression of CKD have not been performed, the health benefits and recommendations for weight loss for the general population would likely apply to this group. In healthy individuals, weight loss of 5% to 10% of body weight lowers blood pressure and cholesterol levels. The means by which patients lose weight is important, and healthy eating patterns and increased physical activity should be emphasized.

In CKD stages I to III, the K/DOQI recommends that energy intake levels support a balanced diet and maintain desirable body weight but does not recommend specific energy-intake amounts.[1] In CKD stages IV to V (GFR <30), specific energy intake amounts are recommended: 35 kcal/kg/d for those younger than 60 years and 30 to 35 kcal/kg/d for those older than 60 years. A 30-kcal/kg diet equates to 2400 to 2900 kcal/d for a 150- to 180-lb patient. Obese patients should be advised to consume lower-energy intake levels. To reduce energy intake, patients should eat a balanced diet that is low in total fat and saturated and trans fats.

Importance of Exercise in Weight Loss Programs

Exercise should be recommended for obese patients with CKD as part of a comprehensive weight-loss therapy and weight-control program. Exercise can be beneficial in obese patients with CKD in controlling comorbidities, such as hypertension, diabetes, CVD, and hyperlipidemia. Therefore, exercise is recommended as part of the National Kidney Foundation's K/DOQI clinical practice guidelines for hypertension and antihypertensive agents in CKD.[3] Specifically, the K/DOQI recommendation for exercise and physical activity is taken from the "Seventh Report of the Joint National Committee on the Prevention, Detection, Evaluation, and Treatment of High Blood Pressure" and suggests moderate-intensity exercise for 30 minutes per day, most days of the week.

Exercise has been shown to modestly contribute to weight loss in overweight and obese adults, decrease abdominal fat, increase cardiorespiratory fitness, and help with maintenance of weight loss. In studies conducted in those with ESRD, data suggest that patients with kidney disease have physiologically similar responses to exercise training when compared with other patient groups.[58,59] Beneficial effects of exercise training have been seen with blood pressure control,[60] physical function,[61,62] and health-related quality of life.[61,62] Studies have shown mixed results on the effects of exercise on anemia,[63,64] lipid levels,[63] and mental health.[61,64]

Before exercise is incorporated into a program, a medical screening should be completed and considerations should be made for coexisting diseases, which includes blood pressure control and volume status, depending on disease severity. Ideally, exercise should be undertaken in combination with behavioral therapy that assesses patients' motivation levels and other factors that contribute to the success of an exercise program. Based on data from the Weight Loss Registry, high levels of physical activity, along with ongoing self-monitoring, restrained eating, and caloric reduction, and comparatively small amounts of television time are factors associated with sustained weight loss.[65,66] Exercise plans will need to be carefully individualized and monitored for each patient, and patients should strive to follow the recommendation by K/DOQI.

ASSESSING USE OF SUPPLEMENTS SUCH AS PHOSPHORUS BINDERS AND BICARBONATE

A common complication of CKD is metabolic acidosis, particularly when GFR decreases to less than 30 mL/min. The consequences of metabolic acidosis include uremic bone disease, protein-energy wasting, impaired glucose homeostasis, and chronic inflammation; it usually manifests as a low serum bicarbonate level. The predominant finding in the literature is that low levels of serum bicarbonate are associated with higher mortality across the spectrum of CKD severity[67–69] with emerging observational epidemiologic data that high levels of serum bicarbonate may negatively affect survival.[70] Trials are needed to determine the effects of various levels of bicarbonate replacement therapy on clinical outcomes that may be predictive of survival.

The use of phosphate binders, as adjunct to reducing dietary phosphorus intake, to manage elevated serum phosphate levels is well recognized. Improved survival has been noted in patients undergoing dialysis treated with phosphate binders when compared with those not receiving them when potentially confounding clinical factors were accounted for.[71] An important consideration regarding the use of phosphate binders is their calcium content given the unsettled debate about the impact of calcium load on clinical outcomes. Additional data from well-conducted clinical trials with clinical outcomes are needed to inform what type of phosphate binder should be used and the best time to initiate therapy.

Evidence suggests that metabolic acidosis contributes to protein-energy malnutrition, as acidosis is associated with increased protein catabolism.[72–74] Clinical trials data suggest that correcting acidosis is associated with increased serum albumin, reduced protein catabolic rate,[75,76] and increases in total essential amino acid concentrations.[77–79] Therefore, good management of CKD involves the assessment of commonly used supplements that may impact nutritional status.

SUMMARY

Dietary modification is recommended in the management of CKD. Individuals with CKD often have significant comorbid conditions, such as high blood pressure, diabetes, CVD, and obesity, for which dietary modification is also recommended. Therefore, dietary considerations in CKD can be numerous, complicated for both the provider and patients; adherence to recommendations is difficult for patients to achieve. The complexity of nutritional advice may confuse patients, delay adoption of recommendations, and increase difficultly of implementation. Furthermore, the effectiveness of dietary therapy is unclear; some recommendations, such as the one for protein intake, are controversial. Furthermore, the guidelines are based on limited evidence, often rated as moderate or uncertain; this may play a role in clinicians' reluctance to give dietary guidance to patients with CKD.

The body of evidence supporting nutrition interventions in CKD is largely derived from observational epidemiologic cohort studies and a few clinical trials. The biggest gaps exist in relation to sodium, potassium, phosphorus, fats, and fiber, whereas there is some consistency about protein intake in those in later stages of CKD. Despite an evidence base that needs to be expanded to include more interventions, the observational epidemiologic evidence suggests it is prudent to address nutrition in CKD; there is evidence of some consistency across the various guidelines. Guiding principles of nutritional management include (1) assessment and monitoring of nutritional status throughout all stages of CKD; (2) creation of an individualized yet comprehensive nutrition plan that meets clinical guidelines and will have favorable effects on CKD and associated comorbidities; and (3) recommendation of meal plans that are feasible, sustainable, and suited for patients' food preferences and needs.

Given the high prevalence of CKD and the tremendous burden for patients, diet/nutrition is a modifiable factor that could help impact a major clinical and public health issue.

REFERENCES

1. National Kidney Foundation. K/DOQI clinical practice guidelines for nutrition in chronic renal failure. Am J Kidney Dis 2000;35(6 Suppl 2):S1–140.
2. National Kidney Foundation. K/DOQI clinical practice guidelines for chronic kidney disease: evaluation, classification and stratification. Am J Kidney Dis 2002; 39(2 Suppl 1):S1–266.
3. National Kidney Foundation. K/DOQI clinical practice guidelines on hypertension and antihypertensive agents in chronic kidney disease. Am J Kidney Dis 2004;43: S1–290.
4. Kidney Disease: Improving Global Outcomes (KDIGO) Anemia Work Group. KDIGO clinical practice guideline for anemia in chronic kidney disease. Kidney Int Suppl 2012;2:279–335.
5. Kidney Disease: Improving Global Outcomes (KDIGO) Blood Pressure Work Group. KDIGO clinical practice guideline for the management of blood pressure in chronic kidney disease. Kidney Int Suppl 2012;2:337–414.
6. Kidney Disease: Improving Global Outcomes (KDIGO) CKD-MBD Work Group. KDIGO clinical practice guideline for the diagnosis, evaluation, prevention, and treatment of chronic kidney disease – mineral and bone disorder (CKD-MBD). Kidney Int Suppl 2009;(113):S1–130.
7. Kidney Disease: Improving Global Outcomes (KDIGO) Lipid Work Group. KDIGO clinical practice guideline for lipid management in chronic kidney disease. Kidney Int Suppl 2013;3:259–305.
8. Appel LJ, Moore TJ, Obarzanek E, et al. A clinical trial of the effects of dietary patterns on blood pressure. DASH Collaborative Research Group. N Engl J Med 1997;336(16):1117–24.
9. Appel LJ, Sacks FM, Carey VJ, et al. Effects of protein, monounsaturated fat, and carbohydrate intake on blood pressure and serum lipids: results of the Omni-Heart randomized trial. JAMA 2005;294(19):2455–64.
10. Estruch R, Ros E, Salas-Salvado J, et al. Primary prevention of cardiovascular disease with a Mediterranean diet. N Engl J Med 2013;368:1279–90.
11. Parillo M, Riccardi G, Pacioni D, et al. Metabolic consequences of feeding a high-carbohydrate, high-fiber diet to diabetic patients with chronic kidney failure. Am J Clin Nutr 1988;48(2):255–9.
12. Rampton DS, Cohen SL, Crammond VD, et al. Treatment of chronic renal failure with dietary fiber. Clin Nephrol 1984;21(3):159–63.

13. Rivellese A, Parillo M, Giacco A, et al. A fiber-rich diet for the treatment of diabetic patients with chronic renal failure. Diabetes Care 1985;8(6):620–1.

14. Lau WL, Kalantar-Zadeh K, Vaziri ND. The gut as a source of inflammation in chronic kidney disease. Nephron 2015;130(2):92–8.

15. Klahr S, Levey AS, Beck GJ, et al. The effects of dietary protein restriction and blood pressure control on the progression of chronic renal disease. Modification of Diet in Renal Disease Study Group. N Engl J Med 1994;330(13):877–84.

16. Friedman AN. High protein diets: potential effects on the kidney in renal health and disease. Am J Kidney Dis 2004;44:950–62.

17. Negoianu D, Golfarb S. Just add water. J Am Soc Nephrol 2008;19(6):1041–3.

18. Hebert LA, Greene T, Levey A, et al. High urine volume and low urine osmolality are risk factors for faster progression of renal disease. Am J Kidney Dis 2003; 41(5):962–71.

19. Campbell KL, Johnson DW, Bauer JD, et al. A randomized trial of sodium-restriction on kidney function, fluid volume and adipokines in CKD patients. BMC Nephrol 2014;15(1):57.

20. Riphagen IJ, Gijsbers L, van Gastel MD, et al. Effects of potassium supplementation on markers of osmoregulation and volume regulation: results of a fully controlled dietary intervention study. J Hypertens 2016;34(2):215–20.

21. Sacks FM, Svetkey LP, Vollmer WM, et al. Effects on blood pressure of reduced dietary sodium and the Dietary Approaches to Stop Hypertension (DASH) diet. DASH-Sodium Collaborative Research Group. N Engl J Med 2001;344(1):3–10.

22. McMahon EJ, Bauer JD, Hawley CM, et al. A randomized trial of dietary sodium restriction in CKD. J Am Soc Nephrol 2013;24(12):2096–103.

23. Mattes RD, Donnelly D. Relative contributions of dietary sodium sources. J Am Coll Nutr 1991;10:383–93.

24. Anderson CA, Appel LJ, Okuda N, et al. Dietary sources of sodium in China, Japan, the United Kingdom, and the United States, women and men aged 40 to 59 years: the INTERMAP study. J Am Diet Assoc 2010;110:736–45.

25. Tikellis C, Pickering RJ, Tsorotes D, et al. Association of dietary sodium intake with atherogenesis in experimental diabetes and with cardiovascular disease in patients with type 1 diabetes. Clin Sci 2013;123:617–26.

26. Miller JA. Renal responses to sodium restriction in patients with early diabetes mellitus. J Am Soc Nephrol 1997;8:749–55.

27. Vallon V, Thomson SC. Renal function in diabetic disease models: the tubular system in the pathophysiology of the diabetic kidney. Annu Rev Physiol 2012;74: 351–75.

28. Cobb LK, Anderson CAM, Elliott P, et al. Methodological issues in cohort studies that relate sodium intake to cardiovascular disease outcomes. Circulation 2014; 129(10):1173–86.

29. Eddington H, Heofield R, Sinha S, et al. Serum phosphate and mortality in patients with chronic kidney disease. Clin J Am Soc Nephrol 2010;5:2251–7.

30. Moe SM, Zidehsarai MP, Chambers MA, et al. Vegetarian compared with meat dietary protein source and phosphorus homeostasis in chronic kidney disease. Clin J Am Soc Nephrol 2011;6(2):257–64.

31. Isakova T, Wahl P, Vargas GS, et al. Fibroblast growth factor 23 is elevated before parathyroid hormone and phosphate in chronic kidney disease. Kidney Int 2011; 79(12):1370–8.

32. Isakova T, Xie H, Yang W, et al. Fibroblast growth factor 23 and risks of mortality and end-stage renal disease in patients with chronic kidney disease. JAMA 2011; 305(23):2432–9.

33. Isakova T, Gutiérrez OM, Smith K, et al. Pilot study of dietary phosphorus restriction and phosphorus binders to target fibroblast growth factor 23 in patients with chronic kidney disease. Nephrol Dial Transplant 2011;26(2):584–91.
34. Isakova T, Barchi-Chung A, Enfield G, et al. Effects of dietary phosphate restriction and phosphate binders on FGF23 levels in CKD. Clin J Am Soc Nephrol 2013;8(6):1009–18.
35. Sigrist M, Tang M, Beaulieu M, et al. Responsiveness of FGF-23 and mineral metabolism to altered dietary phosphate intake in chronic kidney disease (CKD): results of a randomized trial. Nephrol Dial Transplant 2013;28(1):161–9.
36. Hill KM, Martin BR, Wastney ME, et al. Oral calcium carbonate affects calcium but not phosphorus balance in stage 3-4 chronic kidney disease. Kidney Int 2013; 83(5):959–66.
37. Di Iorio B, Di Micco L, Torraca S, et al. Acute effects of very-low-protein diet on FGF23 levels: a randomized study. Clin J Am Soc Nephrol 2012;7(4):581–7.
38. Saltissi D, Morgan C, Knight B, et al. Effect of lipid-lowering dietary recommendations on the nutritional intake and lipid profiles of chronic peritoneal dialysis and hemodialysis patients. Am J Kidney Dis 2001;37:1209–12.
39. Johnson DW, Atai E, Chan M, et al. KHA-CARI guideline: early chronic kidney disease: detection, prevention, and management. Nephrology 2013;18:340–50.
40. Eckel RH, Jakicic JM, Ard JD, et al. 2013 AHA/ACC guideline on lifestyle management to reduce cardiovascular risk: a report of the American College of Cardiology/American Heart Association Task Force on Practice Guidelines. J Am Coll Cardiol 2014;63:2960–84.
41. Proudfoot D, Shanahan CM. Molecular mechanisms mediating vascular calcification: Role of matrix Gla protein. Nephrology 2006;11:455–61.
42. Holden RM, Ross Morton A, Garland JS, et al. Vitamins K and D status in stages 3-5 chronic kidney disease. Clin J Am Soc Nephrol 2010;5:590–7.
43. Teng M, Wolf M, Lowrie E, et al. Survival of patients undergoing hemodialysis with paricalcitol or calcitriol therapy. N Engl J Med 2003;349:446–56.
44. Teng M, Wolf M, Ofsthun MN, et al. Activated injectable vitamin D and hemodialysis survival: a historical cohort study. J Am Soc Nephrol 2005;16:1115–25.
45. Block GA. Therapeutic interventions for chronic kidney disease- mineral and bone disorders: focus on mortality. Curr Opin Nephrol Hypertens 2011;20: 376–81.
46. Menon V, Kopple JD, Wang X, et al. Effect of a very low protein diet on outcomes: long term follow up of the Modification of Diet in Renal Disease (MDRD) Study. Am J Kidney Dis 2009;53(2):208–17.
47. US Renal Data System. USRDS 2004 annual data report. Bethesda (MD): National Institutes of Health; National Institute of Diabetes and Digestive and Kidney Diseases 2004.
48. Johansenn KL, Kutner NG, Young B, et al. Association of body size with health status in patients beginning dialysis. Am J Clin Nutr 2006;83:543–9.
49. Port F, Ashby V, Dhingra R, et al. Dialysis dose and body mass index are strongly associated with survival in hemodialysis patients. J Am Soc Nephrol 2002;13: 1061–6.
50. Kalantar-Zadeh K, Block G, Humphreys MH, et al. Reverse epidemiology of cardiovascular risk factors in maintenance dialysis patients. Kidney Int 2003;63: 793–808.
51. Saladhudeen AK. Obesity and survival on dialysis. Am J Kidney Dis 2003;41: 925–32.
52. Byers T. Body weight and mortality. N Engl J Med 1995;333:723–4.

53. Kalantar-Zadeh K, Abbot K, Salahudeen A, et al. Survival advantages of obesity in dialysis patients. Am J Clin Nutr 2005;81:543–5.

54. Romero-Corral A, Somers VK, Sierra-Johnson J, et al. Accuracy of body mass index in diagnosing obesity in the adult general population. Int J Obes 2008;32: 959–66.

55. Praga M, Hernandez E, Andres A, et al. Effects of body weight loss and catopril treatment on proteinuria associated with obesity. Nephron 1995;70:35–41.

56. Schneider R, Golzman B, Turkot S, et al. Effect of weight loss on blood pressure, arterial compliance, and insulin resistance in normotensive obese subjects. Am J Med Sci 2005;330:157–60.

57. Mokdad AH, Marks JS, Stroup DF, et al. Actual causes of death in the United States, 2000. J Am Med Assoc 2004;291:1238–45.

58. Violan MA, Pomes T, Maldonado S, et al. Exercise capacity in hemodialysis and renal transplant patients. Transplant Proc 2002;34:417–8.

59. Johansen KL, Chertow GM, da Silva M, et al. Determinants of physical performance in ambulatory patients on hemodialysis. Kidney Int 2001;60:1586–91.

60. Anderson JE, Stewart KJ, Hatchett L. Effect of exercise training on interdialytic ambulatory and treatment-related blood pressure in hemodialysis patients. Ren Fail 2004;26:539–44.

61. Painter P, Carlson L, Carey S, et al. Physical functioning and health- related quality-of-life changes with exercise training in hemodialysis patients. Am J Kidney Dis 2000;35:482–92.

62. Painter P, Carlson L, Carey S, et al. Low functioning hemodialysis patients improve with exercise training. Am J Kidney Dis 2000;36:600–8.

63. Goldberg AP, Geltman EM, Hagber JM, et al. Therapeutic benefits of exercise training for hemodialysis patients. Kidney Int 1983;24:S303–9.

64. Shalom R, Blumenthal JA, Williams RS, et al. Feasibility and benefits of exercise training in patients on maintenance dialysis. Kidney Int 1984;25:958–63.

65. Raynor DA, Phelan S, Hill JO, et al. Television viewing and long-term weight maintenance: results from the national weight control registry. Obesity (Silver Spring) 2006;14:1816–24.

66. Astrup A, Madsbad S, Breum L, et al. Effect of tesofensine on bodyweight loss, body composition, and quality of life in obese patients: a randomised, double-blind, placebo-controlled trial. Lancet 2008;372(9653):1906–13.

67. Bommer J, Locatelli F, Satayathum S, et al. Association of predialysis serum bicarbonate levels with risk of mortality and hospitalization in the Dialysis Outcomes and Practice Patterns Study (DOPPS). Am J Kidney Dis 2004;44:661–71.

68. Lowrie EG, Lew NL. Death risk in hemodialysis patients: the predictive value of commonly measured variables and an evaluation of death rate differences between facilities. Am J Kidney Dis 1990;15:458–82.

69. Wu DY, McAllister CJ, Kilpatrick RD, et al. Association between serum bicarbonate and death in hemodialysis patients: is it better to be acidotic or alkalotic? Clin J Am Soc Nephrol 2006;1:70–8.

70. Kovesdy CP, Anderson JE, Kalantar-Zadeh K. Association of serum bicarbonate levels with mortality in patients with non-dialysis-dependent CKD. Nephrol Dial Transplant 2009;24:1232–7.

71. Isakova T, Gutierrez OM, Chang Y, et al. Phosphorus binders and survival on hemodialysis. J Am Soc Nephrol 2009;20:388–96.

72. Ballmer PE, McNurlan MA, Hulter HN, et al. Chronic metabolic acidosis decreases albumin synthesis and induces negative nitrogen balance in humans. J Clin Invest 1995;95:39–40.

73. Lofberg E, Wenerman J, Anderstam B, et al. Correction of acidosis in dialysis patients increases branched chain and total essential amino acid levels in muscle. Clin Nephrol 1997;48:230–7.
74. Bailey JL, Wang X, England BK, et al. The acidosis of chronic renal failure activates muscle proteolysis in rats by augmenting transcription of genes encoding proteins of the ATP dependent ubiquitin-proteasome pathway. J Clin Invest 1996; 97:1447–53.
75. Graham KA, Reaich D, Channon SM, et al. Correction of acidosis in CAPD decreases whole body protein degradation. Kidney Int 1996;49:1396–400.
76. Graham KA, Reaich D, Channon SM, et al. Correction of acidosis in haemodialysis decreases whole body protein degradation. J Am Soc Nephrol 1997;8: 632–7.
77. Kooman JP, Deutz NE, Zijlmans P, et al. The influence of bicarbonate supplementation on plasma levels of branched-chain amino acids in haemodialysis patients with metabolic acidosis. Nephrol Dial Transplant 1997;12:2397–401.
78. Dou L, Brunet P, Dignat-George F, et al. Effect of uremia and haemodialysis on soluble L-selectin and leukocyte surface CD11b and L selectin. Am J Kidney Dis 1998;31:67–73.
79. de Bristo-Ashurst I, Varagunam M, Raftery MJ, et al. Bicarbonate supplementation slows progression of CKD and improves nutritional status. J Am Soc Nephrol 2009;20:2075–84.

Nutrition in Type 2 Diabetes and the Metabolic Syndrome

Michael A. Via, MD[a],*, Jeffrey I. Mechanick, MD[b]

KEYWORDS

- Insulin resistance • Type 2 diabetes prevention • Dietary patterns
- Mediterranean diet • New Nordic Diet

KEY POINTS

- For individuals at risk for type 2 diabetes mellitus (T2D) or the metabolic syndrome (MetS), adherence to an idealized dietary pattern can drastically alter the risk and course of these chronic conditions.
- Target levels of carbohydrate intake should approximate 30% of consumed calories.
- Healthy food choices should include copious fruits, vegetables, and nuts while minimizing foods with high glycemic indices, especially processed foods.

INTRODUCTION

Insulin resistance manifesting as T2D, the MetS, polycystic ovary syndrome, or hypertriglyceridemia, is a major public health problem. Approximately 10% of the United States population is diagnosed with T2D, and the prevalence of MetS is approximately 22% to 30%, depending on the defining criteria used.[1] Modern lifestyles have long been suspected as the major influence of this trend, with the implication that modification of daily routines can prevent or substantially alter the course of these conditions. Prior to the therapeutic use of insulin, lifestyle intervention was the only effective option for the treatment of insulin resistance syndromes. Resistance to insulin is present for years prior to the development of T2D and drives the multiple components of MetS, including increased abdominal girth (waist circumference >102 cm in men and >88 cm in women), hypertension (systolic blood pressure >130 mm Hg and diastolic blood pressure >85 mm Hg), elevated circulating triglycerides (>150 mg/dL), reduced circulating high-density lipoprotein (HDL) levels (<40 mg/dL in men and <50 mg/dL in

[a] Division of Endocrinology and Metabolism, Mount Sinai Beth Israel Medical Center, Icahn School of Medicine at Mount Sinai, 317 East 17th Street, 8th Floor, New York, NY 10003, USA; [b] Metabolic Support, Division of Endocrinology, Diabetes and Bone Disease, Icahn School of Medicine at Mount Sinai, 1192 Park Ave, New York, NY 10128, USA
* Corresponding author.
E-mail address: mvia@chpnet.org

Med Clin N Am 100 (2016) 1285–1302
http://dx.doi.org/10.1016/j.mcna.2016.06.009
0025-7125/16/$ – see front matter © 2016 Elsevier Inc. All rights reserved.
medical.theclinics.com

women), and elevations in serum glucose concentrations (fasting serum glucose >100 mg/dL). Individuals with at least 3 of these 5 components are considered to have MetS, although more precise definitions exist from multiple professional medical organizations (**Table 1**). Current views emphasize MetS as a progressive condition of interrelated pathophysiology, where the aggregate risk is greater than the sum of each individual risk factor.[2]

Several large clinical trials demonstrate the effectiveness of lifestyle modification for the treatment and prevention of T2D and MetS. Despite the wide array of medication classes presently available, lifestyle modification focused on dietary change and enhanced physical activity remains a cornerstone of disease management in T2D, MetS, and other insulin resistance syndromes.

Individuals develop insulin resistance over prolonged periods of time, secondary to alterations in multiple metabolic and energy regulatory pathways. This culminates in hyperglycemia and other metabolic abnormalities, such as hypertriglyceridemia, hypertension, and obesity as well as the emergence of MetS or T2D. Dietary strategies should minimize the pathophysiologic effects of insulin resistance (**Table 2**).

Obesity is the most significant factor contributing to insulin resistance and T2D, and, subsequently, weight loss through dietary caloric restriction has been shown to be the most important treatment in patients with T2D who are overweight or obese. Because obesity is addressed in another article in this issue, this article focuses specifically on other dietary constituents that are related to insulin resistance and T2D.

Altered energy homeostasis in insulin resistance

- Inappropriate glucagon-mediated hepatic glucose release
- Reduced release and activity of glucagon-like peptide-1 (GLP-1)
- Pancreatic β-cell dysfunction via degeneration or transformation to inactive cells
- Delayed and less efficient insulin release
- Inefficient protein synthesis resulting from generalized endoplasmic reticulum stress
- Low-grade systemic inflammation
- Reduced clearance of advanced glycosylated end-products

DIETARY COMPONENTS AFFECTING TYPE 2 DIABETES MELLITUS: CARBOHYDRATES

Carbohydrates, in the form of starch, glycogen, or other polysaccharides, as well as simple sugars (monosaccharides and disaccharides) comprise approximately 40%

Table 1
Definitions of the metabolic syndrome

Organization	Definition of the Metabolic Syndrome
World Health Organization and the European Group for the Study of Insulin Resistance	Insulin resistance and any 2 of the other criteria
National Cholesterol Education Program/ American Heart Association/National Heart, Lung, and Blood Institute	Any 3 of 5 criteria
American Association of Clinical Endocrinologists	Insulin resistance and any of the other criteria
International Diabetes Foundation	Increased waist circumference and any of the other 4 criteria

Criteria: (1) increased abdominal girth; (2) hypertension; (3) elevated triglycerides; (4) low HDL; and (5) elevated blood glucose levels.

Table 2
Summary of clinical evidence

Trial	Study Design	N	Results
Reiser et al,[14] 1979	Crossover	19	Increased fructose intake induces worsened insulin resistance.
Ludwig et al,[21] 1999	Crossover	12	High glycemic index foods account for 53% of postprandial glycemic variance.
ORIGIN[26]	Randomized controlled trial	12,536	No observable effect of 1000 mg daily n-3 PUFA supplementation on glucose homeostasis.
Tanaka et al,[27] 2013	Cohort	978	Increased fruit intake is associated with reduced risk of diabetic retinopathy.
Ganesan et al,[18] 2012	Cohort	1272	Increased fiber intake is associated with reduced risk of diabetic rentinopathy.
DPP[31]	Randomized controlled trial	1079	Intensive lifestyle intervention was superior than metformin in the prevention of T2D.
Look AHEAD[32–35]	Randomized controlled trial	5145	Intensive lifestyle intervention had no observable effect on cardiovascular outcomes in T2D but reduced incidence of retinopathy and nephropathy, improved erectile function, and improved quality of life.
DIRECT[38]	Randomized controlled trial	322	The Mediterranean diet reduced incidence of T2D and improved insulin resistance more effectively than a low-fat diet in subjects with obesity.
PREDIMED[23,40]	Randomized controlled trial	7447	Subjects assigned to the Mediterranean diet had a 30% reduction in cardiovascular events and a 30% reduction in incidence of T2D compared with a low-fat diet.
CASCADE[42]	Randomized controlled trial	224	In addition to the Mediterranean diet, red wine consumption reduced fasting glucose and insulin levels in T2D.
Fritzen et al,[45] 2015	Randomized controlled trial	64	Subjects on the NND had reduced fasting glucose, reduced triglycerides, and greater weight loss than controls.

to 50% of the calories of most diets. Polysaccharides are hydrolyzed within the gastrointestinal tract to glucose monosaccharides for absorption. Most other absorbed dietary monosaccharides are converted to glucose for systemic use.

With few exceptions, circulating glucose is used as the main cellular energy source for generation of adenosine triphosphate. Blood glucose concentration is maintained through multiple regulatory processes with enough versatility to handle large glucose boluses after meals of high carbohydrate content as well as during regular periods of fasting, usually at night. The pathophysiologic mechanisms of T2D, and to a lesser extent those of MetS, disrupt this glycemic regulatory process. At early stages of T2D, postprandial serum glucose concentrations are most affected. As T2D progresses, both fasting and postprandial serum glucose levels become dysregulated. In individuals with T2D, diets with carbohydrate content that is reduced to 30% of total calories and relative increases in protein and fat content demonstrate improved glycemic control and positive nitrogen balance.[3]

Fructose

As a monosaccharide isomer of glucose, fructose is metabolized through many of the same pathways as glucose metabolism with several important caveats.[4,5] Fructose metabolism is not governed by a hormonal control pathway. Moreover, dietary fructose does not induce insulin secretion and nearly all consumed fructose is taken up by hepatocytes. Intracellularly, fructose enters the glycolysis metabolic pathway downstream from the major control and rate-limiting step, leading to dysregulated energy metabolism and fatty acid production.[6]

Detrimental mechanistic effects of fructose
- Does not induce insulin release or affect circulating levels of other energy regulating hormzones
- Nearly complete hepatic uptake of ingested fructose
- Enters cellular metabolism downstream of a key regulatory point
- Stimulates and de novo lipogenesis
- Promotes epigenetic changes that favor abdominal adipocyte growth
- Induces mitochondrial oxidative stress in skeletal myocytes, leading to apotosis

These molecular mechanisms should be considered in conjunction with the availability of fructose in consumed foods.[7] Prior to the industrial production of sugars, dietary sources of fructose included fruits, which generally have a low content of fructose; honey, which is only minimally consumed in agrarian societies; and agave-derived syrups that, historically, were never widely consumed. The high content of fructose as a component of industrially produced sugars, such as sucrose and high-fructose corn syrup, makes this inefficiently metabolized monosaccharide easily obtainable.

Multiple longitudinal and cross-sectional studies demonstrate a strong association between high fructose intake and the development of T2D, MetS, polycystic ovary syndrome, obesity, vascular disease, and hepatosteatosis, among other metabolic conditions.[8–11] Several controlled trials corroborate these findings by comparing the high intake of sucrose, a common source of dietary fructose, with isocaloric diets containing only starch and glucose as carbohydrates. In these trials, subjects given sucrose demonstrated worsened insulin resistance, reduced glucose tolerance, and increased circulating triglyceride levels.[12–14]

In cases of T2D, fructose can be considered a double-edged sword: on the one hand, dietary fructose does not stress the impaired insulin-glucose regulation after immediate consumption. Dietary supplements marketed for use in patients with diabetes that do not meet their nutritional needs take advantage of this property of fructose. Many diabetes-specific supplements add significant amounts of fructose to supply calories in the form of carbohydrates. Over the immediate term, supplemental fructose does not raise serum glucose levels. High-quality prospective studies of these products have not been conducted. Long-term consumption of fructose in high amounts is associated with worsening insulin resistance and T2D.[15] Fructose intake is also associated with the development of common diabetes-associated complications.[16] Dietary fructose should be kept at a minimum in T2D and MetS, which may be achieved by elimination of processed foods and sugar-containing beverages as well as reduction in dessert intake. The World Health Organization recommends that sugar intake, including fructose, be kept at less than 5% of total calorie consumption.[17] Diabetes-specific supplements should be reserved only for patients at high nutritional risk, such as in cases of impaired gastrointestinal function, cancer cachexia, or dementia-associated weight loss.

Fiber

Another class of carbohydrate, dietary fiber, includes polysaccharides and modified polysaccharides that are not easily digested in the stomach or intestine. These substances, produced by plants and fungi, provide structure to intestinal chyme and stool, slow gastric emptying, and delay the absorption of dietary carbohydrates, leading to improved serum glucose concentrations in individuals with diabetes.[18]

Dietary fiber may also serve as an energy source for yeasts and bacteria that reside in the colon that produce short-chain fatty acids (SCFAs) through fiber metabolism. A portion of these SCFAs enters systemic circulation and may contribute 5% to 10% of total calorie intake.

Interactions between the colon microflora and the host have been recognized as influencing systemic metabolism through effects on the inflammatory state and insulin resistance within the host individual.[19] A high intake of dietary fiber promotes a eumetabolic state of colon microflora that can improve glucose metabolism in individuals with T2D and other insulin resistance syndromes.[19]

Physiology of dietary fiber
- Provides bulk and form to stool
- Slows gastric emptying
- Serves as a fuel source of intestinal microbiota
- SCFAs produced from dietary fiber induce release of GLP-1 and reduce hepatic fat accumulation in animal studies.[20]
- Inhibits α-glucosidase, slowing dietary starch and disaccharide hydrolysis
- Impairs absorption of dietary cholesterol

Glycemic Index and Load

The rapidity and extent to which dietary carbohydrates enter circulation in the form of glucose is described as the glycemic index, which is given as the total area delineated by the change in blood glucose concentration over time after food consumption. Foods with a high glycemic index often contain high amounts of monosaccharides or easily digestible polysaccharides and are low in dietary fiber. In T2D, consumption of high glycemic index foods can lead to profound and rapid increases in blood glucose concentrations, worsening the disease state.[21]

Foods are often consumed, however, as part of a meal, mixed with multiple other food items. Mixing can affect the glycemic index of specific foods, commonly dampening and prolonging the degree of glycemic excursion in large mixed meals. In this manner of real-world food consumption, the glycemic load, or simply the total amount of digestible carbohydrates consumed, is the more important factor contributing to postprandial glycemic excursions.

Accordingly, patients with T2D should completely avoid or at least minimize high glycemic index foods and minimize intake of foods that deliver high glycemic loads.

DIETARY FAT

For decades, a low-fat diet has been the standard dietary advice, despite only modest reductions in cardiovascular risk in observational trials. Much of the early scrutiny of dietary fat stems from the association of saturated fatty acid intake with increased low-density lipoprotein (LDL) concentration and atherosclerotic disease. In recent years, this low-fat paradigm has been transformed as metabolic benefits of dietary monounsaturated fatty acids (MUFAs) and polyunsaturated fatty acids (PUFAs) became recognized. Multiple studies demonstrate reduction in LDL cholesterol and improvement in insulin sensitivity in individuals who consume diets high in MUFA and PUFA compared with diets with high saturated fatty acid content.[22] Dietary patterns with significantly higher fat content than traditional low-fat diets, including the Mediterranean diet among others, demonstrate greater improvements in markers of insulin resistance.[23]

Additionally, the use of trans-fats that were typically substituted for saturated fats in processed foods and margarine conveys an even greater cardiometabolic risk than intake of saturated fat. The modern paradigm for fat consumption includes dietary patterns rich in MUFAs and PUFAs that can benefit individuals with T2D and MetS.

Supplementation with n-3 Fatty Acids

As either an alternative to dietary change or an adjunct to a healthy lifestyle, n-3 fatty acids in the form of fish oil capsules are among the commonly consumed dietary supplements. Important drivers of this trend include purported health benefits of n-3 PUFAs and a very low n-3 PUFA content of the typical Western diet. Almost nonexistent regulatory rules, however, coupled with prolonged periods in transit, warehouse storage, and time on the shelf allow many of the fish oil supplements to contain less than 50% of their purported n-3 PUFA content.[24] To overcome this, an individual must consume 6000 mg to 9000 mg of fish oil just to intake 1000 mg of n-3 PUFAs.

Pharmaceutical n-3 PUFAs are available that are more concentrated, more stringently regulated, and deliver a greater amount of PUFAs.[25] These compounds significantly reduce circulating triglyceride levels, which are commonly elevated in T2D and MetS.

As for affecting insulin resistance, simple supplementation with n-3 fatty acids yields disappointing results. In the largest trial to date, 12,536 subjects with T2D, impaired fasting glucose, or impaired glucose tolerance were randomized to receive 1000 mg of n-3 fatty acids, containing mostly docosahexaenoic acid and eicosapentaenoic acid, or olive oil as placebo.[26] After 6 years of follow-up, no differences were noted in fasting glucose, glycosylated hemoglobin A_{1C} (HbA$_{1C}$), blood pressure, cardiovascular events, or death. The only significant difference found was a 14.5-mg/dL reduction in triglyceride levels in the group receiving n-3 fatty acids.

These results suggest that supplementation with n-3 PUFAs is insufficient to alter the course of T2D and MetS. Based on available data, n-3 supplementation should be reserved for the treatment of hypertriglyceridemia. In contrast to supplementation, the modification of an individual dietary pattern to regularly include foods high in n-3 PUFAs is beneficial in T2D and MetS.

DIETARY INTERVENTIONS

Several observational trials have been conducted that show benefits of specific nutritional interventions in T2D. A cohort of 978 Japanese subjects with diabetes assessed by dietary questionnaires showed that high fruit intake was associated with a 52% reduction in incidence of diabetic retinopathy over 8 years of follow-up, despite no change in glycemic control.[27] Another cohort study of 1272 individuals with diabetes living in Sankara Nethralaya, India, demonstrated high dietary fiber consumption is associated with reductions in the incidence of diabetic retinopathy and microalbuminuria.[18] An analysis of the Nurses' Health Study also demonstrates reduced risk of microalbuminuria in association with high fruit, vegetable, nuts, and lean meat intake and increased risk of microalbuminuria in subjects with greater Western diet scores.[28]

Although limited by their observational nature, these studies suggest potential for dietary interventions to affect multiple aspects of T2D.

Although the debate of the optimal diet continues, individual recommendations must consider food preferences, food availability, cultural aspects, and socioeconomic factors in addition to physiologic response.[29] In a landmark trial targeting weight loss in individuals who were overweight or had obesity randomized to 1 of 4 different diets, the specific diet assignment had minimal effect; rather, how closely one adhered to any of the diets was associated with successful weight loss.[30] The impact lifestyle has on the course of insulin resistance depends on individual adherence.

A dietary approach that stresses long-term adherence to lifestyle adjustment should significantly reduce the risk or impact of T2D. The pivotal Diabetes Prevention Program (DPP) provides a basis for intensive dietary and exercise interventions for the prevention of T2D.[31] In this trial, individuals at risk for T2D with impaired fasting glucose or with impaired glucose tolerance were randomized to 1 of 3 groups: those receiving minimal information regarding healthy lifestyle as the control group; those with an intense lifestyle intervention that included frequent contact, monitoring, and feedback by lifestyle coaches and nutritionists, monthly meetings with a dietitian, and 30 minutes of moderately intense cardiovascular exercise for 5 days per week; or those with a prescription for daily metformin. Among the 3 groups that completed 4 years of follow-up, the intensive lifestyle group had a 58% reduction in incidence of T2D compared with the control group and a 31% reduction in incidence of T2D compared with the metformin group. The superior effect of lifestyle intervention to pharmacologic therapy in the DPP highlights the beneficial impact that nutritional approaches have in states of insulin resistance.

More recently, the Look AHEAD (Action for Health in Diabetes) study group published findings from a large trial that investigated an intensive lifestyle intervention used for subjects with excess weight and T2D.[32] In this randomized trial, an intensive protocol similar to that used in the DPP was compared with standard care. During 6 years of follow-up, the intensive lifestyle group had an average of 5-kg weight reduction, improved physical fitness, and a slight but significant improvement in glycemic control. No differences were observed, however, between study groups in the primary trial endpoint of cardiovascular events and death at 11 years.[32] It may be that longer follow-up is required to demonstrate cardiovascular differences in individuals with T2D.

This somewhat disappointing result of the Look AHEAD trial should be contrasted with significant reductions in other complications of T2D. For example, in male subjects with erectile dysfunction at the start of the trial, scores of erectile function improved at 1 year after intensive lifestyle intervention, although no change was noted in men of the control group.[33] Symptoms of depression and quality-of-life scores improved in the intensive group throughout the trial.[34] The incidence of renal dysfunction was reduced by approximately 30% in the intensive group over 10 years of follow-up, providing evidence of reduced microvascular complications.[35] Additionally, the intervention group had an 11% lower rate of hospitalization and was prescribed 6% less medications than the control group.[36] These clinical improvements should be considered as hard endpoints among individuals within the intensive lifestyle group, and they add support to the concept that purposeful interventions in nutrition and physical activity modify the course of T2D.

Lifestyle interventions of the diabetes prevention program and Look-AHEAD
- Frequent contact with lifestyle coaches/nutritionist
- Low-fat, calorie-restricted diet

- Food diary and food reference guide with calorie information
- Measurement of food with cups for portion control
- Regular exercise of moderate intensity

DIETARY PATTERNS

For individuals with T2D, dietary considerations should minimize carbohydrate load, especially fructose; contain high amounts of fiber; and contain a favorable fat content, antioxidants, and vitamins. Most importantly, diet should be palatable for long-term adherence. Dietary patterns consistent with these general principles are briefly described.

The Mediterranean Diet

The Mediterranean diet has long been recognized to promote overall health and improve markers of metabolism.[37] Approximately 30% to 40% of calories are carbohydrate based, and 35% to 40% calories in the form of fats and oils. In a randomized trial in which overweight subjects were given prepared meals daily, those on the Mediterranean diet had the greatest weight loss over the planned 2 years of follow-up compared with a low-fat diet and a very-low-carbohydrate diet.[38] This difference was sustained over a 4-year extension among those who chose to remain in the study.[39] The Mediterranean diet group also had reductions in LDL cholesterol and triglycerides and induced the greatest reduction in fasting glucose and fasting insulin among the subset of subjects with diabetes who were included in the trial.

Components of the Mediterranean diet
- Fruits, 3 to 4 servings per day
- Vegetables, 3 to 4 servings per day
- Poultry
- Fish, 2 to 3 servings per week
- Whole grains
- Olive oil for consumption and food preparation
- Nuts, 5 to 7 nuts per day
- Cheese
- Wine, 1 to 2 glasses per day

To date, the Mediterranean diet is the only diet shown to reduce cardiovascular events and mortality among individuals who are overweight. A large randomized trial that used a low-fat diet as comparison demonstrated an approximate 30% reduction in cardiovascular events and cardiovascular mortality over 6 years.[40] A post hoc analysis of subjects with diabetes who were included in this trial demonstrates an approximate 40% reduction in new-onset retinopathy.[41] Another analysis of the subjects without T2D at baseline showed a 30% reduction in the incidence of T2D in the Mediterranean diet group.[23]

Wine serves as a source of dietary polyphenols, with a 7-fold higher polyphenol content in red wine compared with white wine. A 2-year randomized trial in which 224 subjects with T2D who already were following the Mediterranean diet were provided either 150 mL of red wine, white wine, or water daily and asked to abstain from other alcohol was recently published.[42] Both groups given wine showed reduction in fasting insulin, although only the white wine group had an average reduction in fasting plasma glucose by 18 mg/dL. HDL levels increased by an average of 2 mg/dL in the red wine group. These results are consistent with many other small trials that show improved levels of cholesterol, reduced markers of inflammation, and reduced insulin resistance with moderate consumption of alcohol, mainly wine.[43] Although still controversial, wine is an important component of the Mediterranean diet. These results support moderate wine consumption as beneficial to individuals with diabetes.

The New Nordic Diet

Although the concept for the New Nordic Diet (NND) was developed based on local Scandinavian cuisine, many of the components are similar to the Mediterranean diet, which include intake of copious fruits, vegetables, whole grains, and fish.[44]

Content of the New Nordic Diet
- Organic foods
- Fruits, especially berries
- Vegetables – cabbage, root vegetables, legumes
- Fresh herbs
- Wild mushrooms
- Nuts
- Fish
- Seaweed
- Meats

Currently, there are no large published studies of the NND conducted specifically in subjects with diabetes; however, a recent trial shows promise for treatment of T2D and MetS.[45] This study was performed in Denmark and randomly assigned individuals with obesity to the NND or a typical Danish diet – similar to the Western diet. At 6 months of follow-up, the NND group lost 6 kg compared with a 2-kg weight loss in the control group. Average fasting insulin levels declined by 3 µU/L, fasting glucose decreased by 5 mg/dL, and triglycerides decreased by 18 mg/dL in study subjects assigned to the NND. These improvements in markers of insulin resistance support recommendation of the NND lifestyle intervention in T2D and MetS.

The Ornish Diet

The central principle of the Ornish diet (OD) is a significant reduction or elimination of ingested animal fat and products derived from animal fat. As a result, the OD necessarily includes increased carbohydrates in the form of whole grains. This diet demonstrates significant improvement in circulating LDL levels and is beneficial in the treatment and prevention of atherosclerotic disease.[46]

Ornish diet components
- Fruits
- Vegetables
- Whole grains
- Reduced fish
- Minimal meats

Ornish diet calorie content
15% Daily calories from fat
10% Daily calories from protein
75% Daily calories from complex carbohydrates

The effects of the OD on insulin resistance has not been well characterized. One uncontrolled cohort study included subjects at high risk for cardiovascular disease who were directed to follow the OD as a lifestyle intervention.[47] The subset of subjects with diabetes within the study showed a reduction in average fasting glucose of 16 mg/dL and a 0.4% reduction in HbA_{1C} levels after 3 months of follow-up. Although promising, longer-term follow-up is needed. Although the tradeoff of reduced animal products for increased whole grains seems beneficial in atherosclerotic disease, the increased carbohydrate load of the OD may make this dietary pattern less effective than the Mediterranean diet or NND.[48]

MICRONUTRIENTS

Dietary substances required in small portions daily are classified as micronutrients, which include electrolytes, vitamins, trace elements, and plant alkaloid compounds. The unique chemical and electrical properties of micronutrients drive many of the biochemical processes required for life. Micronutrients that are essential in metabolic pathways affected by T2D, such as glucose metabolism, free radical scavenging, and clearance of advanced glycosylated end products (AGEs), and may have an exaggerated role in individuals with this condition. Still, many of the trials examining the effects of micronutrient supplementation show only minimal benefit.

POTENTIALLY BENEFICIAL MICRONUTRIENTS IN INSULIN RESISTANCE

Chromium (as chromium picolinate 500–1000 μg/d)
- Amplifies insulin signaling
- Induces weight loss and lowers serum glucose levels in some studies

Selenium (approximately 200 μg/d)
- Use in selenoproteins/redox reactions
- Reduces production of AGEs
- May improve insulin resistance

Vitamin D (2000–5000 U/d – targeting normal circulating levels)
- Pancreatic β-cell activity
- Reduces insulin resistance in animal trials
- Minimal effect in T2D and MetS, may be most effective as preventive measure

Chromium

The trace metal chromium is required for intracellular amplification of insulin signaling as a component of the oligopeptide chromodulin. In states of severe chromium deficiency, refractory insulin resistance develops that resolves with chromium supplementation.[49] The Western diet can lead to relative deficiencies of chromium, especially in individuals with obesity. Additionally, chromium wasting has been observed in individuals with T2D due to insulin resistance, which directly affects cellular uptake of chromium.[50]

Several randomized controlled trials in subjects with T2D show a minor benefit on glycemic control and weight loss with chromium supplementation.[51–53] In 1 study, subjects given 600 μg of chromium picolinate daily for 4 months demonstrated significant average reductions of fasting glucose of 17 mg/dL, postprandial glucose of 25 mg/dL, and HbA_{1C} of 0.9% from a baseline of 8.5% compared with placebo.[53] Several other studies, however, fail to demonstrate benefit of chromium supplementation.[52] These mixed clinical results and only minor improvement in insulin resistance suggest that chromium supplementation should not be generally recommended.

Selenium

Selenium is an essential trace element that is incorporated in selenoproteins, including glutathione peroxidase and thyroid peroxidase, that catalyze biochemical redox reactions, often resulting in antioxidant production. Dietary sources of selenium include nuts, meat, eggs, and cereals. As with many micronutrients, individuals with obesity commonly have reduced selenium stores.[54]

In 1 randomized controlled study, subjects with obesity supplemented with 200 µg selenium daily resulted in a 10% reduction in fasting insulin levels.[54] In another study, subjects with gestational diabetes randomized to receive selenium supplementation demonstrated average reductions in fasting plasma glucose by 10 mg/dL and fasting plasma insulin by 1.98 µIU/mL.[55] These few small studies are suggestive that supplementation with selenium, or possibly increasing dietary selenium consumption, has potential to improve glycemic control and insulin resistance in T2D.

Vitamin D

The physiologic role of vitamin D and the multiple purported benefits of vitamin D supplementation remain controversial.[56] High rates of vitamin D insufficiency and deficiency are observed in individuals with T2D and MetS. Within pancreatic β-cells, the presence of vitamin D receptors and 1α-hydroxylase activity, the enzyme responsible for vitamin D activation, suggests a role for vitamin D in glucose homeostasis.[57] 1α-Hydroxylase activity has also been observed in rat adipocytes, again suggesting a role in energy metabolism.[58]

Several randomized studies of vitamin D supplementation at daily doses of 3300 IU to 7000 IU fail to demonstrate weight loss in subjects with obesity.[59–61] Animal models of T2D, however, that are vitamin D deficient show improved β-cell insulin secretion with vitamin D supplementation.[62] Several human trials in subjects who are vitamin D deficient and with impaired glucose tolerance show reduction in insulin resistance with vitamin D supplementation.[63] Most trials of vitamin D supplementation in subjects with diabetes show either no change or very modest improvements in insulin resistance.[64] One trial of vitamin D supplementation in subjects with MetS also demonstrated no improvement in insulin resistance.[65] By these results, vitamin D supplementation seems to have only have a minimal effect on glucose homeostasis and should at best be considered as an adjunct to other therapies.

PLANT POLYPHENOLS

The role of dietary plant polyphenols in health and disease is a subject of controversy. More than 18,000 organic polyphenol compounds have been identified in plant products that are regularly consumed. These substances exhibit diverse biochemical properties, some of which may be beneficial in T2D.

The high polyphenol content of the Mediterranean diet has been hypothesized to impart many of its health benefits.[41] Similarly, high polyphenol content of fruits has been offered as the molecular explanation for reduced diabetic retinopathy associated with high fruit consumption.[27] A review of data from the National Health and Nutrition Examination Survey from 2003 to 2006 demonstrates high dietary polyphenol content associated with improved glycemic control and reduced prevalence of diabetic retinopathy among individuals with T2D.[66] An analysis of the Nurses' Health Study demonstrates that low polyphenol intake, measured by urinary isoflavone levels, is associated with increased risk of T2D.[67]

Cell culture, animal model, and epidemiologic studies hint at the antidiabetic effects of several polyphenol compounds. Further study may identify other individual polyphenols that exhibit specific effects in the prevention and treatment of T2D. It is more likely, however, that through combined mechanisms, the effects of naturally occurring polyphenols are advantageous for the treatment of T2D and MetS. Dietary patterns with high fruit and vegetable content, including the Mediterranean diet and the NND, are rich in polyphenol compounds and may be among the best options in T2D and MetS.

Resveratrol

Resveratrol is a component of grapes, grapeseed oil, and red wine. Multiple studies demonstrate administration of resveratrol improves insulin resistance in animal models of T2D, mainly through activation of sirtuin-1 and adenosine monophosphate–activated kinase activity as well as through reduction in systemic inflammation.[68] Several brief human trials demonstrate improved insulin resistance and a slight reduction in HbA$_{1C}$ levels in subjects with T2D after 4 to 12 weeks of resveratrol supplementation.[69,70] A similar cohort trial demonstrated reduced insulin resistance after 3 months of supplementation in subjects with MetS.[71] Supplemental doses of resveratrol ranged from 5 mg to 500 mg twice daily in the human trials compared with an approximate 5 mg to 20 mg daily intake in a typical Mediterranean diet, depending mainly on the type and source of red wine consumed.[72]

Other short trials in subjects with diabetes fail to show an effect of resveratrol on insulin resistance.[73,74] Still, the compelling evidence from animal studies and the few human trials continue to foster interest in the potential role of resveratrol for T2D and MetS.

Quercetin

The phytonutrient, quercetin, is abundant in onions, fennel, cilantro, capers, and dill, among other richly flavored plants. Supplementation has been shown to reduce fasting glucose levels in streptozotocin treated mice, potentially through inhibition intestinal α-glucosidase.[75,76]

Epigallocatechin Gallate

Epigallocatechin gallate (EGCG) is a flavonoid compound found in grapes, tea, and legumes. In studies of cultured pancreatic β-cells, EGCG improves insulin secretion and mitochondrial activity.[77] In db/db mice, ECGC improves glucose tolerance.[78]

Bilberry Extract

The bilberry extract is rich in anthocyanins, a subclass of flavonoid compounds. In mouse models of T2D, administration of bilberry extract reduced fasting glucose and HbA$_{1C}$ levels.[79]

Naringin and Hesperidin

The naringin and hesperidin flavonoids are bitter-tasting and highly concentrated in citrus fruits, and both have been shown to resolve hyperglycemia in streptozotocin-induced diabetes models and in db/db mice.[80,81]

ENDOCRINE DISRUPTORS

A subset of chemicals that exist in the environment, either naturally or as manufactured industrial compounds, have properties that allow interruption of normal hormone signaling. These endocrine disruptors (EDs) can act as hormones, block hormone activity, or affect the synthesis or catabolism of hormones, with potential to greatly affect the host. Several EDs have been identified that influence metabolism and insulin resistance (**Table 3**).[82–85] These include insecticides, plasticizers, preservatives, and artificial sweeteners, among other compounds. Consumption of artificial sweeteners, with

Table 3 Selected classes of endocrine disruptors that alter energy metabolism		
Compound	**Source**	**Metabolic Effect**
Organotins	Wood preservatives	Adipocyte growth, associated with obesity
Phthalates	Plastics, vinyl, cosmetics	Visceral fat accumulation, associated with obesity, inhibition of PPARα, and PPARγ
DDT, methoxychlor	Pesticides	Associated with obesity
Polybrominated diphenyl esters	Flame retardants	Associated with obesity, impaired lipid metabolism
Saccharine, aspartame	Artificial sweeteners	Induce insulin resistance via altered gut microbiota, possibly activate nutrient sensing receptors eliciting inappropriate insulin release

Abbreviations: DDT, dichlorodiphenyltrichloroethane; PPAR, peroxisome proliferator-activated receptor.

the exception of *Stevia rebaudiana* extracts, promotes insulin resistance though modification of the gastrointestinal microflora.[85]

Both the continuous introduction of novel industrial chemicals and the difficulty in proper study provide formidable obstacles to the complete understanding of the pathophysiologic effects and range of EDs.

RECOMMENDATIONS

Lifestyle has a strong influence on the development and outcome of T2D and MetS. The goal of nutritional intervention should include dietary modifications that promote improved glycemic control and reduce diabetic complications. The most important consideration should be a lifestyle and dietary pattern that a patient chooses to follow over the long term. Common threads among successful diets in T2D include high vegetable and fruit intake, higher protein, and healthy fat intake, along with the avoidance of high carbohydrate loads, high glycemic index foods, and processed foods. These general rules should lead to reduction in the consumption of fructose and saturated fat. Although there is likely to be no single, optimal dietary pattern, the Mediterranean diet and the NND serve as model examples for the successful treatment and prevention of T2D and the MetS.

The addition of micronutrient supplements can be considered but remain controversial and should only be taken as part of a more comprehensive approach to T2D. Avoidance of ED compounds, such as by thoroughly washing foods during preparations or by minimizing use of plastic food containers, may benefit T2D, although strong evidence for this recommendation is not currently available. Similarly, avoidance of artificial sweeteners may also be beneficial, although further study is necessary.

Along with physical activity, dietary modification as part of an intensive lifestyle should be recommended universally to patients with T2D.

Summary of nutritional recommendations
- Follow a healthful dietary pattern, such as the Mediterranean diet or NND
- Maintain lower carbohydrate intake, approximately 30% to 40% of calories
- Consume copious fruits, vegetables, and nuts
- Avoid/minimize high glycemic index foods, such as sugar-containing beverages, desserts, and easily digestible starches, such as white bread and crackers

- Minimize fructose intake by avoiding processed foods
- Take care to minimize ED exposure – wash foods, wash hands, and use organic foods, fertilizers, and cleaning products wherever possible

REFERENCES

1. Miller JM, Kaylor MB, Johannsson M, et al. Prevalence of metabolic syndrome and individual criterion in US adolescents: 2001-2010 National Health and Nutrition Examination Survey. Metab Syndr Relat Disord 2014;12:527–32.
2. Sperling LS, Mechanick JI, Neeland IJ, et al. The cardiometabolic health alliance: working toward a new care model for the metabolic syndrome. J Am Coll Cardiol 2015;66:1050–67.
3. Nuttall FQ, Gannon MC. Effect of a LoBAG30 diet on protein metabolism in men with type 2 diabetes. A Randomized Controlled Trial. Nutr Metab (Lond) 2012;9: 43.
4. Stanhope KL, Schwarz JM, Keim NL, et al. Consuming fructose-sweetened, not glucose-sweetened, beverages increases visceral adiposity and lipids and decreases insulin sensitivity in overweight/obese humans. J Clin Invest 2009;119: 1322–34.
5. Teff KL, Grudziak J, Townsend RR, et al. Endocrine and metabolic effects of consuming fructose- and glucose-sweetened beverages with meals in obese men and women: influence of insulin resistance on plasma triglyceride responses. J Clin Endocrinol Metab 2009;94:1562–9.
6. Lustig RH. Fructose: it's "alcohol without the buzz". Adv Nutr 2013;4:226–35.
7. DiNicolantonio JJ, O'Keefe JH, Lucan SC. Added fructose: a principal driver of type 2 diabetes mellitus and its consequences. Mayo Clin Proc 2015;90:372–81.
8. Maersk M, Belza A, Stodkilde-Jorgensen H, et al. Sucrose-sweetened beverages increase fat storage in the liver, muscle, and visceral fat depot: a 6-mo randomized intervention study. Am J Clin Nutr 2012;95:283–9.
9. Aeberli I, Gerber PA, Hochuli M, et al. Low to moderate sugar-sweetened beverage consumption impairs glucose and lipid metabolism and promotes inflammation in healthy young men: a randomized controlled trial. Am J Clin Nutr 2011;94:479–85.
10. Aeberli I, Hochuli M, Gerber PA, et al. Moderate amounts of fructose consumption impair insulin sensitivity in healthy young men: a randomized controlled trial. Diabetes Care 2013;36:150–6.
11. Stanhope KL, Medici V, Bremer AA, et al. A dose-response study of consuming high-fructose corn syrup-sweetened beverages on lipid/lipoprotein risk factors for cardiovascular disease in young adults. Am J Clin Nutr 2015;101:1144–54.
12. Black RN, Spence M, McMahon RO, et al. Effect of eucaloric high- and low-sucrose diets with identical macronutrient profile on insulin resistance and vascular risk: a randomized controlled trial. Diabetes 2006;55:3566–72.
13. Lewis AS, McCourt HJ, Ennis CN, et al. Comparison of 5% versus 15% sucrose intakes as part of a eucaloric diet in overweight and obese subjects: effects on insulin sensitivity, glucose metabolism, vascular compliance, body composition and lipid profile. A randomised controlled trial. Metabolism 2013;62:694–702.
14. Reiser S, Handler HB, Gardner LB, et al. Isocaloric exchange of dietary starch and sucrose in humans. II. Effect on fasting blood insulin, glucose, and glucagon and on insulin and glucose response to a sucrose load. Am J Clin Nutr 1979;32: 2206–16.

15. Stanhope KL. Sugar consumption, metabolic disease and obesity: the state of the controversy. Crit Rev Clin Lab Sci 2016;53(1):52–67.
16. Hotta N, Kakuta H, Fukasawa H, et al. Effects of a fructose-rich diet and the aldose reductase inhibitor, ONO-2235, on the development of diabetic neuropathy in streptozotocin-treated rats. Diabetologia 1985;28:176–80.
17. WHO. Global action plan for the prevention and control of NCDs 2013-2020. Switzerland: World Health Organization; 2013.
18. Ganesan S, Raman R, Kulothungan V, et al. Influence of dietary-fibre intake on diabetes and diabetic retinopathy: Sankara Nethralaya-Diabetic Retinopathy Epidemiology and Molecular Genetic Study (report 26). Clin Experiment Ophthalmol 2012;40:288–94.
19. Barczynska R, Bandurska K, Slizewska K, et al. Intestinal microbiota, obesity and prebiotics. Pol J Microbiol 2015;64:93–100.
20. den Besten G, Bleeker A, Gerding A, et al. Short-chain fatty acids protect against high-fat diet-induced obesity via a PPARgamma-dependent switch from lipogenesis to fat oxidation. Diabetes 2015;64:2398–408.
21. Ludwig DS, Majzoub JA, Al-Zahrani A, et al. High glycemic index foods, overeating, and obesity. Pediatrics 1999;103:E26.
22. Schwab U, Lauritzen L, Tholstrup T, et al. Effect of the amount and type of dietary fat on cardiometabolic risk factors and risk of developing type 2 diabetes, cardiovascular diseases, and cancer: a systematic review. Food Nutr Res 2014;58.
23. Salas-Salvado J, Bullo M, Estruch R, et al. Prevention of diabetes with Mediterranean diets: a subgroup analysis of a randomized trial. Ann Intern Med 2014;160: 1–10.
24. Ahmed M, Moazzami AA, Andersson R, et al. Varying quality of fish oil capsules: fatty acids and tocopherol. Neuro Endocrinol Lett 2011;32(Suppl 2):37–40.
25. Wang W, Zhu J, Lyu F, et al. Omega-3 polyunsaturated fatty acids-derived lipid metabolites on angiogenesis, inflammation and cancer. Prostaglandins Other Lipid Mediat 2014;113-115:13–20.
26. Bosch J, Gerstein HC, Dagenais GR, et al. n-3 fatty acids and cardiovascular outcomes in patients with dysglycemia. N Engl J Med 2012;367:309–18.
27. Tanaka S, Yoshimura Y, Kawasaki R, et al. Fruit intake and incident diabetic retinopathy with type 2 diabetes. Epidemiology 2013;24:204–11.
28. Lin J, Fung TT, Hu FB, et al. Association of dietary patterns with albuminuria and kidney function decline in older white women: a subgroup analysis from the Nurses' Health Study. Am J Kidney Dis 2011;57:245–54.
29. Hamdy O, Marchetti A, Hegazi RA, et al. The transcultural diabetes nutrition algorithm toolkit: survey and content validation in the United States, Mexico, and Taiwan. Diabetes Technol Ther 2014;16:378–84.
30. Dansinger ML, Gleason JA, Griffith JL, et al. Comparison of the Atkins, Ornish, Weight Watchers, and Zone diets for weight loss and heart disease risk reduction: a randomized trial. JAMA 2005;293:43–53.
31. Diabetes Prevention Program (DPP) Research Group. The Diabetes Prevention Program (DPP): description of lifestyle intervention. Diabetes Care 2002;25: 2165–71.
32. Wing RR, Bolin P, Brancati FL, et al. Cardiovascular effects of intensive lifestyle intervention in type 2 diabetes. N Engl J Med 2013;369:145–54.
33. Wing RR, Rosen RC, Fava JL, et al. Effects of weight loss intervention on erectile function in older men with type 2 diabetes in the Look AHEAD trial. J Sex Med 2010;7:156–65.

34. Rubin RR, Wadden TA, Bahnson JL, et al. Impact of intensive lifestyle intervention on depression and health-related quality of life in type 2 diabetes: the Look AHEAD Trial. Diabetes Care 2014;37:1544–53.

35. Look AHEAD Research Group. Effect of a long-term behavioural weight loss intervention on nephropathy in overweight or obese adults with type 2 diabetes: a secondary analysis of the Look AHEAD randomised clinical trial. Lancet Diabetes Endocrinol 2014;2:801–9.

36. Espeland MA, Glick HA, Bertoni A, et al. Impact of an intensive lifestyle intervention on use and cost of medical services among overweight and obese adults with type 2 diabetes: the action for health in diabetes. Diabetes Care 2014;37: 2548–56.

37. Nordmann AJ, Suter-Zimmermann K, Bucher HC, et al. Meta-analysis comparing Mediterranean to low-fat diets for modification of cardiovascular risk factors. Am J Med 2011;124:841–51.e842.

38. Shai I, Schwarzfuchs D, Henkin Y, et al. Weight loss with a low-carbohydrate, Mediterranean, or low-fat diet. N Engl J Med 2008;359:229–41.

39. Schwarzfuchs D, Golan R, Shai I. Four-year follow-up after two-year dietary interventions. N Engl J Med 2012;367:1373–4.

40. Estruch R, Ros E, Salas-Salvado J, et al. Primary prevention of cardiovascular disease with a Mediterranean diet. N Engl J Med 2013;368:1279–90.

41. Diaz-Lopez A, Babio N, Martinez-Gonzalez MA, et al. Mediterranean diet, retinopathy, nephropathy, and microvascular diabetes complications: a post hoc analysis of a randomized trial. Diabetes Care 2015;38:2134–41.

42. Gepner Y, Golan R, Harman-Boehm I, et al. Effects of initiating moderate alcohol intake on cardiometabolic risk in adults with type 2 diabetes: a 2-year randomized, controlled trial. Ann Intern Med 2015;163:569–79.

43. Brien SE, Ronksley PE, Turner BJ, et al. Effect of alcohol consumption on biological markers associated with risk of coronary heart disease: systematic review and meta-analysis of interventional studies. BMJ 2011;342:d636.

44. Mithril C, Dragsted LO, Meyer C, et al. Guidelines for the new nordic diet. Public Health Nutr 2012;15:1941–7.

45. Fritzen AM, Lundsgaard AM, Jordy AB, et al. New nordic diet-induced weight loss is accompanied by changes in metabolism and AMPK signaling in adipose tissue. J Clin Endocrinol Metab 2015;100:3509–19.

46. Ornish D, Scherwitz LW, Billings JH, et al. Intensive lifestyle changes for reversal of coronary heart disease. JAMA 1998;280:2001–7.

47. Chainani-Wu N, Weidner G, Purnell DM, et al. Changes in emerging cardiac biomarkers after an intensive lifestyle intervention. Am J Cardiol 2011;108:498–507.

48. Gadgil MD, Appel LJ, Yeung E, et al. The effects of carbohydrate, unsaturated fat, and protein intake on measures of insulin sensitivity: results from the OmniHeart trial. Diabetes Care 2013;36:1132–7.

49. Jeejeebhoy KN, Chu RC, Marliss EB, et al. Chromium deficiency, glucose intolerance, and neuropathy reversed by chromium supplementation, in a patient receiving long-term total parenteral nutrition. Am J Clin Nutr 1977;30:531–8.

50. Anderson RA. Chromium and insulin resistance. Nutr Res Rev 2003;16:267–75.

51. Anderson RA, Cheng N, Bryden NA, et al. Elevated intakes of supplemental chromium improve glucose and insulin variables in individuals with type 2 diabetes. Diabetes 1997;46:1786–91.

52. Cefalu WT, Hu FB. Role of chromium in human health and in diabetes. Diabetes Care 2004;27:2741–51.

53. Paiva AN, Lima JG, Medeiros AC, et al. Beneficial effects of oral chromium pico-linate supplementation on glycemic control in patients with type 2 diabetes: a ran-domized clinical study. J Trace Elem Med Biol 2015;32:66–72.

54. Alizadeh M, Safaeiyan A, Ostadrahimi A, et al. Effect of L-arginine and selenium added to a hypocaloric diet enriched with legumes on cardiovascular disease risk factors in women with central obesity: a randomized, double-blind, pla-cebo-controlled trial. Ann Nutr Metab 2012;60:157–68.

55. Asemi Z, Jamilian M, Mesdaghinia E, et al. Effects of selenium supplementation on glucose homeostasis, inflammation, and oxidative stress in gestational dia-betes: Randomized, double-blind, placebo-controlled trial. Nutrition 2015;31:1235–42.

56. Rosen CJ, Taylor CL. Common misconceptions about vitamin D–implications for clinicians. Nat Rev Endocrinol 2013;9:434–8.

57. Ganji V, Zhang X, Shaikh N, et al. Serum 25-hydroxyvitamin D concentrations are associated with prevalence of metabolic syndrome and various cardiometabolic risk factors in US children and adolescents based on assay-adjusted serum 25-hydroxyvitamin D data from NHANES 2001-2006. Am J Clin Nutr 2011;94:225–33.

58. Ching S, Kashinkunti S, Niehaus MD, et al. Mammary adipocytes bioactivate 25-hydroxyvitamin D(3) and signal via vitamin D(3) receptor, modulating mammary epithelial cell growth. J Cell Biochem 2011;112:3393–405.

59. Rosenblum JL, Castro VM, Moore CE, et al. Calcium and vitamin D supplemen-tation is associated with decreased abdominal visceral adipose tissue in over-weight and obese adults. Am J Clin Nutr 2012;95:101–8.

60. Sneve M, Figenschau Y, Jorde R. Supplementation with cholecalciferol does not result in weight reduction in overweight and obese subjects. Eur J Endocrinol 2008;159:675–84.

61. Wamberg L, Kampmann U, Stodkilde-Jorgensen H, et al. Effects of vitamin D supplementation on body fat accumulation, inflammation, and metabolic risk fac-tors in obese adults with low vitamin D levels - results from a randomized trial. Eur J Intern Med 2013;24:644–9.

62. Cade C, Norman AW. Vitamin D3 improves impaired glucose tolerance and insu-lin secretion in the vitamin D-deficient rat in vivo. Endocrinology 1986;119:84–90.

63. Pittas AG, Harris SS, Stark PC, et al. The effects of calcium and vitamin D supple-mentation on blood glucose and markers of inflammation in nondiabetic adults. Diabetes Care 2007;30:980–6.

64. Wamberg L, Pedersen SB, Rejnmark L, et al. Causes of Vitamin D deficiency and effect of Vitamin D supplementation on metabolic complications in obesity: a re-view. Curr Obes Rep 2015;4:429–40.

65. Wongwiwatthananukit S, Sansanayudh N, Phetkrajaysang N, et al. Effects of vitamin D(2) supplementation on insulin sensitivity and metabolic parameters in metabolic syndrome patients. J Endocrinol Invest 2013;36:558–63.

66. Mahoney SE, Loprinzi PD. Influence of flavonoid-rich fruit and vegetable intake on diabetic retinopathy and diabetes-related biomarkers. J Diabetes Complications 2014;28:767–71.

67. Ding M, Franke AA, Rosner BA, et al. Urinary isoflavonoids and risk of type 2 dia-betes: a prospective investigation in US women. Br J Nutr 2015;114:1694–701.

68. Szkudelski T, Szkudelska K. Resveratrol and diabetes: from animal to human studies. Biochim Biophys Acta 2015;1852:1145–54.

69. Timmers S, Konings E, Bilet L, et al. Calorie restriction-like effects of 30 days of resveratrol supplementation on energy metabolism and metabolic profile in obese humans. Cell Metab 2011;14:612–22.

70. Bhatt JK, Thomas S, Nanjan MJ. Resveratrol supplementation improves glycemic control in type 2 diabetes mellitus. Nutr Res 2012;32:537–41.

71. Mendez-del Villar M, Gonzalez-Ortiz M, Martinez-Abundis E, et al. Effect of resveratrol administration on metabolic syndrome, insulin sensitivity, and insulin secretion. Metab Syndr Relat Disord 2014;12:497–501.

72. Bertelli AA, Das DK. Grapes, wines, resveratrol, and heart health. J Cardiovasc Pharmacol 2009;54:468–76.

73. Bashmakov YK, Assaad-Khalil SH, Abou Seif M, et al. Resveratrol promotes foot ulcer size reduction in type 2 diabetes patients. ISRN Endocrinol 2014;2014: 816307.

74. Poulsen MM, Vestergaard PF, Clasen BF, et al. High-dose resveratrol supplementation in obese men: an investigator-initiated, randomized, placebo-controlled clinical trial of substrate metabolism, insulin sensitivity, and body composition. Diabetes 2013;62:1186–95.

75. Kobori M, Masumoto S, Akimoto Y, et al. Dietary quercetin alleviates diabetic symptoms and reduces streptozotocin-induced disturbance of hepatic gene expression in mice. Mol Nutr Food Res 2009;53:859–68.

76. Li YQ, Zhou FC, Gao F, et al. Comparative evaluation of quercetin, isoquercetin and rutin as inhibitors of alpha-glucosidase. J Agric Food Chem 2009;57: 11463–8.

77. Cai EP, Lin JK. Epigallocatechin gallate (EGCG) and rutin suppress the glucotoxicity through activating IRS2 and AMPK signaling in rat pancreatic beta cells. J Agric Food Chem 2009;57:9817–27.

78. Ortsater H, Grankvist N, Wolfram S, et al. Diet supplementation with green tea extract epigallocatechin gallate prevents progression to glucose intolerance in db/db mice. Nutr Metab (Lond) 2012;9:11.

79. Takikawa M, Inoue S, Horio F, et al. Dietary anthocyanin-rich bilberry extract ameliorates hyperglycemia and insulin sensitivity via activation of AMP-activated protein kinase in diabetic mice. J Nutr 2010;140:527–33.

80. Mahmoud AM, Ashour MB, Abdel-Moneim A, et al. Hesperidin and naringin attenuate hyperglycemia-mediated oxidative stress and proinflammatory cytokine production in high fat fed/streptozotocin-induced type 2 diabetic rats. J Diabetes Complications 2012;26:483–90.

81. Zhang Y, Liu D. Flavonol kaempferol improves chronic hyperglycemia-impaired pancreatic beta-cell viability and insulin secretory function. Eur J Pharmacol 2011;670:325–32.

82. Baillie-Hamilton PF. Chemical toxins: a hypothesis to explain the global obesity epidemic. J Altern Complement Med 2002;8:185–92.

83. Valvi D, Mendez MA, Martinez D, et al. Prenatal concentrations of polychlorinated biphenyls, DDE, and DDT and overweight in children: a prospective birth cohort study. Environ Health Perspect 2012;120:451–7.

84. Verhulst SL, Nelen V, Hond ED, et al. Intrauterine exposure to environmental pollutants and body mass index during the first 3 years of life. Environ Health Perspect 2009;117:122–6.

85. Suez J, Korem T, Zeevi D, et al. Artificial sweeteners induce glucose intolerance by altering the gut microbiota. Nature 2014;514:181–6.

Nutrition Interventions for Chronic Liver Diseases and Nonalcoholic Fatty Liver Disease

Carolina Frade Magalhaes Girardin Pimentel, MD, PhD*,
Michelle Lai, MD, MPH

KEYWORDS

- Nonalcoholic liver disease • Nutrition • Diet • Liver disease • Lifestyle intervention
- Liver cirrhosis

KEY POINTS

- Patients suffering from liver disease are susceptible for malnutrition from both overnutrition and undernutrition.
- Nonalcoholic fatty liver disease (NAFLD) has an increasing worldwide prevalence owing to the poor modern diet and the epidemic of obesity.
- NAFLD is closely associated with the metabolic syndrome and cardiovascular disease. Dietary pattern and lifestyle contribute to the development of comorbidities.
- Both weight loss and changes in diet are independently associated with improvement in the liver in NAFLD. A healthy diet is beneficial even when weight reduction is not achieved.
- Patients with decompensated cirrhosis develop undernutrition from increased energy demand, decreased intake and absorption and organ dysfunction.

INTRODUCTION

Liver disease is one of the main causes of hospital admissions worldwide[1] and the 12th leading cause of mortality in many countries.[2] Among all etiologies (toxic–metabolic, viral, autoimmune and genetic disorders), nonalcoholic fatty liver disease (NAFLD) features as the most common cause,[3] with increasing prevalence attributed to the epidemic of metabolic syndrome. Given the high prevalence of NAFLD, this paper focuses on the nutrition interventions in patients with NAFLD, and we also address nutrition issues and interventions in patients who have progressed on to cirrhosis and decompensated liver disease.

Malnutrition is defined as either having not enough or too much nutrients in the diet resulting in health problems. It is a major problem in patients with liver disease,

Disclosure Statement: The authors have nothing to disclose.
Gastroenterology, Liver Center, Beth Israel Deaconess Medical Center, Harvard University, 110 Francis St, Boston, MA 02115, USA
* Corresponding author.
E-mail address: carolinapimentel.gastro@gmail.com

Med Clin N Am 100 (2016) 1303–1327
http://dx.doi.org/10.1016/j.mcna.2016.06.010
0025-7125/16/© 2016 Elsevier Inc. All rights reserved.

in the forms of both overnutrition and undernutrition. Although NAFLD is caused by excessive intake in certain nutrients, patients with chronic liver disease are at risk of other forms of malnutrition owing to both disease-specific impairment (ie, reduced fat-soluble vitamins in cholestatic disorders) and as a consequence of organ dysfunction. An estimated 65% to 90% of patients with advanced liver disease suffer from undernutrition.[4,5] Addressing the malnutrition can result in disease reversal, prevent disease progression, or improve prognosis and quality of life (QOL) in a large proportion of these patients. Nutrition evaluation and interventions should be part of the management of every patient with NAFLD or advanced liver disease.

Nonalcoholic Fatty Liver Disease

NAFLD is spectrum of disease characterized by fat deposits in the liver in the absence of significant alcohol consumption. The spectrum ranges from simple steatosis, thought to be a benign condition, to the more severe form, nonalcoholic steatohepatitis (NASH), which is thought to lead to liver cirrhosis, hepatocellular carcinoma (HCC), and to be associated with cardiovascular disease and higher risk of both liver-related and overall mortality.[3] It is the most common cause of liver disease worldwide with prevalences ranging from 25% to 45%.[6] In the United States, the prevalence of NAFLD is estimated to be up to 49% and of NASH to be 12%.[7] Although the prevalence of other liver diseases has been stable over the last 20 years, that of NAFLD has increased remarkably along with the prevalence of the metabolic syndrome and diabetes.[8] NAFLD is considered the hepatic manifestation of the metabolic syndrome and is strongly linked to obesity. An estimated 80% of patients with obesity have NAFLD.[9] The natural history of NAFLD varies and depends on the severity of the liver damage and population risk factors, such as obesity and diabetes.[10] Although simple steatosis is thought to have a benign course, NASH, the severe end of the disease spectrum characterized by inflammation, hepatocyte ballooning, and apoptosis, is thought to be a progressive disease in which patients are at risk of developing liver cirrhosis and HCC.[11,12] Of patients with NASH, 15% to 20% will develop end-stage liver disease within 10 to 20 years, with NASH projected to become the leading indication for liver transplantation in the next decade (**Fig. 1**).[3,13] In addition to the increased risk of liver-related complications and mortality, patients with NASH have an increased risk of cardiovascular disease and overall mortality.[14] Given the high worldwide prevalence of NAFLD, the social impact (reduced QOL, morbidity, and mortality), and substantial costs of managing the complications from NASH, early intervention is vital. Given the prevalence of the disease, primary care providers will play a key role in this early intervention.

Obesity is a worldwide problem, with prevalence rates almost doubling in the last 3 decades.[15] According to the World Health Organization,[16] in 2014, more than 30% of the United States population were obese and more than 60% overweight. The number of individuals who are overweight worldwide in 2015 is estimated to exceed 2.3 billion. Furthermore, 15% of all Western population and 35% of patients with obesity will develop steatohepatitis (NASH).[17] This pandemic disease is attributed to both the increased amounts of processed foods high in fructose, sodium, and saturated fats, and the increasingly sedentary lifestyle.[18] Obesity is considered a chronic state of low-grade inflammation, being associated with complications such as the metabolic syndrome, type 2 diabetes, hypertension, and cardiovascular disease.[19] It has also been linked with increased risks of certain cancers, such as colon, breast, endometrium, kidney, esophagus, stomach, pancreas, and gallbladder.[20,21] The

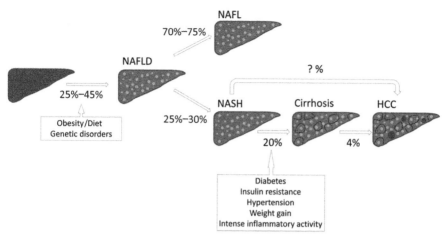

Fig. 1. Phases involved in the progression of nonalcoholic fatty liver disease (NAFLD). It is estimated that 25% to 45% of general population have NAFLD and among them that 70% to 75% will develop NAFL (isolated steatosis with or without nonspecific inflammation), a more benign form. 25% to 30% has the more severe form of the disease, nonalcoholic steatohepatitis (NASH), and are at risk of developing liver cirrhosis (in 20% of cases) and hepatocellular carcinoma (HCC; approximately 4% of cirrhotic patients). Recent literature suggests that HCC may directly develop from NASH even in the absence of cirrhosis. (*Data from* Rinella ME. Nonalcoholic fatty liver disease. JAMA 2015;313(22):2263; and Piscaglia F, Svegliati-baroni G, Barchetti A, et al. Clinical patterns of hepatocellular carcinoma in nonalcoholic fatty liver disease: a Multicenter Prospective Study. Hepatology 2016;63:827–38.)

combination of obesity, insulin resistance, and NASH is also thought to increase the risk of HCC.[22]

The Role of Malnutrition in the Development of Nonalcoholic Fatty Liver Disease

The pathophysiology of NAFLD and NASH is complex, and not completely understood. Three mechanisms thought to result in liver fat accumulation include (1) excessive delivery of free fatty acids (FFA) from lipolysis of superficial and visceral fat depots (60%), (2) increased de novo hepatic lipogenesis from impairment of the beta-oxidation of FFA and diminished export of FFA from the liver owing to reduced synthesis or secretion of very low density lipoprotein (30%), and (3) increased dietary intake (10%).[17,23]

Although dietary fat intake accounts for the lowest proportion of liver fat accumulation, progressive weight gain leads to decreased adiponectin and increased insulin resistance leading to enhanced peripheral lipolysis, increased delivery of FFA to liver and enhanced de novo lipogenesis. This results in a vicious cycle responsible for the development and progression of NAFLD.

The dietary pattern can directly influence NAFLD progression because it is associated with insulin resistance, FFA cell influx, de novo lipogenesis, and oxidative stress in the liver.[24] Patients with NAFLD consume higher amounts of saturated fats, cholesterol, fructose, and lower amounts of polyunsaturated fatty acids (PUFA), fiber, and antioxidants (vitamins C and E).[25,26] This dietary pattern results in overnutrition, which leads to progressive insulin resistance, hepatic injury, and liver dysfunction. Modification of the macronutrients in a diet (reduced fat or carbohydrate), even

Table 1
Proposed mechanisms in which dietary pattern promotes fat liver accumulation

Diet Pattern	Mechanism/Consequence	Reference
High-fat diet	Higher FFA delivery from diet inducing release of cathepsin B by hepatocytes, promoting TNFα secretion and inhibition of insulin action and mitochondrial dysfunction	Carter-Kent et al,[27] 2008
	Increased adipose tissue promotes adipocyte lipolysis and higher FFA delivery owing to a reduction in adiponectin plasma levels, preventing lipid clearance in plasma and increasing β-oxidation in muscles.	Xu et al,[28] 2003
	The accumulation of fat metabolites secondary to HFD stimulates the secretion of IL-6, TNFα, triggering several signal transduction pathways (PKC, JNK, and kappa β-kinase inhibitor) causing hepatic insulin resistance.	Postic and Girard,[29] 2008
	Patients with NAFLD present an impaired postprandial TG response, increasing TG uptake by the liver inducing hepatic fat deposition. In addition, TG production in 3 times higher in these patients.	Assy et al,[30] 2009
High carbohydrate diet	It is the major source for liver production of FFA in patients with NAFLD. In this group, it accounts for 30% of FFA production, in contrast with only 5% in normal livers.	Neuschwander-Tetri,[31] 2013
High fructose diet	Decreased function of PPARα, leading to reduced hepatic lipid oxidation and hepatic steatosis. Also, increases NF-κβ expression inducing oxidative stress and increases hepatic fibrosis.	Roglans et al,[32] 2007; Wei et al,[33] 2007
High glucose diet	Stimulates lipogenic genes in the liver (JNK) contributing to liver fat accumulation and inflammation. Also, increases visceral adipose tissue.	Wei et al,[33] 2007
High glycemic index diet	Enhance the hepatic influx of glucose exceeding the ability of glycogen production, conducting carbohydrates to TG synthesis through de novo lipogenesis within hepatocytes. May also augment oxidative stress and inflammation process.	Liu et al,[34] 2000; Hu et al,[35] 2006

Abbreviations: FFA, free fatty acid; HFD, high-fat diet; JNK, c-JUN NH2-terminal kinase-1; NF-κβ, nuclear factor kappa-light-chain-enhancer of activated B cells; PKC, serine/threonine kinases (protein kinase C); PPAR-α, peroxisome proliferator-activated receptor α; TNF-α, tumor necrosis factor-alpha.
Data from Refs.[28-36]

without weight reduction, results in a beneficial effect on NAFLD progression.[24] **Table 1** presents the proposed mechanisms in which dietary patterns promote liver fat accumulation.

Liver Cirrhosis and Malnutrition Associated with Liver Cirrhosis

Liver cirrhosis is the end result from chronic liver damage from many liver diseases, including NAFLD. Cirrhosis is defined by hepatocyte damage and transformation of the liver parenchyma into fibrotic tissue and regenerative nodules. Patients who have progressed to cirrhosis are at risk of developing undernutrition. With progressive deterioration of liver function, patients develop clinical decompensation with ascites, bacterial spontaneous peritonitis, hepatorenal syndrome, gastrointestinal bleeding, or HCC.[36] Although patients with compensated cirrhosis have a mean survival of 50% at 10 years, those with decompensated liver cirrhosis have a much shorter life expectancy, 20% in 5 years.[37] It is important to prevent liver deterioration in patients with compensated cirrhosis. Addressing both overnutrition in the early phases of NAFLD and NASH and undernutrition in cirrhosis has an enormous impact on the QOL and prognosis of patients with liver disease.[38]

Patients with decompensated cirrhosis develop undernutrition as a result of liver dysfunction, poor oral intake and absorption, and increased protein and caloric needs. Because the liver is responsible for the metabolism of a variety of nutrients including synthesis of glucose (gluconeogenesis), cholesterol metabolism (synthesis and fatty acid oxidation), protein breakdown (amino acid oxidation and ureagenesis), and bile production (important for absorption of fats and fat-soluble vitamins), patients with severe liver disease are prone to developing malnutrition resulting from impairment of these functions (**Table 2**). In addition to hepatic dysfunction, clinical complications that prohibit adequate food intake or

Table 2
Role of liver in metabolism

Nutrient Group Select	Liver Functions
Protein	Synthesis of plasma proteins (transferrin, albumin, ceruloplasmin, etc) Deamination of amino acids to make urea Transamination and synthesis of amino acids Oxidation of amino acids
Carbohydrates	Gluconeogenesis Glycogenesis Glycogenolysis
Fat	Production of bile for emulsion, absorption and fat storage Synthesis of cholesterol and triglycerides Uptake and oxidation of fatty acids Synthesis of lipoproteins
Vitamins	Uptake and storage of multiple vitamins (A, D, E, B_{12}, K) Enzymatic activation of vitamins (B_6, B_1, D, folic acid) Vitamin transport (A, B_{12}, etc) through carrier proteins synthesized by liver
Minerals	Storage site for multiple minerals (zinc, iron, copper, etc)

From Manne V, Saab S. Impact of nutrition and obesity on chronic liver disease. Clin Liver Dis 2014;18:207; with permission.

absorption, such as large volume ascites, chronic diarrhea, reduced intestinal absorption owing to wall edema, loss of appetite, multiple hospital admissions, and infections, also contribute to a wide spectrum of nutrition deficiencies in patients with cirrhosis. Patients with ascites have increased protein and caloric needs secondary to a hypermetabolic state and protein loss in repeated paracentesis[39] (**Table 3**).

Nutrition evaluation and interventions are important in the management of patients with NAFLD and other chronic liver diseases. We discuss the main goals of nutrition interventions in patients with NAFLD and chronic liver disease, how to perform a nutrition evaluation, and present a review of available data regarding nutrition interventions in these patients.

MANAGEMENT GOALS

Given the strong association between dietary pattern and NAFLD, nutrition intervention is the main treatment currently available to modify the disease process. The main goals of this therapy are:

- Improvement or resolution of NAFLD;
- Improvement in QOL;

Table 3
Select nutrient deficiencies and their relation to liver disease

Nutrient Group	Relation to Liver	Some Associated Signs/ Symptoms
Protein	Decreased synthesis and transportation in liver disease Increased breakdown	Muscle wasting Edema/ascites
Fat	Decreased absorption in liver disease	Scaly skin Soft/brittle nails
Vitamin B$_1$ (thiamine)	Increased requirement in liver disease, especially alcoholic liver disease	Cheilosis
Vitamin B$_6$ (pyridoxine)	Increased degradation in liver disease	Weakness
Vitamin B$_{12}$ (cyanocobalamin)	Malabsorption seen in liver disease	Neuropathy
Folate	Deficiency seen in liver disease	Anemia
Fat-soluble vitamins (A, D, E, K)	Malabsorption in liver disease	Night blindness Keratosis Osteoporosis Neuropathy Increased risk of bleeding
Zinc	Malabsorption and increased requirement in liver disease, thought to be a risk factor for encephalopathy	Risk of infections Taste and smell change Slow wound healing
Magnesium	Deficiency seen in liver disease	Taste changes

From Manne V, Saab S. Impact of nutrition and obesity on chronic liver disease. Clin Liver Dis 2014;18:207; with permission.

- Improvement in outcomes during hospital admission, surgery, and liver transplantation of malnourished patients with liver cirrhosis; and
- Prevention of development or worsening of metabolic syndrome and cardiovascular complications.

Several studies have demonstrated dietary interventions in patients with NAFLD and liver cirrhosis to be safe and cost effective. Data have shown that 7% to 10% of body weight reduction either in patients with NAFLD, from nutrition intervention and other lifestyle modification decreases hepatic steatosis, inflammation and fibrosis, with improvement or resolution of NAFLD, especially when in early phases of the disease.[40,41]

Weight reduction has also been shown to improve QOL in patients who are obese, have NAFLD, and have a reduced QOL at baseline.[42,43] QOL is not only important for well-being, but also directly impacts adherence to treatment. One of the main challenges is weight loss maintenance because many patients regain their weight. A goal directly assigned to help solving this challenge is highly desirable.

Patients with decompensated liver cirrhosis have a dramatically decreased QOL owing to frequent hospital admissions, complications such as chronic fatigue, ascites, and encephalopathy, and progressive undernutrition. Although there are no data available on the impact of nutrition intervention on QOL in these patients, controlling their ascites with a low sodium diet can improve symptoms and increase oral intake. In these patients, nutrition intervention has been shown to improve the outcomes after liver transplant. Studies have reported that patients with cirrhosis and undernutrition have much higher rates of complication after surgery, with delay hospital discharge, higher rates of infections, higher insurance costs, and greater morbidity and mortality.[5,44]

NAFLD is linked directly to insulin resistance, the metabolic syndrome, and increased cardiovascular disease. By incorporating diet and physical activity into the treatment plan, it is possible to reduce rates of associated comorbidities, especially diabetes and coronary disease, the main cause of mortality in this group of patients.

EVALUATION

A practical evaluation of nutrition status consists of (1) evaluation of dietary habits and physical activity, (2) performing anthropometric measurements, and (3) obtaining laboratory studies. Reporting by patients of their dietary pattern and lifestyle is subjective and subject to recall bias. To increase accuracy, we recommend that patients complete a food diary or a calorie counter mobile app to help patients keep a more careful record of their dietary habits to review with the physician. In reviewing the patient's lifestyle and making recommendations for intervention, we propose a mnemonic "PREVENTION" to help the clinician remember the key points of lifestyle intervention. This tool is present as part of an algorithm proposed to the evaluation of nutrition status in patients with NAFLD (**Fig. 2**).

Anthropometric measurements include weight, body mass index, skinfold thickness, handgrip strength, and mid-arm and waist circumference. The body weight is the easiest noninvasive measure of nutrition status in clinical practice, but does not distinguish between muscle mass, body fat, ascites, or edema. Patients with decompensated cirrhosis have progressive subcutaneous fat loss and muscle wasting, which predict higher rates of hospital admissions and mortality.[44] Skinfold thickness and mid-arm circumference measurements help to assess muscle mass, and waist circumference measurement helps to assess fat mass. Waist circumference, however, is not accurate and is not useful in patients with ascites. Although these are simple measurements that can be done in the office, they can be unreliable in the presence of ascites and edema.[23,38] Although a computed tomography scan measurement of

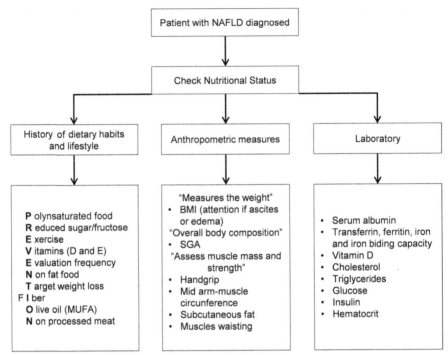

Fig. 2. Nutrition assessment in liver patients. BMI, body mass index; MUFA, monounsaturated fatty acids; NAFLD, nonalcoholic fatty liver disease; SGA, Subjective Global Assessment.

psoas thickness is the most accurate,[45] it is more costly and not practical. The applicability of handgrip and mid-arm muscle circumference in patients with liver disease is described in some studies,[46] and provide a reasonable estimate of muscle wasting during a primary care visit. The interpretation and limitation of these and other tests are presented in **Table 4**.

The Subjective Global Assessment is a commonly used multidimensional nutrition assessment tool,[47] that provides an overall evaluation of nutrition status. Some disadvantages regarding its use are the lack of studies evolving patients with liver disease and the dependence on a certain level of clinical judgment. Some studies reported the use of Subjective Global Assessment in liver cirrhosis, but not in NAFLD.[5,23,48]

Laboratory evaluation is detailed in **Fig. 2**. Serum albumin is used to assess both the liver synthetic function and nutrition status, vitamin D deficiency is very prevalent and is discussed in greater depth elsewhere in this paper. The lipid panel, glucose, and insulin levels assess components of the metabolic syndrome and risk for cardiovascular disease. Hematocrit and iron studies assess for iron deficiency anemia. A high ferritin is often seen as NASH and is a marker of inflammation.

INTERVENTION

Although there is no established protocol regarding that is the optimal nutrition recommendation to be followed by patients with NAFLD and liver disease, data supports the following:

- Weight reduction for patients who are overweight or obese;
- Reducing sugar intake;

Table 4
The most common measurements for weight, muscle, and fat and their interpretation

Measurement	What Does It Evaluate?	How to Perform It	Interpretation	Limitations
BMI	Fat mass	BMI = Weight/(Height)^2	Underweight (<18.5 kg/m^2), normal weight (18.5–24.99 kg/m^2), overweight (25.0–29.99 kg/m^2), and obesity (>30.0 kg/m^2)	Overestimated values in patients with ascites and edema
SGA[47]	Overall body composition	Use information from history (last 6 mo) and physical examination (**Table 5**)	There is no scores, interpretation based on clinical evaluation. Patients are classified as: A – well-nourished B – moderately malnourished C – severely malnourished	Not validated in liver patients and requires an experienced examiner. Most studies use for evaluate undernutrition, not for obesity.
Handgrip strength	Muscle mass	Evaluate strength by holding a dynameter	Malnourished patients, presenting reduced muscle mass, have reduced values during this maneuver.	Not validated in liver cirrhosis.
Mid arm muscle circumference	Muscle mass	Measurement of mid arm diameter	Values <185 and <160 mm denote moderate and severe undernutrition, respectively[46]	Difficult evaluation in patients with ascites and edema.
Waist circumference	Fat mass and CV risk	Related to cardiovascular risk and central obesity.	Female <88 mm Male <102 mm	Overestimated values in patients with ascites and edema. Validated in nonliver patients.
Subcutaneous fat	Fat mass	Inspection of reduced subcutaneous fat under chin and temporal areas.	The presence of those clinical findings during physical examination suggests undernutrition.	Highly subjective and influenced by fluid overloaded states.
Muscle wasting (abdominal CT)	Muscle mass	CT perfumed using TPMT measurement	TPMT/height <0.84[45] suggests loss of muscle mass and predicts mortality	Just a few studies evaluated cirrhotic patients. More studies are needed to established practical cutoffs in liver patients.

Abbreviations: BMI, body mass index; CT, computed tomography; CV risk, cardiovascular risk; SGA, Subjective Global Assessment; TPMT, transversal psoas muscle thickness.

Table 5
Subjective Global Assessment questionnaire

History	Physical Examination
Weight change in 6 mo	Loss of subcutaneous fat in triceps and chest
Dietary change (starvation, full liquid diet, hypocaloric, and suboptimal liquid diet)	Muscle wasting in deltoids and quadriceps
Presence or absence of nausea, vomiting, and diarrhea for the last 2 wk	Ankle edema
Functional status	Sacral edema
Evaluation of individual nutrition requirements	Ascites

Data from Detsky A, McLaughlin J, Baker J, et al. What is Subjective Global Assessment of nutritional status? Nutr Hosp 2008;23(4):400–7.

- Restriction of simple carbohydrate and high glycemic carbohydrate;
- Restriction of total and saturated fat; and
- Diet rich in fiber and healthy fats (olive oil, a monounsaturated fatty acid) and omega 3 PUFA.

Weight reduction of 5% results in improvement in hepatic steatosis and a 7% to 10% reduction results in significant improvement in steatosis, inflammation, and hepatocyte ballooning liver histology.[40,41,49] Gradual weight loss is recommended (1-2 lb/wk or 0.5-1 kg/wk); greater rates of weight loss (>2 lb/wk or 1 kg/wk) has been shown to worsen disease.[50,51] Avoidance of high carbohydrate (simple carbohydrate and high glycemic carbohydrate) and fat (restriction of total and saturated fat) is associated with improvement in metabolic and hepatic parameters, and a reduction in steatosis and liver enzymes. It highlights the importance on "quality" and "healthy" diet, even without weight loss. The beneficial effect of weight loss, however, seems to be associated independently with reduction in steatosis, improvement in metabolic parameters, and transaminases, regardless of which macronutrient is restricted (carbohydrate or fat). It is likely that the combination of a good quality diet combined with a reduction in weight loss is the preferred recommendation.[9,17] **Table 6** compares the key studies that investigated specific diets for NAFLD patients, as well as their outcomes and impact in disease progression. Regardless of the type of diet, weight loss is able to prevent disease progression and improve inflammatory markers in patients with NAFLD.

Some studies have investigated the role of other dietary constituents in the prevention of NAFLD progression. The most studied components are coffee, fiber, olive oil (rich in monounsaturated fatty acid), and omega 3 PUFA. **Table 7** summarized the recent evidence that support the use of those dietary components in NAFLD management.

In addition to macronutrients, some micronutrients (vitamins and minerals) have been studied as possible coadjuvant therapies during nutrition intervention. Because of their antioxidant properties, different supplements have been studied in NAFLD therapy. The most studied micronutrient is vitamin E, considered an antioxidant substance. The PIVENS trial[79] randomized 247 patients with biopsy-proven NASH in nondiabetic patients to receive vitamin E 800 IU, pioglitazone 30 g, or placebo. There was significant improvement in steatosis and inflammation on histology and transaminases reduction in both the vitamin E or pioglitazone groups compared with placebo, but pioglitazone did not achieve the pretest expected significant P value. However, patients need to be advised that vitamin E is related to unfavorable changes in plasma lipoproteins, possibly increasing all-cause mortality and to increased risk of prostate cancer.[80] In addition, there are insufficient data to recommend vitamin E for patients with NASH with diabetes or cirrhosis.[81]

Although vitamin C has antioxidant properties, prior studies assessing its role in patients with NAFLD could not demonstrate any beneficial result.[82] Vitamin D deficiency, in contrast, is associated with NAFLD and hepatic inflammation. Vitamin D has direct antiinflammatory actions on macrophages and B and T helper cells, increases adiponectin secretion, and reduces stellate cells proliferation. Patients with NASH have significantly lower vitamin D levels when compared with controls and patients with NAFLD, with vitamin D levels were directly associated with liver histology.[83] Murine studies showed that increased vitamin D concentration was associated with decrease inflammation, apoptosis, and fibrosis in liver biopsy. However, there are no trials that have been done to assess if vitamin D supplementation can result in improvement in patients with NAFLD. We recommend checking vitamin D levels, using serum 25(OH)vitamin D measurement, every 6 months and supplementation for patients with vitamin levels less than 30 ng/mL.[84]

There are data in patients without liver disease to suggest that coffee may lower the risk of developing NAFLD and the metabolic syndrome. Furthermore, regular consumption is correlated negatively with hepatic fibrosis and seems to be a protective factor.[54–56] The exact mechanism of action is not completely understood. More studies are required to define dose range and long-term benefits in NAFLD before knowing what dose to recommend.

Based on the data presented, we present our recommendations for nutrition intervention and monitoring in NAFLD in **Box 1**. One way to remember the general areas of nutrition intervention is the mnemonic presented in **Fig. 2**.

As discussed, patients with decompensated cirrhosis face undernutrition from a combination of increased nutrition demand from being in a hypercatabolic state and decreased intake and absorption.[85–87] The goals of nutrition intervention in these patients is to stop muscle wasting, prevent hypoglycemia, control ascites, and improve outcomes during liver-related decompensation as well as after liver transplantation. **Table 8** details our recommendations for nutrition interventions in patients with liver cirrhosis to meet these goals. Some patients also have disease-specific malnutrition owing to excess or impaired absorption of specific micronutrients, requiring extra attention during nutrition management.

MAINTENANCE

Although there is no doubt about the beneficial impact of weight reduction in NAFLD, achieving and maintaining weight loss is challenging and often unsuccessful with 1 study showing 80% of patients failed to lose at least 5% body weight during the follow-up period.[91] A retrospective review of 924 outpatients with NAFLD showed that frequent clinical encounters ($\geq$3 visits in the period of 1 year) were associated with weight reduction, especially among individual with a high baseline body mass index. The benefit of intensive monitoring was also demonstrated by another trial, when, among 152 patients, those randomized to receive moderate intensive lifestyle intervention (6 session/10 weeks), instead of 3 sessions/4 weeks, presented a higher reduction in liver enzymes and weight loss.[92] We therefore recommend more frequent visits, especially in patients with high body mass index, NASH, or obesity-related comorbidities. Providing more support to patients in the form of a multidisciplinary approach (physician, dietitian, exercise physiologist, and

Table 6
Diets and NAFLD impact

Author	Dietary Patterns	Time	n	Weight Loss	Assessment	Overall Outcomes
Utzschneider et al,[66] 2013	Isoenergetic for both groups. SF 7%, LGI <55, LSAT 23% vs high fat 24%, HSAT 43%, HGI >70). Comparison between both diets.	4 wk	35	Stable	MRI	LSAT decreased significantly lipid parameters but not liver fat. Insulin and HOMA did not change.
Van der Meer et al,[67] 2008	High-fat high energy diet (280 g fat/d). No controls.	3 d	15	Not evaluated	MRI	Increase hepatic TG compared with baseline.
Westerbacka et al,[68] 2005	HFD (56%), CHO 31%, protein 13%, SFA 28%, MUFA 16%, PUFA 5% vs LFD 16%, CHO 61%, protein 19%, SFA 5%, MUFA 5%, PUFA 4%	2 wk	10	Stable	MRI	Reduced liver fat by 20% in LFD and increased 35% during HFD.
Kontogianni et al,[69] 2014	High vs low MD score. NAFLD vs healthy patients.		73	Not evaluated	Liver elastography and histology	High adherence to MD did not prevent NAFLD but is associated with less IR and less severe disease in NAFLD patients.
Ryan et al,[58] 2013	MD × control (low saturated and unsaturated fat). All subjects were submitted to both diets.	3 mo	30	Both reduced weight (P<.05)	MRI	MD decreased more hepatic steatosis and insulin sensitivity.

Study	Diet	Duration	N	Weight	Measure	Results
de Luis et al,[70] 2012	LFD (1): CHO 53%, Fat 27%, protein 20% LCD (2): CHO 38%, Fat 26% Diets were compared between 30 NAFLD and 112 controls.	3 mo	142	Both diets led to similar weight reduction.	Laboratory	Reduction in transaminases, improvement in insulin resistance.
Haufe et al,[71] 2011	All patients obese. Hypocaloric (decrease by 30% from baseline, 1200 kcal/d). Patients were submitted to one of diet: LCD: <90 g CHO, ≥30% fat, 0.8 g/kg protein LFD: fat ≤ 20%, protein 0.8 g/kg, the remaining CHO	6 mo	170	Both diets led to similar weight reduction.	MRI	Both diets had the same benefit on intrahepatic lipid accumulation.
Ryan et al,[72] 2007	Hypocaloric diet and: LFD: CHO 60%, fat 25%, protein 15% LCD: CHO 40%, Fat 45%, protein 15%	16 wk	52	Both diets led to similar weight reduction.	Laboratory	LCD decreased ALT and plasma glucose greater than LFD, despite equal weight loss.
Tendler et al,[73] 2007	VLCD (<20 g/d), normocaloric and supplement	6 mo	5	Weight reduction of 11%	Histology	Reduced liver steatosis and inflammation and improvement in AST, ALT, insulin, and glucose.
Huang et al,[49] 2005	Hypocaloric, CHO 40%–45%, fat 30%–35%	12 mo	23	Weight reduction of 3%	Histology and laboratory (ALT, AST, glucose and TG)	Neither significant change in histology nor in laboratory.

(continued on next page)

Table 6
(continued)

Author	Dietary Patterns	Time	n	Weight Loss	Assessment	Overall Outcomes
Ueno et al,[40] 1997	15 follow the diet and no instruction was given to 10 patients. Hypocaloric (25 kcal/kg, CHO 50%, fat 30%) and physical activity	3 mo	25	Weight reduction of 10% in the diet group and 3.4% in controls	Histology and laboratory	Reduction of steatosis in biopsy, and also reduction of ALT, AST, glucose and cholesterol.
Harrison et al,[41] 2009	All patients were obese and submitted and submitted hypocaloric diet (1400 kcal/d) divided into 2 groups: (1) diet + vitamin E + orlistat; (2) diet + vitamin E	36 wk	50	1. -8.3% 2. -6.0% ($P = .36$)	Histology	Similar weight reduction. Weight loss >5% was associated with steatosis reduction and >9% also a reduction in inflammation and ballooning. Both reduced ALT and AST.
Promrat et al,[74] 2010	All patients were obese and submitted to (1) intensive lifestyle: moderate hypocaloric, 25% fat, and exercise, or (2) just structured education	48 wk	31	Weight reduction of 9% in the intervention group and 0.2% in control	Histology	Reduction in NAS was greater in the intervention group than control (−2.4 vs −1.4, $P<.01$). Patients with >7% weight loss reduced more steatosis (−0.9), inflammation (−0.6) and ballooning (−0.7).

Study	Intervention	Duration	N	Results	Method	Conclusion
Rodriguez-Hernández et al,[75] 2011	LCD (31 obese patients) vs LFD (28 obese patients)	6 mo	59	Weight reduction in LCD group was 5.7% and in LFD, 5.5%	Laboratory	Decrease of aminotransferase levels in obese women is related to body weight reduction, irrespective of type of diet.
Elias et al,[76] 2010	All NAFLD patients submitted to hypocaloric (reduction of 500–1000 kcal/d), CHO 55%, fat 30%, protein 15%	6 mo	31	Adherent, weight reduction of >5% (17 patients) Nonadherent weight loss <5% (14 patients)	CT and laboratory	Group (1) present significant greater reduction of ALT, AST, GGT, HOMA_IR < visceral fat and hepatic density on CT
Lin et al,[77] 2009	VLCD: (1) 400 kcal/d or (2) 800 kcal/d	12 wk	132	Weight reduction in group (1) 9.14% and (2) 8.98%	Laboratory	There was no additional benefit in prescribing the more restrictive diet intervention.
Razavi Zade et al,[78] 2016	Both diets had: CHO 52%–55%, protein 16%–18%, fat 30%. DASH diet was also rich of fruits, vegetables, whole grains, low-fat dairy products, low SF, cholesterol and refined grains.	8wk	60	Weight reduction was higher in DASH group (−3.8 vs −2.1; $P = .006$)	Laboratory	DASH diet was better when compared with the control diet, regarding weight reduction, ALT, AST, triglycerides, insulin, and inflammatory markers.

Abbreviations: ALT, alanine aminotransferase; AST, aspartate aminotransferase; CH, carbohydrate; CHO, cholesterol; CT, computed tomography; DASH, Dietary Approaches to Stop Hypertension; GGT, gamma-glutamyl transferase; HEI, health eating index; HFD or LFD, high or low fat diet; HGI or LGI, high or low glycemic index; HOMA, Homeostasis Model Assessment; HOMA_IR, Homeostasis Model Assessment–insulin resistance; HSAT or LSAT, high or low saturated fat diet; IR, insulin resistance; LCD, low carbohydrate diet; MD, Mediterranean diet; MDS, Mediterranean diet score; MUFA, monunosaturated fatty acid; NAFLD, nonalcoholic fatty liver disease; NAS, NAFLD activity score; PUFA, polyunsaturated fatty acid; SF, saturated fat; SFA, saturated fatty acid; TG, triglyceride; VLCD, very low carbohydrate diet.

Data from Refs.[51–82]

Table 7
The role of supplements in NAFLD management

Substance	Where to Find?	Possible Mechanism of Action	Studies (Pros and Cons)	Recommendation
Coffee and caffeine	Coffee drink	Caffeine modulates expression of genes related to fatty synthesis in the liver. Coffee polyphenols have antioxidant properties.[52,53]	Can reduce the risk of NAFLD, and also a metabolic syndrome. Consumption of regular coffee was an independent protective factor for fibrosis (OR = 0.75, 95% CI),[54] and present an inverse relationship between regular coffee consumption and hepatic fibrosis.[55] Coffee intake was lower than in controls, but no association was observed between protective effect and oxidative stress markers.[56]	No clear recommendation about amount per day.
MUFA	Olive oil	Increase levels of HDL and lower TG, also improve glycemic control in patients with diabetes.	One trial showed significant greater steatosis reduction in the high-MUFA-diet group (-27% vs 5%; $P<.05$).[57] Diet enrich of MUFA decrease liver fat content.[58]	Try to substitute as much as possible SFA for MUFA.
PUFA (omega 3)	Oily fish, chia seeds, flaxseeds, canola oil, walnuts, and eggs	Induce a reduction in liver steatosis by upregulation of PPAR-α, increased FA oxidation ad reduced lipogenesis. Also, it has antiinflammatory and insulin-sensitizing effects.	Patients with NAFLD have reduced ω3FA and ω3/ω6 ratio. Increased ω3 is associated with reduced risk of CVD,[59] HCC,[60] and steatosis by MRI or US. No significant effect on liver function test.[61]	Increase consumption of ω3 on diet. There is no consent regarding ideal dose.

| Fiber | Oatmeal, vegetables, fruits, nuts | Increased satiety, incretin secretion, absorption rate of CHO and protein, and modulation of gut microbiota.[62] | Whole-grain intake was associated with reduced CVD (RR = 0.79) and DM (RR = 0.74).[63] | There is no studied in patients with NAFLD. |
| Choline/betaine | Red meat, eggs, dairy products | Mitochondrial lipid stabilization and VLDL production. | One trial fail to demonstrate benefit in 55 patients.[64] Increased cardiovascular events in patients in use of choline metabolites.[65] | Not recommended |

Abbreviations: CHO, carbohydrate; CI, confidence interval; CVD, cardiovascular disease; DM, diabetes mellitus; FA, fatty acid; HCC, hepatocellular carcinoma; HDL, high-density lipoprotein cholesterol; MS, metabolic syndrome; MUFA, monosaturated fatty acid; NAFLD, nonalcoholic fatty liver disease; OR, odds ratio; PPAR-α, peroxisome proliferator-activated receptor α; PUFA, polyunsaturated fatty acid; RR, relative risk; SFA, saturated fatty acid; TG, triglycerides; US, ultrasound imaging; VLDL, very low density lipoprotein.
Data from Refs.[56–69]

Box 1
Recommendation for nutrition, lifestyle, and monitoring in patients with NAFLD

- Decrease calorie intake of about 500 to 1000 per day for patients who are overweight or obese.
- Reduction of total kcal per day to less than 30 kcal/kg.
- Target weight loss of 0.5 kg/week.
- Reduction on total fat intake of 30%.
- Prefer n-3 PUFA and MUFA instead of saturated fatty acids.
- Reduction of carbohydrates of 40% to 45% (restriction of simple and high glycemic carbohydrate).
- Avoid food high in fructose (sucrose – table sugar, corn syrup, honey, fruit juice concentrate or corn syrup solids).
- Limit red meat consumption.
- Vitamin E 800 IU daily (if nondiabetic and noncirrhotic).
- Vitamin D supplementation (if vitamin D levels <30 ng/mL).
- Physical activity, at least 150 min/week (moderate intensity aerobic) or 75 min/week (vigorous intensity aerobic).
- Use self-monitoring tools, diet, and exercise logs.
- Clinical visits at least 4 times a year.
- Reevaluation of nutrition status every year in stabilized patients.

Abbreviations: MUFA, monounsaturated fatty acids; NAFLD, nonalcoholic fatty liver disease; PUFA, polyunsaturated fatty acids.

---

psychologist) would likely be beneficial. The role of the psychologist is particularly important to address emotional eating and the high anxiety rates that likely contribute to unsuccessful weight reduction and poor adherence.[93] Patients should be encouraged to use support in the forms of other tools such as group meetings and diaries or mobile apps designed to record food intake and daily physical activity. The diaries and mobile apps may also serve as a measurement for clinicians to evaluate adherence.

Patients with decompensated liver cirrhosis with ascites or edema frequently complain about early satiety, nausea, vomiting, and diarrhea, and are unable to maintain a positive calorie balance. We recommend frequent small calorie-dense meals, including nighttime snacks for better tolerability and to avoid hypoglycemia and oxidative stress during starvation. Patients with ascites and edema should be on a 2 g/d sodium restriction.

Physical activity is undoubtedly an important strategy to improve weight loss maintenance and QOL. It is not the focus of this review, but readers should remember to include exercise recommendations during lifestyle intervention counseling. It is imperative to explain to patients that exercise is highly beneficial in reducing the risk of type 2 diabetes, insulin resistance, hypertension, dyslipidemia, impaired fasting glucose, and the metabolic syndrome.[94] It should be considered a part of treatment for those individuals.

Based on data regarding maintenance, primary providers should focus on the points presented in **Box 2** to avoid loss of adherence and weight gain.

Table 8
Recommendation in liver cirrhosis

Disease	Recommendation	Explanation
Liver cirrhosis	Do not restrict protein. Provide 1.2–1.5 g/kg/d (compensated) or 0.5 g/kg/d (if acutely decompensated). Incorporate "healthy" sources of protein (Greek yogurt, grilled or baked chicken). Avoid hypoglycemia. Smaller and frequent snacks and late-night snack.[88]	Protein–energy malnutrition has a negative impact. Patients are in a catabolic state requiring extra resources of calories and nutrients. Even patients with HE has better outcomes not avoiding protein resources.[87] Limited glycogen stores increase the risk of hypoglycemia. Fat oxidation and protein catabolism occurs early in starvation.[89]
	Restrict salt intake (2 g/d). Worsening of reduced food intake after this restriction. Alert for inadvertent ingestion of salt (drinks rich in salt, like soda, condiments). Avoid fluid restriction.	Patients decompensated in ascites present water retention secondary to hyperstimulate RAAS.[39] Salt restriction is the first step in ascites management. Hyponatremia is rare (<1.2%) and fluid restriction could precipitate hypovolemia or hypoperfusion.
	Maintain an intake of 35–40 kcal/kg/d.	Undernutrition is frequent in end-stage liver disease, owing to hypercatabolic state, and has a negative effect on liver-related complications and transplantation.[90]

Abbreviations: HE, hepatic encephalopathy; RAAS, renin–angiotensin–aldosterone system.
Data from Refs.[50–54]

Box 2
Points to be followed to help maintenance

- A clear explanation to patients about the benefits related to weight loss and physical activity. Provide clinical information and possible impact on disease evolution.

- Intensive monitoring for those who need 5% or more of weight loss – plan approximately 4 visits per year.

- Evaluate anxiety and depression, and provide clinical management or psychological consultation, avoiding 1 risk factor related to nonadherence.

- Frequently reassess dietary intake. Do not trust only on retrospective self-reports. Provide log or electronic food intake monitoring.

- Ancillary support: stress management, dietitian support, group meeting, and mobile apps.

- Recommend physical activity, at least 150 minutes per week of moderate intensity cardiovascular exercise or 75 minutes per week of vigorous intensity.

SUMMARY

Nutrition intervention is key in the management of patients with advanced cirrhosis and also in the treatment and prevention of NAFLD and its associated diseases and resulting complications. A thorough nutrition evaluation and intervention plan should be part of the management of patients with malnutrition, whether it is undernutrition or overnutrition. Although behavioral modification in the form of nutrition intervention requires time and effort on the part of health care providers, the benefits to the patients are immense. Strategies to prevent nonadherence should be established during clinical visits. Benefits from a healthy dietary pattern and physical activity outweigh disease modification, providing a better QOL and survival free of comorbidities.

REFERENCES

1. Mokdad AA, Lopez AD, Shahraz S, et al. Liver cirrhosis mortality in 187 countries between 1980 and 2010: a systematic analysis. BMC Med 2014;12(1):145.
2. Lozano R. Global and regional mortality from 235 causes of death for 20 age groups in 1990 and 2010: a systematic analysis for the Global Burden of Disease Study 2010. Lancet 2012;380(9859):2095–128.
3. Rinella ME. Nonalcoholic fatty liver disease. JAMA 2015;313(22):2263.
4. Lautz H, Selberg O, Korber J, et al. Protein calorie malnutrition in liver cirrhosis. Clin Investig 1992;70(6):478–86.
5. DiCecco S, Wieners E, Wiesner R, et al. Assessment of nutritional status of patients with end-stage liver disease undergoing liver transplantation. Mayo Clin Proc 1989;64(1):95–102.
6. Bellentani S, Scaglioni F, Marino M, et al. Epidemiology of non-alcoholic fatty liver disease. Dig Dis 2010;28(1):155–61.
7. Williams CD, Stengel J, Asike MI, et al. Prevalence of nonalcoholic fatty liver disease and nonalcoholic steatohepatitis among a largely middle-aged population utilizing ultrasound and liver biopsy: a prospective study. Gastroenterology 2011;140(1):124–31.
8. Mozundar A, Liguori G. Persistent increase of prevalence of metabolic syndrome among U.S. adults: NHANES III to NHANES 1999-2006. Diabetes Care 2011; 34(1):1–4.
9. Barrera F, George J. The role of diet and nutritional intervention for the management of patients with NAFLD. Clin Liver Dis 2014;18(1):91–112.
10. Anty R, Iannelli A, Patouraux S, et al. Alimentary pharmacology and therapeutics a new composite model including metabolic syndrome, alanine aminotransferase and cytokeratin-18 for the diagnosis of non-alcoholic steatohepatitis in morbidly obese patients. Aliment Pharmacol Ther 2010;32:1315–22.
11. Adams LA, Sanderson S, Lindor KD, et al. The histological course of nonalcoholic fatty liver disease: a longitudinal study of 103 patients with sequential liver biopsies. J Hepatol 2005;42(1):132–8.
12. Starley BQ, Calcagno CJ, Harrison SA. Nonalcoholic fatty liver disease and hepatocellular carcinoma: a weighty connection. Hepatology 2010;51(5):1820–32.
13. Wong RJ, Cheung R, Ahmed A. Nonalcoholic steatohepatitis is the most rapidly growing indication for liver transplantation in patients with hepatocellular carcinoma in the U.S. Hepatology 2014;59(6):2188–95.
14. Ong JP, Younossi ZM. Epidemiology and natural history of NAFLD and NASH. Clin Liver Dis 2007;11(1):1–16.
15. Finucane MM, Stevens GA, Cowan MJ, et al. National, regional, and global trends in body-mass index since 1980: systematic analysis of health examination

surveys and epidemiological studies with 960 country-years and 9·1 million participants. Lancet 2011;377(9765):557–67.

16. World Health Organization. Obesity and overweight. Geneva (Switzerland): World Health Organization; 2014. p. 311. Available at: http://www.who.int/mediacentre/factsheets/fs311/en/http://www.who.int/mediacentre/factsheets/fs311/en/.

17. Ferolla SM. Dietary approach in the treatment of nonalcoholic fatty liver disease. World J Hepatol 2015;7(24):2522.

18. Swinburn BA, Sacks G, Hall KD, et al. The global obesity pandemic: shaped by global drivers and local environments. Lancet 2011;378(9793):804–14.

19. Fontaine KR, Redden DT, Wang C, et al. Years of life lost due to obesity. J Am Med Assoc 2003;289(2):187–93.

20. Milić S, Lulić D, Stimac D. Non-alcoholic fatty liver disease and obesity: biochemical, metabolic and clinical presentations. World J Gastroenterol 2014;20(28): 9330–7.

21. Welzel TM, Graubard BI, Zeuzem S, et al. Metabolic syndrome increases the risk of primary liver cancer in the United States: a study in the SEER-Medicare database. Hepatology 2011;54(2):463–71.

22. Bechmann LP, Hannivoort RA, Gerken G, et al. The interaction of hepatic lipid and glucose metabolism in liver diseases. J Hepatol 2012;56(4):952–64.

23. Purnak T, Yilmaz Y. Liver disease and malnutrition. Best Pract Res Clin Gastroenterol 2013;27(4):619–29.

24. Asrih M, Jornayvaz FR. Diets and nonalcoholic fatty liver disease: the good and the bad. Clin Nutr 2014;33(2):186–90.

25. Musso G. Dietary habits and their relations to insulin resistance and postprandial lipemia in nonalcoholic steatohepatitis. Hepatology 2003;37(4):909–16.

26. Ouyang X, Cirillo P, Sautin Y, et al. Fructose consumption as a risk factor for non-alcoholic fatty liver disease. J Hepatol 2008;48(6):993–9.

27. Carter-Kent C, Zein NN, Feldstein AE. Cytokines in the pathogenesis of fatty liver and disease progression to steatohepatitis: implications for treatment. Am J Gastroenterol 2008;103(21):1036–42.

28. Xu A, Wang Y, Keshaw H, et al. The fat-derived hormone adiponectin alleviates alcoholic and nonalcoholic fatty liver diseases in mice. J Clin Invest 2003; 112(1):91–100.

29. Postic C, Girard J. Contribution of de novo fatty acid synthesis to hepatic steatosis and insulin resistance: lessons from genetically engineered mice. J Clin Invest 2008;118(3):829–38.

30. Assy N, Nassar F, Nasser G, et al. Olive oil consumption and non-alcoholic fatty liver disease. World J Gastroenterol 2009;15(15):1809–15.

31. Neuschwander-Tetri BA. Carbohydrate intake and nonalcoholic fatty liver disease. Curr Opin Clin Nutr Metab Care 2013;16(4):446–52.

32. Roglans N, Vilà L, Farré M, et al. Impairment of hepatic STAT-3 activation and reduction of PPARα activity in fructose-fed rats. Hepatology 2007;45(3):778–88.

33. Wei Y, Wang D, Topczewski F, et al. Fructose-mediated stress signaling in the liver: implications for hepatic insulin resistance. J Nutr Biochem 2007;18(1):1–9.

34. Liu S, Willett WC, Stampfer MJ, et al. A prospective study of dietary glycemic load, carbohydrate intake, and risk of coronary heart disease in US women 1–3. Am J Clin Nutr 2000;71:1455–61.

35. Hu Y, Block G, Norkus EP, et al. Relations of glycemic index and glycemic load with plasma oxidative stress markers. Am J Clin Nutr 2006;84(1):70–7.

36. Liou IW. Management of end-stage liver disease. Med Clin North Am 2014;98(1): 119–52.

37. Ginés P, Quintero E, Arroyo V, et al. Compensated cirrhosis: natural history and prognostic factors. Hepatology 1987;7(1):122–8.

38. Manne V, Saab S. Impact of nutrition and obesity on chronic liver disease. Clin Liver Dis 2014;18(1):205–18.

39. Runyon BA. Management of adult patients with ascites due to cirrhosis: an update. Hepatology 2009;49(6):2087–107.

40. Ueno T, Sugawara H, Sujaku K, et al. Therapeutic effects of restricted diet and exercise in obese patients with fatty liver. J Hepathol 1997;27(16):103–7.

41. Harrison SA, Fecht W, Brunt EM, et al. Orlistat for overweight subjects with nonalcoholic steatohepatitis: a randomized, prospective trial. Hepatology 2009;49(1): 80–6.

42. Tapper EB, Sengupta N, Hunink MGM, et al. Cost-effective evaluation of nonalcoholic fatty liver disease with NAFLD fibrosis score and vibration controlled transient elastography. Am J Gastroenterol 2015;110(9):1298–304.

43. Tapper E, Lai M. Weight loss results in significant improvements in quality of life for patients with nonalcoholic fatty liver disease: a prospective cohort study. Hepatology 2016;63:1184–9.

44. Montano-Loza AJ. Muscle wasting: a nutritional criterion to prioritize patients for liver transplantation. Curr Opin Clin Nutr Metab Care 2014;17(3):219–25.

45. Durand F, Buyse S, Francoz C, et al. Prognostic value of muscle atrophy in cirrhosis using psoas muscle thickness on computed tomography. J Hepatol 2014;60(6):1151–7.

46. Collins S. Using middle upper arm circumference to assess severe adult malnutrition during famine. JAMA 1996;276(5):391–5.

47. Detsky A, McLaughlin J, Baker J, et al. What is Subjective Global Assessment of nutritional status? Nutr Hosp 2008;23(4):400–7.

48. Álvares-da-Silva MR, Reverbel da Silveira T. Comparison between handgrip strength, Subjective Global Assessment, and prognostic nutritional index in assessing malnutrition and predicting clinical outcome in cirrhotic outpatients. Nutrition 2005;21:113–7.

49. Huang MA, Greenson JK, Chao C, et al. One-year intense nutritional counseling results in histological improvement in patients with nonalcoholic steatohepatitis: a pilot study. Am J Gastroenterol 2005;100(5):1072–81.

50. Keating SE, Hackett DA, George J, et al. Exercise and non-alcoholic fatty liver disease: a systematic review and meta-analysis. J Hepatol 2012;57(1):157–66.

51. Chavez-Tapia NC, Tellez-Avila FI, Barrientos-Gutierrez T, et al. Bariatric surgery for non-alcoholic steatohepatitis in obese patients. Cochrane Database Syst Rev 2010;(1):CD007340.

52. Anese M, Nicoli MC. Antioxidant properties of ready-to-drink coffee brews. J Agric Food Chem 2003;51:942–6.

53. Murase T, Misawa K, Minegishi Y, et al. Coffee polyphenols suppress diet-induced body fat accumulation by downregulating SREBP-1c and related molecules in C57BL/6J mice. Am J Physiol Endocrinol Metab 2011;300(1):E122–33.

54. Anty R, Marjoux S, Iannelli A, et al. Regular coffee but not espresso drinking is protective against fibrosis in a cohort mainly composed of morbidly obese European women with NAFLD undergoing bariatric surgery. J Hepatol 2012;57(5): 1090–6.

55. Molloy JW, Calcagno CJ, Williams CD, et al. Association of coffee and caffeine consumption with fatty liver disease, nonalcoholic steatohepatitis, and degree of hepatic fibrosis. Hepatology 2012;55(2):429–36.

56. Birerdinc A, Stepanova M, Pawloski L, et al. Caffeine is protective in patients with non-alcoholic fatty liver disease. Aliment Pharmacol Ther 2012;35(1): 76–82.

57. Bozzeto L, Prinster A, Costagliola L, et al. Liver fat is reduced by an isoenergetic MUFA diet in a controlled randomized study in type 2 diabetic patients. Diabetes Care 2012;35:1429–35.

58. Ryan MC, Itsiopoulos C, Thodis T, et al. The Mediterranean diet improves hepatic steatosis and insulin sensitivity in individuals with non-alcoholic fatty liver disease. J Hepatol 2013;59(1):138–43.

59. Joensen AM, Overvad K, Dethlefsen C, et al. Marine n-3 polyunsaturated fatty acids in adipose tissue and the risk of acute coronary syndrome. Circulation 2011;124(11):1232–8.

60. Sawada N, Inoue M, Iwasaki M, et al. Consumption of n-3 fatty acids and fish reduces risk of hepatocellular carcinoma. Gastroenterology 2012;142(7):1468–75.

61. Parker HM, Johnson NA, Burdon CA, et al. Omega-3 supplementation and non-alcoholic fatty liver disease: a systematic review and meta-analysis. J Hepatol 2012;56(4):944–51.

62. Papathanasopoulos A, Camilleri M. Dietary fiber supplements: effects in obesity and metabolic syndrome and relationship to gastrointestinal functions. Gastroenterology 2010;138(1):65–72.e1-2.

63. Ye E, Chacko S, Chou E, et al. Greater whole-grain intake is associated with lower risk of type 2 diabetes, cardiovascular disease, and weight gain. J Nutr 2012; 142(7):1304–13.

64. Abdelmalek MF, Sanderson SO, Angulo P, et al. Betaine for nonalcoholic fatty liver disease: results of a randomized placebo-controlled trial. Hepatology 2009;50: 1818–26.

65. Koeth RA, Wang Z, Levison BS, et al. Intestinal microbiota metabolism of l-carnitine, a nutrient in red meat, promotes atherosclerosis. Nat Med 2013;19(5): 576–85.

66. Utzschneider KM, Bayer-Carter JL, Arbuckle MD, et al. Beneficial effect of a weight-stable, low-fat/low-saturated fat/low-glycaemic index diet to reduce liver fat in older subjects. Br J Nutr 2013;109(6):1096–104.

67. van der Meer RW, Hammer S, Lamb HJ, et al. Effects of short-term high-fat, high-energy diet on hepatic and myocardial triglyceride content in healthy men. J Clin Endocrinol Metab 2008;93(7):2702–8.

68. Westerbacka J, Lammi K, Häkkinen AM, et al. Dietary fat content modifies liver fat in overweight nondiabetic subjects. J Clin Endocrinol Metab 2005;90(5): 2804–9.

69. Kontogianni MD, Tileli N, Margariti A, et al. Adherence to the Mediterranean diet is associated with the severity of non-alcoholic fatty liver disease. Clin Nutr 2014; 33:678–83.

70. de Luis D, Izaola A, Sagrado M, et al. Effect of two different hypocaloric diets in transaminases and insulin resistance in nonalcoholic fatty liver disease and obese patients. Hepatology 2012;53(1):730–5.

71. Haufe S, Engeli S, Kast P, et al. Randomized comparison of reduced fat and reduced carbohydrate hypocaloric diets on intrahepatic fat in overweight and obese human subjects. Hepatology 2011;53(5):1504–14.

72. Ryan MC, Abbasi F, Lamendola C, et al. Serum alanine aminotransferase levels decrease further with carbohydrate than fat restriction in insulin-resistant adults. Diabetes Care 2007;30(5):1075–80.

73. Tendler D, Lin S, Yancy WS, et al. The effect of a low-carbohydrate, ketogenic diet on nonalcoholic fatty liver disease: a pilot study. Dig Dis Sci 2007;52(2): 589–93.

74. Promrat K, Kleiner DE, Niemeier HM, et al. Randomized controlled trial testing the effects of weight loss on nonalcoholic steatohepatitis. Hepatology 2010;51(1): 121–9.

75. Rodríguez-Hernández H, Cervantes-Huerta M, Rodríguez-Moran M, et al. Decrease of aminotransferase levels in obese women is related to body weight reduction, irrespective of type of diet. Ann Hepatol 2011;10(4):486–92.

76. Elias MC, Parise ER, de Carvalho L, et al. Effect of 6-month nutritional intervention on non-alcoholic fatty liver disease. Nutrition 2010;26:1094–9.

77. Lin W-Y, Wu C-H, Chu N-F, et al. Efficacy and safety of very-low-calorie diet in Taiwanese: a multicenter randomized, controlled trial. Nutrition 2009;25(11–12): 1129–36.

78. Razavi Zade M, Telkabadi MH, Bahmani F, et al. The effects of DASH diet on weight loss and metabolic status in adults with non-alcoholic fatty liver disease: a randomized clinical trial. Liver Int 2016;36:563–71.

79. Sanyal AJ, Chalasani N, Kowdley K, et al. Pioglitazone, vitamin E, or placebo for nonalcoholic steatohepatitis. N Engl J Med 2010;362(18):1675–85.

80. Bjelakovic G, Nikolova D, Gluud L, et al. Mortality in randomized trials of antioxidant supplements for primary and secondary prevention systematic review and meta-analysis. JAMA 2007;297(8):842–57.

81. Ahmed A, Wong RJ, Harrison SA. Nonalcoholic fatty liver disease review: diagnosis, treatment, and outcomes. Clin Gastroenterol Hepatol 2015;13(12): 2062–70.

82. Harrison S. Vitamin E and vitamin C treatment improves fibrosis in patients with nonalcoholic steatohepatitis. Am J Gastroenterol 2003;98(11):2485–90.

83. Targher G, Bertolini L, Scala L, et al. Associations between serum 25-hydroxyvitamin D3 concentrations and liver histology in patients with non-alcoholic fatty liver disease. Nutr Metab Cardiovasc Dis 2007;17(7):517–24.

84. Kwok RM, Torres DM, Harrison SA. Vitamin D and nonalcoholic fatty liver disease (NAFLD): is it more than just an association? Hepatology 2013;58:1166–74.

85. Merli M, Riggio O, Romiti A, et al. Basal energy production rate and substrate use in stable cirrhotic patients. Hepatology 1990;12(1):106–12.

86. Muller M, Boker K, Selberg O. Are patients with liver cirrhosis hypermetabolic? Clin Nutr 1994;13(3):131–44.

87. Johnson TM, Overgard EB, Cohen AE, et al. Nutrition assessment and management in advanced liver disease. Nutr Clin Pract 2013;28(1):15–29.

88. Toshikuni N, Arisawa T, Tsutsumi M. Nutrition and exercise in the management of liver cirrhosis. World J Gastroenterol 2014;20(23):7286–97.

89. Kachaamy T, Bajaj JS. Diet and cognition in chronic liver disease. Curr Opin Gastroenterol 2011;27:174–9.

90. Fialla AD, Israelsen M, Hamberg O, et al. Nutritional therapy in cirrhosis or alcoholic hepatitis: a systematic review and meta-analysis. Liver Int 2015;35(9): 2072–8.

91. Douketis JD, Macie C, Thabane L, et al. Systematic review of long-term weight loss studies in obese adults: clinical significance and applicability to clinical practice. Int J Obes 2005;29(10):1153–67.

92. St George A, Bauman A, Johnston A, et al. Effect of a lifestyle intervention in patients with abnormal liver enzymes and metabolic risk factors. J Gastroenterol Hepatol 2009;24:399–407.

93. Stewart KE, Levenson JL. Psychological and psychiatric aspects of treatment of obesity and nonalcoholic fatty liver disease. Clin Liver Dis 2012;16(3): 615–29.
94. Haskell WL, Lee I, Pate RR, et al. Physical activity and public health: updated recommendation for adults from the American College of Sports Medicine and the American Heart Association. Circulation 2007;116(9):1081–93.

Nutrition Intervention in Cancer

David Heber, MD, PhD*, Zhaoping Li, MD, PhD

KEYWORDS

● Nutrition ● Cancer treatment ● Cancer prevention ● Malnutrition ● Cancer

KEY POINTS

● Nutrition intervention supports the patient with malnutrition secondary to cancer and its treatment.
● Nutrition intervention has been used in the primary and secondary prevention of common forms of cancer.
● The cancer patient is vulnerable and easily subject to nutritional claims for curing cancer from unqualified and sometimes dangerous practitioners.

INTRODUCTION

Nutrition intervention supports the patient with malnutrition secondary to cancer and its treatment and more recently has been used in the primary and secondary prevention of common forms of cancer.[1] During the emotional stress of dealing with a cancer risk or diagnosis at any stage, patients derive increased quality of life and a sense of control over their lives as the result of receiving supportive advice on diet and lifestyle. Therefore, the use of nutrition intervention in cancer patients is justified in the absence of absolute proof of efficacy as long as it is done safely and with the consent of the cancer patient. As will be repeatedly emphasized here, the cancer patient is vulnerable and easily subject to nutritional claims for curing cancer from unqualified and sometimes dangerous practitioners. Patient's families also read a great deal about the promise of nutrition for cancer in the popular press and must be educated as to its real and potential benefits for each patient's situation.

As the number of cancer survivors who have successfully completed therapy increases, together with a growing population of patients with ongoing preventive pharmacology based on small molecule pharmacotherapy, the demand for nutrition counseling to decrease risk of cancer recurrence or for general health is becoming

The authors do not have any commercial or financial conflicts of interest to disclose.
Department of medicine, Center for Human Nutrition, David Geffen School of Medicine at UCLA, Warren Hall, Room 12-217, 900 Veteran Avenue, Los Angeles, CA 90095, USA
* Corresponding author.
E-mail address: dheber@mednet.ucla.edu

more prevalent. The evidence base for nutrition intervention in these patients is drawn from a combination of extensive epidemiologic inference from association studies of the relationship of nutrition and physical activity to cancer and extensive animal studies showing cellular and molecular mechanisms of the interaction. There are limited nutrition intervention studies in humans, but the general advice given for cancer prevention is also beneficial in reducing the risks of other common age-related chronic diseases, such as diabetes and heart disease. In the absence of proven benefits of nutrition intervention in this population, the interventions should be based on generally accepted macronutrient ranges according to the Institute of Medicine guidelines and be based on results of clinical trials, which show a lack of adverse events when the nutrition interventions have been used.

MALNUTRITION AND CANCER

At the time of diagnosis, 80% of patients with upper gastrointestinal cancers and 60% of patients with lung cancer have significant weight loss,[2,3] defined as at least a 10% loss of body weight in the prior 6 months.[4] In addition, malnutrition is a common complication of patients undergoing chemotherapy, radiation, or surgery for cancer.

This common problem in cancer patients has been recognized as a significant contributor to morbidity and mortality in cancer. Malnutrition is associated with a decreased quality of life in cancer patients, and significant weight loss is a biomarker of poor prognosis in cancer patients.[3] Nutrition intervention can help cancer patients maintain body weight and nutrition stores, offering relief from symptoms and improving their quality of life.[5] Poor nutrition practices, which can lead to undernutrition, can contribute to the incidence and severity of treatment side effects and increase the risk of infection and mortality in cancer patients.[6]

Anorexia, nausea, vomiting, diarrhea, constipation, stomatitis, mucositis, dysphagia, alterations in taste and smell, pain, depression, and anxiety all occur as complications of malnutrition in cancer patients.[7] Nutrition screening can be used to detect malnutrition early and reduce the risk for malnutrition. Nutrition screening is an important component in the development of standards of quality of care in oncology practices and in general medical and surgery practices caring for cancer patients and their families.[3]

Although weight loss is traditionally associated with cancer in the minds of professionals and the public, weight gain can occur as the result of chemotherapy treatment for early-stage cancers, possibly resulting from decreases in lean body mass and resting metabolism.[8] This is especially common in postmenopausal women with breast cancer who have sarcopenic obesity after treatment. Sarcopenic obesity is found to be a risk factor for breast cancer progression.[9] Obesity has also been associated with increased mortality in prostate cancer.[10] The nutrition of cancer patients should be assessed throughout the continuum of care to reflect changing objectives of nutrition intervention.

TUMOR-HOST INTERACTION AND PROTEIN-ENERGY MALNUTRITION

Protein-energy malnutrition (PEM) is the most common secondary diagnosis in individuals with cancer. PEM results most commonly from inadequate intake of macronutrients needed to meet energy requirements. In addition to reduced food intake, several associated abnormalities can combine to worsen malnutrition, including reduced absorption of macronutrients secondary to changes in the gastrointestinal tract. Altered taste sensation can contribute to anorexia, whereas physical barriers to the ingestion or digestion of food are common in head and neck cancer patients and patients with gastrointestinal cancer such as pancreatic and esophageal cancers. Cancer-induced metabolic abnormalities secondary to inflammation affect the metabolism of the major nutrients including glucose and protein. Such abnormalities may include glucose intolerance and insulin resistance, increased lipolysis, and increased whole-body protein turnover.[11] PEM leads to progressive wasting, weakness, and debilitation, as protein synthesis is reduced and lean body mass is lost, often leading to death.[3]

Anorexia, the loss of appetite or desire to eat, is typically present in 15% to 25% of all cancer patients at diagnosis and may also occur as a side effect of treatments. Anorexia is an almost universal side effect in individuals with widely metastatic disease[12,13] secondary to chemotherapy and radiation therapy side effects, which lead to taste and smell changes, nausea, and vomiting. Surgical treatments such as esophagectomy and gastrectomy, may produce early satiety and lead to reduced food intake.[4] Common psychological factors in cancer patients, such as depression, loss of hope, anxiety, and morbid thoughts, may be enough to bring about anorexia and result in PEM.[2] Evidence-based recommendations have been published describing various approaches to the problems of cancer-related fatigue, anorexia, depression, and dyspnea.[14] Other systemic or local effects of cancer or its treatment that may affect nutritional status include sepsis, malabsorption, maldigestion, and intestinal obstruction.[11]

NUTRITION SCREENING

Nutrition intervention in cancer care embodies prevention of disease, treatment, cure, or supportive palliation. Prudence should always be exercised when considering alternative or unproven nutritional therapies for 2 reasons. First, these diets or supplements may prove harmful. Second, these diets may delay prudent and effective therapies, as was the case for Steve Jobs who had a treatable tumor of the pancreas (an insulinoma) that was not diagnosed promptly because of the use of ineffective herbal treatments for many months. On the other hand, some physicians provide patients with anticancer dietary supplements while not emphasizing diet and lifestyle changes. Proactive nutritional care can prevent or reduce the complications typically associated with the treatment of cancer.[15]

Whether the goal of cancer treatment is cure or palliation, early detection of nutritional problems and prompt intervention are essential. Nutrition screening and nutrition assessment should be instituted by all the members of the health care team caring for the cancer patient, including physicians, nurses, registered dietitians, social workers, and psychologists.[7] The Prognostic Nutrition Index,[16,17] delayed hypersensitivity skin testing, institution-specific guidelines, and anthropometrics are all tools that can be used effectively to identify patients at nutritional risk. The selection of nutrition screening tools must be individualized and interpreted in light of clinical factors, as the various biomarkers can be affected by immune incompetence, inflammation, and hydration status.[18]

The Patient-Generated Subjective Global Assessment (PG-SGA) is a simple and inexpensive approach to identifying individuals at nutritional risk and in triaging cancer patients for nutritional intervention.[3,19] The PG-SGA is based on an earlier protocol called the Subjective Global Assessment (SGA).[20] With the PG-SGA, the individual or caretaker complete sections on weight history, food intake, symptoms, and function. Bioelectrical impedance analysis (BIA) is also used to assess nutritional status, as determined by body composition.[21] Single BIA measures show body cell mass, extracellular tissue, and fat as a percentage of ideal, whereas sequential measurements can be used to show body composition changes over time. BIA is increasingly becoming available in ambulatory settings, and its use should be encouraged. With estimation of lean body mass, estimates of resting energy expenditure can be made by multiplying lean body mass by 14. This calculation can guide nutritional interventions for weight gain or weight loss. The goals of nutrition intervention include:

1. Preserving or increasing lean body mass
2. Reducing fatigue and improving quality of life
3. Correcting specific nutrition deficiencies
4. Improving tolerance of cancer therapy
5. Reducing side effects and complications related to nutrition
6. Enhancing immunity and decreasing the risk of infection
7. Promoting recovery and healing

SELECTING APPROPRIATE METHODS OF NUTRITION CARE

The first rule of nutrition intervention is to use the gut when it is available, and the preferred method of nutrition support is via the oral route using food. Dietary modifications can be made with the help of a registered dietitian to reduce the symptoms associated with cancer treatments. Appetite stimulants may be used to enhance the enjoyment of foods and to facilitate weight gain in the presence of significant anorexia.[22] Suggestions for appetite improvement include the following.[23]

1. Establish a daily menu and record food intake.
2. Eat small, frequent, high-calorie meals.
3. Arrange for help in preparing meals.
4. Add extra protein and calories to food.
5. Prepare and store small portions of favorite foods.
6. Consume one-third of daily protein and calorie requirements at breakfast.
7. Snack between meals with nuts or other healthy foods when possible.
8. Seek foods that appeal to the sense of smell.
9. Be creative with desserts.
10. Experiment with different foods.
11. Perform frequent mouth care to relieve symptoms and decrease unpleasant tastes.

Supplemental enteral nutrition in the form of protein powders added to foods or liquid nutritional supplement between meals are indicated when the gastrointestinal tract is functional, but oral intake may be insufficient to meet nutritional needs. Individual characteristics of patients who can benefit from nutrition intervention include:

1. Significant weight loss defined as less than 80% of preillness usual weight or recently experienced unintentional weight loss of more than 10% of usual weight
2. Clinical malabsorption owing to digestive disease, short bowel syndrome, or side effects of cancer therapy
3. Intestinal obstruction, fistulas, or draining abscesses
4. Absence of significant food intake for more than 5 days

DELIVERY OF ENTERAL NUTRITION

Enteral nutrition is often needed in patients with cancers of the head and neck regions, esophagus, and stomach. Nasogastric tubes and such tubes that extend into the duodenum or jejunum are best suited for short-term support (<2 weeks).[24] Enteral feeding into the jejunum is appropriate for patients at risk of aspiration. However, if the patient is at high risk of aspirating, enteral nutritional support is contraindicated, and parenteral nutrition should be considered. Moreover, patients with mucositis or esophagitis, and those who are immunocompromised and have herpetic, fungal, or candida lesions in the mouth or throat may not be able to tolerate the presence of a nasogastric tube.

Percutaneous endoscopic gastrostomy tubes and percutaneous endoscopic jejunostomy tubes are needed for long-term enteral feedings for more than 2 weeks. Enteral nutrition can be delivered at different rates and durations. Bolus feedings that mimic meals are preferable because this method requires less time and equipment, offers greater flexibility to the patient, and enables normal physiologic and hormonal mechanisms to operate.[24]

When administering bolus or intermittent enteral feeding, the following steps should be followed:

1. Determine the calorie, nutrient, and free-water requirements to plan the feeding schedule. Dehydration will occur if adequate water is not included in the formulation, typically at 1 mL per calorie administered.
2. Administer bolus feedings 3 to 6 times per day. It is possible to give 250 to 500 mL over 10 to 15 minutes as long as the patient tolerates these amounts without undue gastric distension.
3. Bolus feeding is only to be used when a nasogastric tube is in the stomach. Bolus feeding is contraindicated when feedings are delivered into the duodenum or jejunum, as gastric distention and dumping syndrome can occur.
4. Administer the bolus feeding using a gravity drip from a bag or syringe or a slow push with the syringe.
5. Change the amount of formula given at a time, the type of formula, or added ingredients in the formula if diarrhea, a common side effect of this type of infusion, is encountered.

When instituting continuous or cyclic enteral feeding, the following steps should be followed:

1. Determine the caloric/nutrient and free-water requirements to plan rate and timing recommendations whether continuous or cyclic infusions.
2. Use a controlled enteral feeding pump that provides reliable, constant infusion rates to decrease the risk of gastric retention.
3. Initiate feeding into the stomach at rates of 25 to 30 mL/h and start at 10 mL/h into the jejunum (10 mL/h), and then increase rates as tolerated every 4 to 6 hours until the rate needed to deliver the required caloric/nutrient needs is reached.
4. If continuous feeding is used, it can be run at night to allow greater flexibility for the patient. In addition, night feeding can be combined with bolus feedings during the day to provide a more normal lifestyle for the patient.

Once the infusion method has been determined, a formula is selected. When a formula is being chosen, the institution nutrition formulary for available preparations, modular formulas, and additions such as glutamine or fiber should be considered. Consideration should also be given to the patient's medical condition, gastrointestinal function, and financial resources. Enteral formulas from elemental preparations of predigested nutrients to more complete and complex formulas that mimic oral nutrition intake are available. More information on specific formulas and their ingredients and properties can be obtained from the manufacturers. There are also specialized formulas designed for specific disease conditions, including diabetes mellitus and compromised renal function, but the additional benefits of these formulas may not justify their cost, and the need for these should be carefully considered.

PARENTERAL NUTRITION

Parenteral nutrition is only required in patients who are unable to use the oral or enteral route. If the gut is working, use it. Nutrients provided through the enteral route nourish the gut epithelium and provide better overall nutrition and involve the gut peptides, which enhance insulin action. Patients with obstruction, intractable nausea vomiting, short-bowel syndrome, or ileus may require parenteral nutrition, but there are no advantages to cancer care simply because total parenteral nutrition (TPN) is perceived to be a more aggressive form of nutrition than enteral nutrition. Additional reasons to use TPN in the cancer population are severe diarrhea/malabsorption, severe mucositis or esophagitis, high-output gastrointestinal fistulas that cannot be bypassed by enteral intubation, or severe preoperative malnutrition.[24] The decision to use parenteral nutrition in patients with advanced cancer is difficult. The widespread use of TPN as was done in the 1970s and 1980s is not advised, as there is no evidence of improved survival in patients with advanced cancer.[25,26] Most data point to the same conclusion: health care providers should not prescribe parenteral nutrition to patients with advanced, incurable cancer. A meta-analysis summarized findings from 15 clinical trials. Parenteral nutrition led to inferior survival, lower tumor response rates, and increased infection rate. The increased infection rate persisted even after catheter-related sepsis was excluded. This observation bolsters recommendations from recent, guidelines that suggest parenteral nutrition may not be in the best interest of patients with advanced, incurable cancer.[27]

DIET AND CANCER PREVENTION: THE ROLE OF COLORFUL FRUITS AND VEGETABLES

International studies of the food habits of several different populations over the last 40 years have clearly documented the diversity of human dietary patterns and defined those associated with a lower risk of chronic diseases including common forms of cancer.[28] Compared with the diet of Americans, dietary patterns including a consistently higher intake of fruits, vegetables, whole grains, and plant proteins such as soy are associated with a markedly reduced risk of cancer. In the nutritional science and epidemiologic literature, these dietary patterns have often been characterized as simply low-fat, high-fiber diets, or the intake of vegetables was quantitated as a single phytochemical such as β-carotene.[29] Such simplified terminologies led to the concept that fiber or phytochemical supplementation could reproduce the benefits of the healthy dietary patterns they represented.

The idea that a dietary pattern conferred its benefits through a single component led to trials that purported to test one component of the diet in an American population while all other variables were held constant. When research based on these flawed concepts was conducted, the expected benefits were not realized for fiber supplementation[30] or β-carotene supplementation.[31] This finding led to a series of publications resulting from intervention trials, which have been interpreted as evidence that nutrition simply does not work in cancer prevention. On the other hand, findings from international studies suggest that for some cancers of the aerodigestive tract, a 50% reduction in risk is associated with intakes of 400 to 600 g/d of fruits and vegetables.[28] The challenge for nutrition scientists is to translate this scientific information into dietary guidelines that result in healthful changes in dietary patterns.

Over the last 200 years, a series of uniquely American foods have been developed through adaptation from other cultures: pizza made with oil added to the crust and large amounts of melted cheese, potato chips, corn chips, peanut butter, hot dogs, hamburgers made with beef fat flavoring, and profitable soft drinks made with corn sugar and artificial flavors.[32] Westernized Chinese food is among the highest-fat foods in America because it was adapted from low-fat Chinese versions to meet American tastes. Moreover, refried beans or frijoles have added lard or vegetable oil in the Mexican-American adaptation of beans eaten in Mexico and South America without added fat. Special offers of larger portions delivering an extra 800 kcal for only an additional 39 cents have made fast food restaurants especially popular with teenagers, low-income Americans, and the elderly. These foods have displaced the fruits, vegetables, and whole grains recommended in the US Dietary Guidelines, and consumers have increasingly reduced their commitments to cooking healthy meals and eating as a family over the last few decades.

We are now separated from the system that enabled us to select foods according to color and taste. Humans and a few primate species have trichromatic color vision so that they are able to distinguish red from green.[33] All other mammals have dichromatic vision and cannot distinguish between the 2 colors. One hypothesis for the evolution of this visual ability was that it conferred an advantage by enabling primates to distinguish red fruits from the green background of forest leaves. Today colors are still used to promote food choices, as most fast food restaurants package their beige French fries in a red cardboard package. Contrasting colors have been shown to be one of the key factors in food selection by Drewnowski.[34] A new method for selecting fruits and vegetables based on colors keyed to the content of phytochemicals is described as a way of translating the science of phytochemical nutrition into dietary guidelines for the public. Most Americans eat only 2 to 3 servings of fruits and vegetables per day without regard to the phytochemical contents of the foods being eaten. Certain phytochemicals give fruits and vegetables their colors and also indicate their unique physiologic roles. All of the colored phytochemicals that absorb light in the visible spectrum have antioxidant properties. In artificial membrane systems, it is possible to show synergistic interactions of lutein and lycopene in antioxidant capacity, and there are well-known antioxidant interactions of vitamin C and vitamin E based on their solubility in hydrophilic and hydrophobic compartments of cells.

However, many phytochemicals have other functions beyond acting as antioxidants. For example, lycopene stabilizes the connexin 43 gene product that is essential for gap junction communication[35] while also interacting with vitamin D in the differentiation of HL-60 leukemia cells.[36] In breast cancer cells, lycopene can interfere with insulinlike growth factor 1–stimulated tumor cell proliferation.[37] Lycopene levels in the blood are associated with a reduced risk of prostate cancer,[38] and lycopene administration may reduce proliferation and increase apoptosis in human prostate tissue in which lycopene is the predominant carotenoid.[39] Lutein is concentrated in the retina, where it may help prevent macular degeneration, the most common preventable form of age-related blindness.[40] Other studies have found that lycopene, α-carotene, and β-carotene are associated with a reduced risk of lung cancer.[41] Based on a recent review of functional properties of foods[42] and research from our laboratories showing that it is relatively simple to influence circulating levels of lycopene with administration of only 177 mL (6 fluid ounces) of mixed vegetable juice daily,[43] we developed a color code for a book aimed at helping consumers change dietary patterns to include more fruits and vegetables by including one serving from each of 7 color groups each day selected based on the family of phytochemicals they contain (What Color Is Your Diet? Harper-Collins, 2001)[44] (**Table 1**).

Although the color method is superior to the current system of simply encouraging increased fruit and vegetable intake, it does not account for actual phytochemical delivery to the consumer. Today, there is no labeling law that enables fruit and vegetable manufacturers to list the phytochemicals in their products. Fruits and vegetables are developed and grown less for their flavor and nutritional content and more to

Table 1
The color code relationship to families of phytochemicals

Color	Phytochemical	Fruits and Vegetables
Red	Lycopene	Tomatoes and tomato products such as juice, soups, and pasta sauces
Red-purple	Anthocyanins and polyphenols	Grapes, blackberries, red wine, raspberries, blueberries
Orange	α-Carotene and β-Carotene	Carrots, mangos, pumpkin
Orange-yellow	β-Cryptoxanthin and flavonoids	Cantaloupe, peaches, tangerines, papaya, oranges
Yellow-green	Lutein and zeaxanthin	Spinach, avocado, honeydew melon
Green	Glucosinolates and indoles	Broccoli, bok choi, kale
White-green	Allyl sulfides	Leeks, garlic, onion, chives

accommodate the need to transport these products over long distances and extend their shelf life once they get to market. Finally, research in this area needs to continue on the greater than 25,000 phytochemicals provided by fruits and vegetables, including those that do not have color, such as isoprenoids.[45] These important phytochemicals are widely distributed among different plant species, but the delivery of phytochemicals and their effects on biomarkers relevant to cancer prevention need to be documented.

OBESITY AND CANCER

Obesity is defined as excess body fat, so studies examining the association between body mass index and height/weight ratio, may underestimate the effects of obesity on common forms of cancer. Unfortunately, body mass index is the only practical measure for large-scale epidemiologic studies. In 2003, a study that included more than 900,000 American adults followed up with the healthy study participants for 16 years and found the heaviest participants were more likely to develop and die from cancer than participants who were at a healthy weight.[46] The results were interpreted as showing that excess fat "could account for 14% of all deaths from cancer in men and 20% of those in women."

An important consideration when assessing the epidemiology linking obesity to cancer pathogenesis is the growing recognition that obesity is a heterogeneous condition. Among US adults, for example, approximately 30% of individuals who are obese are considered metabolically healthy, whereas approximately 23% of normal-weight adults are defined as metabolically unhealthy.[47] Thus, the body weight that is predictive of cancer progression and mortality is likely to be influenced by many covariants, including genetics, aerobic fitness and daily physical activity, age, and an individual's metabolic and endocrine profile. The assessment of such phenotypic traits is important in providing insights into the causal role of obesity-related metabolic abnormalities on prostate cancer progression.

The scientific understanding of fat cell function has shifted from purely a cellular fat and energy storage site to one that has both endocrine and metabolic importance over the last few decades. This understanding has led to several mechanisms implicated in how obesity drives cancer prevalence and cancer deaths. Currently, there are 4 categories into which these mechanisms fall—increased lipids and lipid signaling, inflammatory responses, insulin resistance, and adipokines.

Adipose tissue is a complex organ that consists of multiple cell types including adipocytes, adipocyte progenitor cells, mesenchymal stem cells, endothelial cells, and various resident and infiltrating immune cells.[48] It is unlikely that adipose tissue expansion per se is responsible for the development of obesity-associated complications, but complications become evident when adipocyte hypertrophy occurs in the absence of appropriate neovascularization.[49] Adipocytes are active endocrine cells responsible for the biosynthesis and secretion of a many hormones and cytokines that have a variety of biological functions.[50] Screening studies have identified approximately 170 adipokines including adiponectin, leptin, retinol-binding protein 4, pigment epithelium–derived factor, visfatin, vascular endothelial growth factor, transforming growth factor β and various acute phase reactants.[51] Protein secretion from adipocytes is modulated by a variety of processes including transcription, translation, posttranslational modifications, and secretion through classical and various nonclassical pathways.[52] Dysfunction of the expanded adipose tissue is postulated to significantly alter the adipokine secretion profile in obesity, in turn, altering endocrine and paracrine/autocrine signaling that is postulated to impact both the systemic circulation or local tumor microenvironment in obese patients.

Adipose tissue can become infiltrated with macrophages, neutrophils, T cell and B cells, and mast cells during the development of obesity.[49] Hence, low-grade or subclinical chronic inflammation may provide a permissive or protumorigenic endocrine or paracrine environment in obese individuals. It has long been recognized that inflammation is a predisposing factor for cancer initiation and progression, and chronic inflammation is now regarded as an enabling characteristic of human cancer.[53]

Adipose tissue also expresses the estrogen-metabolizing enzyme, aromatase. Low testosterone in aging men is typically combined with higher estrogen levels, comparable to the level detected in postmenopausal women.[54] Sarcopenic obesity with excess body fat is found to be a risk factor for progression of breast cancer in postmenopausal women. Estradiol levels (and aromatase activity) are positively correlated with body fat mass and, more specifically, to subcutaneous abdominal fat but not to visceral fat.[55]

Although there is a gathering body of research in this field, our knowledge of the interrelationship between obesity and cancer development or progression is limited. Understanding the endocrine and metabolic pathways that play roles in disease progression and malignancy is important for identifying potential therapeutic avenues to slow cancer growth and metastasis.

REFERENCES

1. Heber D, Blackburn G, Milner J. Nutritional oncology. 2nd edition. San Diego (CA): Acadmemic Press; 2006.
2. Bruera E. ABC of palliative care. Anorexia, cachexia, and nutrition. BMJ 1997; 315(7117):1219–22.
3. McMahon K, Decker G, Ottery FD. Integrating proactive nutritional assessment in clinical practices to prevent complications and cost. Semin Oncol 1998;25(2 Suppl 6):20–7.
4. Rivadeneira DE, Evoy D, Fahey TJ III, et al. Nutritional support of the cancer patient. CA Cancer J Clin 1998;48(2):69–80.
5. American Cancer Society. Nutrition for the person with cancer:a guide for patients and families. 2015. [Ref Type: Internet Communication]. http://www.cancer.org/acs/groups/cid/documents/webcontent/002903-pdf.pdf.

6. Vigano A, Watanabe S, Bruera E. Anorexia and cachexia in advanced cancer patients. Cancer Surv 1994;21:99–115.

7. Tchekmedyian NS, Halpert C, Ashley J, et al. Nutrition in advanced cancer: anorexia as an outcome variable and target of therapy. JPEN J Parenter Enteral Nutr 1992;16(6 Suppl):88S–92S.

8. Harvie MN, Campbell IT, Baildam A, et al. Energy balance in early breast cancer patients receiving adjuvant chemotherapy. Breast Cancer Res Treat 2004;83(3): 201–10.

9. Prado CM, Baracos VE, McCargar LJ, et al. Sarcopenia as a determinant of chemotherapy toxicity and time to tumor progression in metastatic breast cancer patients receiving capecitabine treatment. Clin Cancer Res 2009;15(8):2920–6.

10. Hsing AW, Sakoda LC, Chua S Jr. Obesity, metabolic syndrome, and prostate cancer. Am J Clin Nutr 2007;86(3):s843–57.

11. Heber D, Byerley LO, Chi J, et al. Pathophysiology of malnutrition in the adult cancer patient. Cancer 1986;58(8 Suppl):1867–73.

12. Langstein HN, Norton JA. Mechanisms of cancer cachexia. Hematol Oncol Clin North Am 1991;5(1):103–23.

13. Shills M. Nutrition and diet in cancer management. Modern nutrition in health and disease. Baltimore (MD): Williams & Wilkins; 1999. p. 1317–47.

14. Tisdale MJ. Cancer cachexia. Anticancer Drugs 1993;4(2):115–25.

15. Dewys WD, Begg C, Lavin PT, et al. Prognostic effect of weight loss prior to chemotherapy in cancer patients. Eastern Cooperative Oncology Group. Am J Med 1980;69(4):491–7.

16. Dempsey DT, Mullen JL. Prognostic value of nutritional indices. JPEN J Parenter Enteral Nutr 1987;11(5 Suppl):109S–14S.

17. Dempsey DT, Mullen JL, Buzby GP. The link between nutritional status and clinical outcome: can nutritional intervention modify it? Am J Clin Nutr 1988; 47(2 Suppl):352–6.

18. Sarhill N, Mahmoud FA, Christie R, et al. Assessment of nutritional status and fluid deficits in advanced cancer. Am J Hosp Palliat Care 2003;20(6):465–73.

19. Bauer J, Capra S, Ferguson M. Use of the scored Patient-Generated Subjective Global Assessment (PG-SGA) as a nutrition assessment tool in patients with cancer. Eur J Clin Nutr 2002;56(8):779–85.

20. Ottery FD. Rethinking nutritional support of the cancer patient: the new field of nutritional oncology. Semin Oncol 1994;21(6):770–8.

21. Lukaski HC. Requirements for clinical use of bioelectrical impedance analysis (BIA). Ann N Y Acad Sci 1999;873:72–6.

22. Seligman PA, Fink R, Massey-Seligman EJ. Approach to the seriously ill or terminal cancer patient who has a poor appetite. Semin Oncol 1998;25(2 Suppl 6): 33–4.

23. Ottery FD. Supportive nutrition to prevent cachexia and improve quality of life. Semin Oncol 1995;22(2 Suppl 3):98–111.

24. Heys SD, Walker LG, Smith I, et al. Enteral nutritional supplementation with key nutrients in patients with critical illness and cancer: a meta-analysis of randomized controlled clinical trials. Ann Surg 1999;229(4):467–77.

25. Bozzetti F. Effects of artificial nutrition on the nutritional status of cancer patients. JPEN J Parenter Enteral Nutr 1989;13(4):406–20.

26. Chlebowski RT. Critical evaluation of the role of nutritional support with chemotherapy. Cancer 1985;55(1 Suppl):268–72.

27. Jeffcoat R, Kirkwood S. Implication of histidine at the active site of exo-beta-(1-3)-D-glucanase from Basidiomycete sp. QM 806. J Biol Chem 1987;262(3):1088–91.

28. Glade MJ. Food, nutrition, and the prevention of cancer: a global perspective. American Institute for Cancer Research/World Cancer Research Fund, American Institute for Cancer Research, 1997. Nutrition 1999;15(6):523–6.
29. Garewal HS, Schantz S. Emerging role of beta-carotene and antioxidant nutrients in prevention of oral cancer. Arch Otolaryngol Head Neck Surg 1995;121(2): 141–4.
30. Alberts DS, Martinez ME, Roe DJ, et al. Lack of effect of a high-fiber cereal supplement on the recurrence of colorectal adenomas. Phoenix Colon Cancer Prevention Physicians' Network. N Engl J Med 2000;342(16):1156–62.
31. The effect of vitamin E and beta carotene on the incidence of lung cancer and other cancers in male smokers. The Alpha-Tocopherol, Beta Carotene Cancer Prevention Study Group. N Engl J Med 1994;330(15):1029–35.
32. Schlosser E. Fast food nation. Boston: Houghton Mifflin; 2001.
33. Dominy NJ, Lucas PW. Ecological importance of trichromatic vision to primates. Nature 2001;410(6826):363–6.
34. Drewnowski A. From asparagus to zucchini: mapping cognitive space for vegetable names. J Am Coll Nutr 1996;15(2):147–53.
35. Stahl W, von LJ, Martin HD, et al. Stimulation of gap junctional communication: comparison of acyclo-retinoic acid and lycopene. Arch Biochem Biophys 2000; 373(1):271–4.
36. Amir H, Karas M, Giat J, et al. Lycopene and 1,25-dihydroxyvitamin D3 cooperate in the inhibition of cell cycle progression and induction of differentiation in HL-60 leukemic cells. Nutr Cancer 1999;33(1):105–12.
37. Karas M, Amir H, Fishman D, et al. Lycopene interferes with cell cycle progression and insulin-like growth factor I signaling in mammary cancer cells. Nutr Cancer 2000;36(1):101–11.
38. Gann PH, Ma J, Giovannucci E, et al. Lower prostate cancer risk in men with elevated plasma lycopene levels: results of a prospective analysis. Cancer Res 1999;59(6):1225–30.
39. Kucuk O, Sarkar FH, Sakr W, et al. Phase II randomized clinical trial of lycopene supplementation before radical prostatectomy. Cancer Epidemiol Biomarkers Prev 2001;10(8):861–8.
40. Mares-Perlman JA, Fisher AI, Klein R, et al. Lutein and zeaxanthin in the diet and serum and their relation to age-related maculopathy in the third national health and nutrition examination survey. Am J Epidemiol 2001;153(5):424–32.
41. Heber D. Colorful cancer prevention: alpha-carotene, lycopene, and lung cancer. Am J Clin Nutr 2000;72(4):901–2.
42. Milner JA. Functional foods: the US perspective. Am J Clin Nutr 2000;71(6 Suppl): 1654S–9S.
43. Heber D, Yip I, Go VLW, et al. Plasma carotenoids profiles in prostate cancer patients after dietary intervention [Ref Type: Abstract]. FASEB J 2000;14.
44. Heber D. What color is your diet? Harper-Collins; 2002.
45. Elson CE. Novel lipids and cancer. Isoprenoids and other phytochemicals. Adv Exp Med Biol 1996;399:71–86.
46. Calle EE, Rodriguez C, Walker-Thurmond K, et al. Overweight, obesity, and mortality from cancer in a prospectively studied cohort of U.S. adults. N Engl J Med 2003;348(17):1625–38.
47. Wildman RP, Gu D, Muntner P, et al. Trends in overweight and obesity in Chinese adults: between 1991 and 1999-2000. Obesity (Silver Spring) 2008;16(6): 1448–53.

48. Khandekar MJ, Cohen P, Spiegelman BM. Molecular mechanisms of cancer development in obesity. Nat Rev Cancer 2011;11(12):886–95.

49. Rutkowski JM, Davis KE, Scherer PE. Mechanisms of obesity and related pathologies: the macro- and microcirculation of adipose tissue. FEBS J 2009;276(20): 5738–46.

50. Galic S, Oakhill JS, Steinberg GR. Adipose tissue as an endocrine organ. Mol Cell Endocrinol 2010;316(2):129–39.

51. Crowe S, Wu LE, Economou C, et al. Pigment epithelium-derived factor contributes to insulin resistance in obesity. Cell Metab 2009;10(1):40–7.

52. Zadra G, Photopoulos C, Loda M. The fat side of prostate cancer. Biochim Biophys Acta 2013;1831(10):1518–32.

53. Hanahan D, Weinberg RA. Hallmarks of cancer: the next generation. Cell 2011; 144(5):646–74.

54. Colangelo LA, Ouyang P, Liu K, et al. Association of endogenous sex hormones with diabetes and impaired fasting glucose in men: multi-ethnic study of atherosclerosis. Diabetes Care 2009;32(6):1049–51.

55. Vermeulen A, Kaufman JM, Goemaere S, et al. Estradiol in elderly men. Aging Male 2002;5(2):98–102.

Nutrition Interventions for Obesity

Jamy D. Ard, MD[a],*, Gary Miller, PhD[b], Scott Kahan, MD, MPH[c]

KEYWORDS

- Obesity • Dietary therapy • Energy balance • Weight loss
- Maintenance of weight loss • Weight-reducing diet

KEY POINTS

- Obesity is a complex, chronic disease that requires a period of negative energy deficit followed by restoration of energy balance to successfully reduce body weight.
- Multiple dietary strategies have been shown to be effective for reducing body weight. The particular components of the dietary strategy, including macronutrient balance, amount of energy deficit, and foods/food types, can have an impact on adherence and comorbid risk factors.
- Maintenance of weight loss of 3% or more of body weight can lead to significant improvements in risk factors. Specific guidance should be provided on strategies that are most effective for weight loss maintenance to help sustain risk factor improvements and reduce body weight.

INTRODUCTION

Obesity is among the most prevalent chronic diseases in the United States and much of the world, contributing to substantial morbidity, mortality, and health care expenditures. Nearly every health care professional has to manage obesity or comorbid conditions related to obesity. The most recent NHANES (National Health and Nutrition Examination Survey) data show that 36.5% of American adults fit the definition of obesity.[1] Prevalence of obesity is significantly higher in certain subgroups, with Hispanic Americans and African Americans having rates of 42.5% and 47.8%, respectively.[2] Globally, approximately 600 million people have obesity, with more of the world's inhabitants overweight than underweight, and most of the world's population living in countries where overweight and obesity cause more deaths than underweight.[3]

---

[a] Department of Epidemiology and Prevention, Wake Forest School of Medicine, Winston Salem, NC, USA; [b] Department of Health and Exercise Science, Wake Forest University, Winston Salem, NC, USA; [c] Department of Health Policy and Management, Milken Institute School of Public Health, George Washington University, Washington, DC, USA
* Corresponding author.
E-mail address: jard@wakehealth.edu

Med Clin N Am 100 (2016) 1341–1356
http://dx.doi.org/10.1016/j.mcna.2016.06.012
0025-7125/16/$ – see front matter © 2016 Elsevier Inc. All rights reserved.

medical.theclinics.com

Although the causes of obesity are multifactorial, the common pathway is a sustained state of positive energy balance, leading to an increase in fat mass. The excess accumulation and storage of adipose tissue that defines obesity leads to a wide array of comorbid conditions. To successfully treat obesity, the primary tenet of nutrition therapy is to create a negative energy balance, leading to reduction of fat stores that are being used as a source of energy. Weight loss of 3% or more of body weight can lead to clinically meaningful improvements in risk factors associated with obesity. This article provides an overview of obesity and its classification, dietary strategies for treatment, expected outcomes and challenges, and considerations for successful maintenance of weight loss. It discusses specific nutrition considerations for patients with obesity and common comorbid conditions, and addresses several popular claims for diets and weight loss supplements.

Background and Classification

Obesity is a condition of excess accumulation and storage of adipose tissue, which is a metabolically active tissue that has many bodily functions in addition to energy storage, including hormone synthesis and thermoregulation. Obesity is associated with nearly 200 comorbid conditions, including cardiometabolic disorders (eg, type 2 diabetes, cardiovascular disease, hypertension, dyslipidemia), gastrointestinal disorders (eg, gallbladder disease, pancreatitis, esophageal reflux), mechanical disorders (eg, osteoarthritis of weight-bearing joints, hypoventilation), numerous cancers, and mental health conditions (eg, depression), as well as functional limitations and decreased health-related quality of life.[4]

Obesity is most commonly defined by body mass index (BMI; body weight [kg [/height [meters] squared) greater than or equal to 30 kg/m^2. For adults, a normal BMI is defined as 18.5 to 25 kg/m^2, overweight as BMI 25 to 29.9 kg/m^2, and obesity as BMI greater than or equal to 30 kg/m^2, with severe obesity defined as BMI greater than or equal to 40 kg/m^2 (**Table 1**). BMI is highly correlated with total body fat, based on studies of body composition using various techniques in the general population, and is positively associated with morbidity and mortality.[5-7] However, BMI has several limitations. First, BMI does not distinguish fat from lean mass. BMI can underestimate body fat in older adults, because people tend to lose lean mass and accumulate fat mass with age; conversely, very lean individuals with high muscle mass, such as highly trained athletes, have less body fat than predicted by calculated BMI.[8] Next, as with any attempt to categorize a continuous phenomenon, the association with other disease risks in the lower ranges of abnormal BMI (ie, overweight) are not as consistent on an individual level.[7] In addition, BMI does not account for body fat distribution, which can alter risk associations. Visceral adipose tissue, most commonly found in

Table 1
BMI classification

Weight Classification	BMI (kg/m^2)
Underweight	<18.5
Normal weight	18.5–24.9
Overweight	25–29.9
Obesity class 1	30–34.9
Obesity class 2	35–39.9
Obesity class 3	40+

truncal/abdominal obesity, is metabolically active tissue and a promoter of systemic inflammation and insulin resistance via secretion of adipokines, which increases risk for cardiovascular disease, type 2 diabetes, and carcinogenesis.[9,10] Subcutaneous fat accumulation is generally associated with lower metabolic risk, although some evidence suggests that subcutaneous fat accumulation in the abdominal area may contribute to insulin resistance and inflammation.[11,12]

Several proposed obesity classifications combine anthropometric and clinical criteria to define obesity and obesity risk. These staging systems, such as the Edmonton Obesity Staging System and the American Association of Clinical Endocrinologists staging algorithm, include obesity comorbid conditions and functional limitations to provide a broader classification scheme of obesity[13,14] (**Table 2**). Preliminary data suggest that staging systems may have higher correlation with morbidity and mortality risk, compared with BMI alone, and therefore may aid clinicians in determining appropriate intensity of treatment strategies for each individual (ie, patients with higher stages of obesity are likely to be at greater risk of morbidity and mortality from obesity and thus may be more appropriate candidates for aggressive obesity treatment modalities, compared with lower stage patients), although further research is necessary.[15]

DIETARY STRATEGIES FOR OBESITY TREATMENT
Creating an Energy Deficit

Weight loss requires inducing and sustaining a state in which total energy expenditure is greater than energy intake (ie, an energy deficit), resulting in the use of stored fat as a source of energy. Although this principle is often communicated to patients in a message of eat less and exercise more, understanding the multifactorial contributions to weight gain and the rationale and nuances of evidence-based strategies can lead to more effective treatment and counseling. This article focuses on nutritional contributions to energy balance and other nutritional considerations for obesity management.

In adults, the primary components for total daily energy expenditure (TDEE) include resting metabolic rate (RMR), energy expenditure of activity (AEE), and thermic effect of food (TEF). For sedentary individuals, RMR represents roughly two-thirds of TDEE

Table 2
Edmonton Obesity Staging System

Stage	Obesity-related Medical Risk Factors/Comorbidities	Obesity-related Physical Symptoms/Comorbidities or Functional Limitations	Obesity-related Mental Health or Psychosocial Symptoms/Comorbidities
0	None	None	None
1	Mild/subclinical (eg, borderline hypertension, IFG)	Mild (eg, fatigue, dyspnea on exertion)	Mild
2	Established (eg, hypertension, type 2 diabetes)	Moderate	Moderate
3	End-organ damage (eg, CAD, CHF)	Significant	Significant
4	Severe/end stage	Severe	Severe

Abbreviations: CAD, coronary artery disease; CHF, congestive heart failure; IFG, impaired fasting glucose.

with AEE comprising 15% to 25% and the TEF contributing ~8% of TDEE. The energy balance equation is a thermodynamic process that incorporates both TDEE and energy intake. With a sustained positive balance (ie, energy intake greater than energy expenditure), overweight and obesity develop. In contrast, a prolonged negative energy balance with energy expenditure being greater than energy intake changes the energy balance to negative and leads to weight loss.

Reducing daily energy intake to create an energy deficit can be accomplished through several types of dietary changes. These changes include reducing portion sizes, using meal replacement products to reduce dietary choice and caloric intake, choosing more nutrient-dense and less energy-dense foods, or altering macronutrient composition, glycemic index/load, meal frequency, or eating pattern. Controlling portion sizes is often achieved through use of prepackaged foods, such as meal replacements. Prepackaged foods are commonly in the form of shakes or bars, but may also include meals of whole foods that are allocated in set portions (eg, frozen meals or preprepared meals). These foods are regularly promoted as a low-calorie product and several studies have shown their effectiveness for weight loss.[16–18] Altering food choices to limit high-energy foods, such as sugar-sweetened beverages and high-fat and high-sugar baked goods, and replacing these with foods that are lower in energy and higher in micronutrients, water, and fiber increases satiety and reduces energy density. The notion that humans eat a certain volume of food, independent of total energy content, led to the strategy to increase food volume through reducing energy density.[19–21] In the short term, consuming a food with a low energy density, such as soup or salad, before a meal reduces total energy intake for a single meal and for multiple meals when consumed over 1 to 2 days.[22–25] Furthermore, counseling to reduce energy density through increasing fruit and vegetable intake, along with decreasing fat intake, showed greater weight loss than was seen in a group that was only instructed on reducing fat intake.[26] This evidence formed the basis for the 2010 Dietary Guidelines recommendation to follow an eating pattern with a low energy density to manage body weight.

The role of macronutrients and other dietary factors

Unique combinations of macronutrient levels are often prescribed for weight loss. Because proteins, carbohydrates, and lipids have different effects on energy metabolism, appetite, and satiety, it is intuitive to consider that altering the proportion of macronutrients in diets with similar total calories will cause weight loss and body composition changes. Furthermore, the energy density of the diet may be changed in isocaloric diets differing in macronutrient composition. Because of the finite capacity for storing protein and carbohydrate in the body, and the nearly limitless capacity for fat storage, the body must have an ability to acutely regulate protein and carbohydrate balance.[27] How dietary macronutrient content affects the body's energy balance depends to some extent on the energy state of the body (ie, in a negative, positive, or neutral energy balance). In carefully controlled feeding studies, there is no significant difference in weight loss when reducing fat or carbohydrate content of the diet as long as there is similar total energy reduction. In contrast, during ad libitum intake, there are differences in weight loss between high-fat versus low-fat diets.[28–30] This difference is attributed to the higher diet-induced thermogenesis and lower energy intake with carbohydrates and proteins versus fat.[31,32]

Manipulating dietary protein levels (25%–35% of energy as protein) has been favored as a dietary strategy for weight loss and post–weight-loss regain. High-protein diets are thought to increase diet-induced thermogenesis, as well as reduce energy intake through altering satiety hormones, both of which promote a negative energy balance.[33–36] In ecological studies and randomized controlled trials, high-protein diets have favorable weight management outcomes.[37–40] However, clinically meaningful weight loss can occur across a broad range of macronutrient compositions, particularly varying proportions of carbohydrates and fats, which are the most commonly varied among dietary recommendations and claims.[41] In a study that examined 4 diets that varied in content of fat (20%–40%), protein (15%–25%), and carbohydrates (35%–65%), there was similar weight loss among the interventions over a 2-year period. There were no differences in hunger and satiety ratings for all diets.

It is well known that there is a wide interindividual variation in weight loss between dietary strategies. The variation in response can potentially be mitigated by identifying factors that modify the effect of a given dietary intervention. For example, evidence from subgroup analyses suggests that the weight loss response on high-carbohydrate or low-carbohydrate diets is related to insulin sensitivity, with a better response seen with a low-carbohydrate versus a high-carbohydrate diet in insulin-resistant, but not insulin-sensitive, individuals.[42–44] Despite these findings, most of the current evidence suggests that the average weight loss responses to a wide range of dietary macronutrient patterns and other dietary manipulations are similar and generally a function of compliance and the energy restriction achieved.[7] One relevant example based on the recent popularization of the concept is the use of low-glycemic-index/low-glycemic-load diets for weight loss. Low-glycemic-index foods produce a lesser and more gradual increase in blood glucose levels, leading to less stimulation of insulin secretion.[45] Glycemic load is calculated as the total carbohydrate of the food (grams) multiplied by the glycemic index value of the food divided by 100. One of the CALERIE (Comprehensive Assessment of Long term Effects of Reducing Intake of Energy) trials assessed a high-glycemic-load diet compared with a low glycemic load diet in the setting of a 30% calorie restriction.[46] After a feeding period of 6 months, both groups self-administered assigned dietary plans for an additional 6 months. There were no differences in weight loss at 12 months for both groups (8% for high vs 7.8% for low).[46] Future research needs to address variable responses in the setting of different diet compositions and nutrient profiles, and in different genetic and biological makeups.

Ultimately, the future direction of obesity intervention will be to prescribe personalized nutrient profiles to match the specific needs of individual patients. Interindividual responses to specific foods create an opportunity to design prescriptions that lead to optimized outcomes compared with general guidelines.[47] The targets for individualization could include specific dietary patterns (eg, low glycemic load or decreased sugar intake), exclusion of certain nutrients (eg, gluten), specific dietary supplements, nutritional alteration of the microbiome, or consideration of biological factors (eg, degree of insulin sensitivity). Because the targets involved in energy homeostasis are myriad, the keys to unlocking the interaction between the nutrient environment and energy balance may ultimately include genotyping, metabolomics, and proteomics to direct nutrient therapy. However, these concepts are currently in the domain of potential future use as research and technology improve. At present, the most promising nutrition consideration for obesity is managing energy balance.

MODIFYING DIET COMPOSITION TO ADDRESS ASSOCIATED RISK FACTORS

Dietary patterns and compositions can be used to address specific cardiometabolic risk factors in the context of a weight-reducing diet. In this manner, a specific dietary pattern leads to a specific type of response in the cardiometabolic profile, allowing targeted intervention. For example, a low-carbohydrate, high-fat diet has been associated with significant improvements in triglycerides, high-density lipoprotein cholesterol, and blood glucose levels in people with type 2 diabetes.[48,49] The DASH (Dietary Approaches to Stop Hypertension) dietary pattern, which features high intakes of fruits, vegetables, low-fat dairy, and whole grains, has been used as the basis of a weight reduction diet targeted for people with greater than normal blood pressure and stage I hypertension. In the Pounds Lost clinical trial, specific patterns of improvements in cardiometabolic risk factors were evident across 4 diets that varied in fat (20%–40%), protein (15%–25%), and carbohydrate (35%–65%) content.[41] The highest carbohydrate diet had the greatest decrease in low-density lipoprotein level, whereas the lowest carbohydrate diet had the greatest increase in high-density lipoprotein level. The high-protein diet had the largest decrease in fasting serum insulin level. Consistent with these results, Shai and colleagues[50] showed improvements in blood lipids with low-fat and low-carbohydrate dietary interventions, but the low-carbohydrate diet had a greater reduction in the ratio between total cholesterol and high-density lipoprotein. Note that they also found more favorable cardiometabolic effects in individuals with diabetes in patients on a Mediterranean diet pattern versus low-fat diet. Thus, specific dietary recommendations may have more to do with goals for improvements in obesity-associated comorbid conditions than any expected differences in average weight loss from the dietary pattern.

Consistent with these results, most weight loss claims of popular diets are unsubstantiated, as was recently codified by the obesity management guidelines led by the National Heart, Lung, and Blood Institute and published jointly by the American Heart Association, American College of Cardiology, and The Obesity Society.[7] As part of an in-depth systematic review process, a key question was included about which is the best diet for weight loss. Seventeen popular diets were reviewed, including the American Heart Association Step 1, ADA diet, low-carbohydrate and Atkins-type diets, low-fat diets, low-glycemic-index diets, vegetarian and vegan diets, DASH diets, Zone diets, and Mediterranean diets. There was no clearly superior dietary approach, beyond finding a pattern that leads to moderately reduced caloric intake. Importantly, the guidelines recommend respecting patients' preferences; thus, personal preference, rather than diet claims, are a key factor in macronutrient dietary prescription. Moreover, generally healthful dietary recommendations, and eliminating or minimizing sugar-sweetened beverages, should be considered for any dietary approach.

PROMOTING ADHERENCE WITH AN APPROPRIATE DIETARY PRESCRIPTION

Overall, trials comparing a wide variety of macronutrient distributions have found weight loss success in nearly all types of hypocaloric diets.[51] This finding suggests adherence to a reduced energy diet as the main driving force for weight loss success.[41,52,53] Thus, finding a diet that is palatable and fits with the lifestyle of the individual is a key to effective weight loss. For some, this may be achieved with a high-carbohydrate diet, whereas others may prefer a high-fat or high-protein diet. This approach is consistent with the Pounds Lost findings, by Sacks and colleagues,[41] discussed earlier, which showed that adhering to the macronutrient intake goal with a hypocaloric diet was associated with increased weight loss. In this study, group means for satisfaction with the diet, as well as satiety and hunger, were not different across 4 groups that had different target intakes for protein, fat, and carbohydrates. Importantly, there was a loss in dietary adherence over the 1-year follow-up period, showing the difficulty in long-term adherence to a dietary plan that is different from the person's habitual diet.

EXPECTED WEIGHT LOSS OUTCOMES

Similar to the management of many other chronic diseases, the goal of obesity treatment is to improve health and long-term risk, not necessarily to rid the body of obesity (eg, a treatment goal of diabetes management is to improve glycemic control to achieve a hemoglobin A1c level <7%, not necessarily to achieve a normal hemoglobin A1c level). There is strong evidence for health and comorbidity improvement with small weight losses. Sustained weight loss of 3% to 5% of initial body weight is likely to improve triglyceride levels, glycemic control, and risk of developing type 2 diabetes.[7] Sustained loss of 5% to 10% of initial body weight generally ameliorates or improves numerous other comorbid conditions and risk factors (eg, blood pressure, hepatic steatosis, urinary incontinence), although improvements in some risk factors and obesity-associated conditions (eg, low-density lipoprotein [LDL] cholesterol, sleep apnea, nonalcoholic steatohepatitis) may require greater weight losses for meaningful clinical improvement.[7,54–56]

As described earlier, reduction of body fat is accomplished by negative energy balance via changes in energy intake or expenditure. Expected rate of weight loss is traditionally estimated by reduced energy intake and/or increased energy expenditure by 3500 kcal to lose 450 g (1 pound). Thus, a 500 kcal/d energy deficit would theoretically lead to 450 g/wk of body weight loss. However, this general rule does not account for dynamic physiologic adaptations during weight loss, such as alterations in resting energy expenditure and increased muscle efficiency, thereby overestimating weight loss results.

These compensatory adaptations make evolutionary sense in that they counter sustained negative energy balance related to famine. More complex mathematical models have been developed that account for these metabolic adjustments during negative energy balance. In one such model, Hall and colleagues[57] predict greater than 10 kg difference in weight loss using the static linear model of the 3500-kcal rule versus their dynamic model, which incorporates energy expenditure changes with weight loss. Thus, when using the 3500-kcal/450 g value, patients typically experience less rapid weight loss and may fail to reach their expected weight loss goals, even for those strictly adhering to their target behavioral goals. On average, weight losses of up to 8 kg have been observed at 1 year in behavioral interventions that include a prescribed energy deficit diet combined with frequent behavioral counseling and a prescription for increased physical activity.[7] The weight loss nadir is generally observed at about 6 months of intervention with maintenance of weight loss achieved with continued intervention through 12 months. The nadir at 6 months is commonly observed as a weight loss plateau, and is, in part, attributed to these metabolic adaptations to energy expenditure in the setting of persistent low energy intake.

In light of these physiologic adaptations that occur with weight loss, in addition to the obesogenic environment that makes sustained decreases in dietary intake difficult to maintain over long periods, it is important to manage expectations and communicate realistic expectations for both the rate of expected weight loss and long-term weight loss goals. Several studies of individuals beginning weight loss programs show that weight loss expectations wildly exceed what is realistic. For example, in one study of 60 patients beginning a clinical trial of behavioral weight loss, subjects reported mean goal weight loss of 33% of initial body weight; an amount that exceeds the average weight loss with bariatric surgery.[58] At a minimum, health care providers should proactively work with patients to negotiate realistic weight loss and behavioral goals, informed by the type of strategy used (eg, very-low-calorie diets [VLCDs] using meal replacement products generally lead to faster initial rates of weight loss, whereas a food-based deficit diet may require a longer period to achieve a similar weight loss) and life circumstances (ie, realistic weight loss may be lower during periods of life transition, such as job changes). Importantly, goal setting should include non–weight-specific goals (eg, improvements in physical functioning, risk factors, quality-of-life indices).

TROUBLESHOOTING AND COMMON COMPLICATIONS
Limited Weight Loss

Patients with less than their expected weight loss are a challenging consideration. The clinician's role is to systematically review key components of the intervention, with the goal of reinforcing consistent use of evidence-based tools that are effective for promoting sustained adherence to behaviors that promote a negative energy balance. With any behavioral intervention, it can be expected that the level of engagement and degree of adherence will decline over time on average.[59] However, brief and focused interactions can help patients refocus efforts and lead to modifications in the prescription that enhance weight loss.

Self-monitoring is the most common tool that can be easily used to help identify deviations from the dietary prescription or areas for adjustment. Patients should generally be encouraged to self-monitor dietary intake on a daily basis because this is one of the behaviors that are most commonly associated with achieving clinically meaningful weight loss.[60] A brief review of 1 to 2 weeks of food records can help the clinician identify deviations that might not be readily obvious to the patient. Deviations most often seen in clinical practice include skipping prescribed meals and snacks, longer intervals between eating episodes, and incorrect diet composition. A more thorough review can also reveal inadequate portion control and underestimation of calorie intake.

When none of these common patterns of deviation from the prescribed dietary intake is obvious, refining the dietary prescription may be necessary. Decreasing the calorie prescription is often the first consideration. Other than reducing portion sizes or eating episodes, calories can often be reduced by using meal replacements or substituting less-energy-dense food options for more-calorie-dense foods (eg, whole fruit for dried fruit snacks). These options preserve the nutrient density of the prescription while allowing maintenance of satiation. Altering macronutrient balance is a second level of adjustment that can be attempted in cases of limited weight loss. The food record can be the basis for making this adjustment; clinicians can recommend changes that are substantively different from the current macronutrient intake that is resulting in limited weight loss. For example, the clinician could recommend that a patient shift approximately 10% of calories from the group that represents the highest percentage of calorie intake into 2 other macronutrient groups (eg, shift 10% of carbohydrate calories into lean protein and unsaturated fat).

Weight Loss Plateau

As noted previously, many behavioral interventions for obesity have a weight loss nadir at approximately 6 months. When patients report maintenance of behaviors that previously resulted in weight loss but are no longer able to achieve reductions in weight, this represents a weight loss plateau. At this point, the negative energy balance is diminished largely because of metabolic adaptations in energy expenditure resulting from the previously discussed compensatory mechanisms designed to protect against loss of body mass. RMR decreases substantially with energy restriction, and, because it is the largest component of TDEE, this has a significant effect on the resulting energy balance.[61–63] RMR declines as body mass decreases, because less energy is required for movement and maintenance. Furthermore, the decrease in RMR with weight loss can be attributed to alterations in hormones and the autonomic nervous system that conserve energy. Energy restriction also reduces physical activity energy expenditure in weight-dependent activities, resulting in fewer calories burned for a given task.[61] For example, a 100-kg patient who previously burned 100 calories when walking 1.6 km (1 mile) would now burn fewer calories after a 10% weight reduction because of improved exercise efficiency and decreased workload.

Basic Considerations for Dealing with a Weight Loss Plateau

Many of the same techniques used to address limited weight loss can also be implemented to help patients work through a weight loss plateau (eg, altering macronutrient balance, portion controls, meal replacements). Ultimately, the goal is to find the new combination of energy intake and activity energy expenditure that leads to an energy deficit that is sufficient to resume weight loss. Although further calorie restriction may seem an obvious target, this strategy has limitations. Further reduction of calories may only force more aggressive adaptation at this point, sending signals to the brain that the low-calorie environment is persistent and even more severe. Alternatively, clinicians typically elect to increase calories in small increments ($\sim$100 calories/d) along with alterations in the exercise program that circumvent the efficiencies recently gained with ongoing training. This approach leads to a higher energy flux state, which has been hypothesized to be more favorable for allowing expenditure of stored excess energy as heat; the primary adaptation that is altered in the weight loss plateau.[64]

Risks Associated with Weight Reduction Strategies

Although the benefits of weight reduction generally outweigh the risks, clinicians should be aware of potential complications and advise patients when precautions are necessary. Rapid weight loss, defined as greater than 1.5 kg/wk, has been associated with an increased risk of symptomatic gallstones.[65] VLCDs (ie, <800 kcal/d), which are associated with higher rates of weight loss, were thought to lead to gallstones in 10% to 25% of participants.[66] The largest report to date of 3320 consecutively enrolled patients in a VLCD commercial weight-loss program in Sweden showed that the incidence of gallstones was higher compared with matched controls on a low-calorie diet (LCD), but that the overall risk of gallstones requiring hospital care was low (152 per 10,000 person years for the VLCD compared with 44 for the LCD).[67] Differences in contemporary rates of symptomatic gallstones in people attempting to lose weight may be a result of higher dietary fat intakes in many modern weight loss strategies relative to the very low fat intakes that dominated in the 1980s and 1990s. These very low fat intakes may have contributed to bile stasis because fat intake decreased below a threshold needed to stimulate gallbladder contraction.[68]

Other medical concerns that are seen more frequently in high-risk patients include symptoms, such hypoglycemia and hypotension, resulting from the overtreatment of comorbid conditions. Individuals with type 2 diabetes and hypertension are at risk for adverse events if medication management is not done expectantly. Individuals on insulin or oral hypoglycemics such as sulfonylureas should have medications adjusted based on initial level of glycemic control and degree of calorie restriction. Antihypertensive medications can lead to postural hypotension along with symptoms of lightheadedness and dizziness if blood pressure decreases in response to the weight reduction intervention. In addition, antihypertensive regimens with significant amounts of diuretics can increase the risk of dehydration in patients with more rapid weight loss responses to calorie restriction, especially if sodium intake is decreased concomitantly.

Less serious but more commonly occurring side effects of weight loss and reduced calorie intake can include hair loss, changes in bowel patterns and habits, muscle cramping, and fatigue. Hair loss is generally a function of the duration and intensity of exposure to a low calorie intake. This type of hair loss, known as telogen effluvium, is a reactive response to lower energy intake and generally recovers spontaneously within 6 months of restoring energy balance (ie, during maintenance).[69] Changes in bowel habits are typically associated with changes in dietary fiber content and can be mitigated by supplementing fiber if the dietary plan is lower (eg, a lower-carbohydrate dietary plan). Cramping and fatigue are often related and can be associated with minor electrolyte disturbances such as low levels of sodium, calcium, or magnesium. These symptoms are more likely to occur when electrolytes are not replaced adequately after strenuous exercise routines, when the patient is taking diuretics, or when insensible losses are high because of warm temperatures.

WEIGHT MAINTENANCE STRATEGIES

The compensatory changes that occur in response to weight loss also make it more challenging to maintain weight loss long term. Ultimately, successful weight loss maintenance is a function of engaging in a consistent pattern of increased physical activity while maintaining a dietary pattern and energy intake that is appropriate for the new, lower body weight.

Benefits of Physical Activity in Weight Maintenance

Metabolic benefits occur from exercise training that facilitate weight loss maintenance. The preservation of lean body mass during dietary restriction is the most commonly mentioned factor that benefits weight loss maintenance. The level of calories burned during physical activity is related to weight loss at long-term (18–36 months) follow-up.[70,71] Women who achieved at least a 10% weight loss after 24 months of behavioral weight loss therapy reported activity energy expenditure of 1515 kcals/wk, compared with fewer than 500 kcals/wk in those achieving less than 0% to 5% weight loss at 24 months.[71] The recent 2014 obesity guidelines from American College of Cardiology/American Heart Association/The Obesity Society also suggest that exercise reduces weight regain with VLCDs.[7] These same guidelines prescribe at least 150 minutes of aerobic physical activity per week for weight loss with 200 to 300 min/wk for maintaining lost weight or reducing weight regain. However, most of these data are from secondary analyses from randomized controlled trials or from observational studies and do not fully answer the question of the role for physical activity in weight loss maintenance or the regain of lost weight. Several investigations have shown that, when programs are compared with varying combinations of low or high amounts of activity and exercise intensity, there is minimal impact on weight loss and weight loss maintenance.[71,72]

Role of Diet Composition in Weight Maintenance

Over the long-term, most individuals struggle with maintaining their lost weight. It has been theorized that diet composition may be critical in weight loss maintenance. Because the energy efficiencies of metabolic pathways vary, macronutrient content may influence energy expenditure, as well as dietary adherence.[73] This theory was tested in a crossover feeding trial of 3 isocaloric diets that varied in fat, carbohydrate, and glycemic load during the weight maintenance period following a 10% to 15% weight loss in overweight and obese young adults.[74] Reductions in energy expenditure (RMR and TDEE) from the pre–weight-loss period baseline were greatest in a low-fat diet compared with a very-low-carbohydrate diet, with the low-glycemic-index diet being intermediate between the two. Furthermore, leptin and triiodothyronine (T3) levels were lowest, and insulin sensitivity was highest, in the very-low-carbohydrate diet compared with the low-fat diet. Moreover, the differences in energy expenditure with the diets are not from lower T3 levels, because the lowest T3 level was seen with the diet that had the least decline in energy expenditure.

The DIOGENES (Diet, Obesity and Genes) dietary study also comprehensively studied the impact of varying protein intakes and glycemic loads on weight maintenance following 8 weeks of weight loss induced by an 800 kcal/d diet.[38] Participants were provided with food for the first 6 months, followed by self-administered plans supported by a dietitian for the remaining 6 months. The high-protein groups (23%–28% of calories) regained 2 kg less at 12 months than the groups consuming low-protein diets (10%–15% of calories).[75] However, there was no consistent effect of the assigned dietary glycemic index on maintenance of weight loss. These results show that metabolic effects during weight loss maintenance differ based on macronutrient content, with protein intake showing the most consistent effects on promoting successful weight loss maintenance.

DIETARY SUPPLEMENTS FOR WEIGHT LOSS

Dietary supplements should be mentioned in any discussion of weight interventions. Herbal and dietary supplements for weight loss can be attractive, because they commonly promise near-miraculous benefits, seemingly without risk. Despite increasing sales and use of over-the-counter (OTC) weight loss products, there are minimal, if any, data supporting benefits for weight management.[76–78] Unlike US Food and Drug Administration (FDA)–approved treatments, dietary supplements are not required to be proved effective, and few have rigorous clinical trial evidence assessing efficacy and safety. When scientific studies are conducted, the results are disappointing. A 2004 systematic review of 25 clinical trials covering 10 popular supplements showed "no evidence beyond a reasonable doubt that any specific dietary supplement was effective for reducing body weight."[79] A 2010 review of published systematic reviews for 9 popular weight loss supplements concluded that none are supported by sound evidence.[80] However, there are 2 OTC options to consider for weight management. The first is the FDA-approved OTC version of orlistat, a prescription medication that was initially approved by the FDA in 1999. Several studies support the utility of orlistat for long-term weight management. One study showed that orlistat (at prescription dose of 120 mg, which is twice the dose available OTC) in combination with a behavioral weight loss intervention based on the Diabetes Prevention Program leads to 10% body weight loss over 1 year, maintenance of most of this weight loss through 4 years, and 45% decreased development of diabetes.[81] Various versions of fiber supplements may also be reasonable to use as dietary supplementation. Fiber-related supplements may support weight control by increasing satiety or slowing digestion. The most commonly used fiber supplement is psyllium, which has been shown to cause small weight losses and improvements in some cardiovascular risk factors.[82] At recommended levels, the risk of adverse effects is low.

SUMMARY

Obesity is an extremely common disorder with a complex cause. The ongoing epidemic has spurred significant advances in the understanding of nutritional approaches to treat obesity. Although the primary challenge is to introduce a dietary intake that creates an energy deficit, clinicians should also consider targeted risk factor modification with specific manipulation of the nutrient profile of the weight-reducing diet. These strategies are broadly effective in producing clinically significant weight loss and associated improvements in cardiometabolic risk factors. Future research is needed to better understand how to personalize nutrient prescriptions further to promote optimal risk modification and maintenance of long-term energy balance in the weight-reduced state.

REFERENCES

1. Ogden CL, Carroll MD, Fryar CD, et al. Prevalence of obesity among adults and youth: United States, 2011-2014. NCHS Data Brief 2015;(219):1–8.
2. Ogden CL, Carroll MD, Kit BK, et al. Prevalence of childhood and adult obesity in the United States, 2011-2012. JAMA 2014;311(8):806–14.
3. World Health Organization. 2015. Available at: www.who.int/mediacentre/factsheets/fs311/en/. Accessed January 19, 2016.
4. Yuen MM, Kahan S, Kaplan LM, et al. A systematic review and evaluation of current evidence reveals 195 obesity-associated disorders. Poster: The Obesity Society 2016, in press.
5. Garrow JS, Webster J. Quetelet's index (W/H2) as a measure of fatness. Int J Obes 1985;9(2):147–53.
6. Prospective Studies C, Whitlock G, Lewington S, et al. Body-mass index and cause-specific mortality in 900 000 adults: collaborative analyses of 57 prospective studies. Lancet 2009;373(9669):1083–96.
7. Jensen MD, Ryan DH, Apovian CM, et al. 2013 AHA/ACC/TOS guideline for the management of overweight and obesity in adults: a report of the American College of Cardiology/American Heart Association Task Force on Practice Guidelines and The Obesity Society. Circulation 2014;129(25 Suppl 2):S102–38.
8. Villareal DT, Apovian CM, Kushner RF, et al, American Society for Nutrition, NAASO, The Obesity Society. Obesity in older adults: technical review and position statement of the American Society for Nutrition and NAASO, The Obesity Society. Obes Res 2005;13(11):1849–63.
9. Kershaw EE, Flier JS. Adipose tissue as an endocrine organ. J Clin Endocrinol Metab 2004;89(6):2548–56.
10. Lee MJ, Wu Y, Fried SK. Adipose tissue heterogeneity: implication of depot differences in adipose tissue for obesity complications. Mol Aspects Med 2013;34(1):1–11.
11. Snijder MB, Zimmet PZ, Visser M, et al. Independent and opposite associations of waist and hip circumferences with diabetes, hypertension and dyslipidemia: the AusDiab Study. Int J Obes Relat Metab Disord 2004;28(3):402–9.
12. Patel P, Abate N. Role of subcutaneous adipose tissue in the pathogenesis of insulin resistance. J Obes 2013;2013:489187.
13. Sharma AM, Kushner RF. A proposed clinical staging system for obesity. Int J Obes 2009;33(3):289–95.
14. Garvey WT, Garber AJ, Mechanick JI, et al. American Association of Clinical Endocrinologists and American College of Endocrinology position statement on the 2014 advanced framework for a new diagnosis of obesity as a chronic disease. Endocr Pract 2014;20(9):977–89.
15. Padwal RS, Pajewski NM, Allison DB, et al. Using the Edmonton Obesity Staging System to predict mortality in a population-representative cohort of people with overweight and obesity. CMAJ 2011;183(14):E1059–66.
16. Heymsfield SB. Meal replacements and energy balance. Physiol Behav 2010; 100:90–4.

17. Miller GD, Nicklas BJ, Davis C, et al. Intensive weight loss program improves physical function in older obese adults with knee osteoarthritis. Obesity (Silver Spring) 2006;14:1219–30.
18. Rock CL, Flatt SW, Sherwood NE, et al. Effect of a free prepared meal and incentivized weight loss program on weight loss and weight loss maintenance in obese and overweight women: a randomized controlled trial. JAMA 2010;304:1803–10.
19. Stubbs RJ, Harbron CG, Murgatroyd PR, et al. Covert manipulation of dietary fat and energy density: effect on substrate flux and food intake in men eating ad libitum. Am J Clin Nutr 1995;62:316–29.
20. Stubbs RJ, Ritz P, Coward WA, et al. Covert manipulation of the ratio of dietary fat to carbohydrate and energy density: effect on food intake and energy balance in free-living men eating ad libitum. Am J Clin Nutr 1995;62:330–7.
21. Kral TV, Roe LS, Rolls BJ. Combined effects of energy density and portion size on energy intake in women. Am J Clin Nutr 2004;79:962–8.
22. Bell EA, Castellanos VH, Pelkman CL, et al. Energy density of foods affects energy intake in normal-weight women. Am J Clin Nutr 1998;67:412–20.
23. Bell EA, Rolls BJ. Energy density of foods affects energy intake across multiple levels of fat content in lean and obese women. Am J Clin Nutr 2001;73:1010–8.
24. Rolls BJ, Bell EA, Thorwart ML. Water incorporated into a food but not served with a food decreases energy intake in lean women. Am J Clin Nutr 1999;70:448–55.
25. Rolls BJ, Roe LS, Meengs JS. Salad and satiety: energy density and portion size of a first-course salad affect energy intake at lunch. J Am Diet Assoc 2004;104:1570–6.
26. Ello-Martin JA, Roe LS, Ledikwe JH, et al. Dietary energy density in the treatment of obesity: a year-long trial comparing 2 weight-loss diets. Am J Clin Nutr 2007;85:1465–77.
27. Flatt JP. Importance of nutrient balance in body weight regulation. Diabetes Metab Rev 1988;4:571–81.
28. Samaha FF, Iqbal N, Seshadri P, et al. A low-carbohydrate as compared with a low-fat diet in severe obesity. N Engl J Med 2003;348:2074–81.
29. Stern L, Iqbal N, Seshadri P, et al. The effects of low-carbohydrate versus conventional weight loss diets in severely obese adults: one-year follow-up of a randomized trial. Ann Intern Med 2004;140:778–85.
30. Foster GD, Wyatt HR, Hill JO, et al. A randomized trial of a low-carbohydrate diet for obesity. N Engl J Med 2003;348:2082–90.
31. Astrup A, Ryan L, Grunwald GK, et al. The role of dietary fat in body fatness: evidence from a preliminary meta-analysis of ad libitum low-fat dietary intervention studies. Br J Nutr 2000;83(Suppl 1):S25–32.
32. Thomas CD, Peters JC, Reed GW, et al. Nutrient balance and energy expenditure during ad libitum feeding of high-fat and high-carbohydrate diets in humans. Am J Clin Nutr 1992;55:934–42.
33. Halton TL, Hu FB. The effects of high protein diets on thermogenesis, satiety and weight loss: a critical review. J Am Coll Nutr 2004;23:373–85.
34. Paddon-Jones D, Westman E, Mattes RD, et al. Protein, weight management, and satiety. Am J Clin Nutr 2008;87:1558S–61S.
35. Abete I, Astrup A, Martinez JA, et al. Obesity and the metabolic syndrome: role of different dietary macronutrient distribution patterns and specific nutritional components on weight loss and maintenance. Nutr Rev 2010;68:214–31.
36. Pesta DH, Samuel VT. A high-protein diet for reducing body fat: mechanisms and possible caveats. Nutr Metab 2014;11:53.

37. Due A, Toubro S, Skov AR, et al. Effect of normal-fat diets, either medium or high in protein, on body weight in overweight subjects: a randomised 1-year trial. Int J Obes Relat Metab Disord 2004;28:1283–90.

38. Larsen TM, Dalskov S-M, van Baak M, et al. Diets with high or low protein content and glycemic index for weight-loss maintenance. N Engl J Med 2010;363: 2102–13.

39. Ankarfeldt MZ, Angquist L, Stocks T, et al. Body characteristics, [corrected] dietary protein and body weight regulation. Reconciling conflicting results from intervention and observational studies? PLoS One 2014;9:e101134.

40. Wycherley TP, Moran LJ, Clifton PM, et al. Effects of energy-restricted high-protein, low-fat compared with standard-protein, low-fat diets: a meta-analysis of randomized controlled trials. Am J Clin Nutr 2012;96:1281–98.

41. Sacks FM, Bray GA, Carey VJ, et al. Comparison of weight-loss diets with different compositions of fat, protein, and carbohydrates. N Engl J Med 2009; 360:859–73.

42. Pittas AG, Das SK, Hajduk CL, et al. A low-glycemic load diet facilitates greater weight loss in overweight adults with high insulin secretion but not in overweight adults with low insulin secretion in the CALERIE Trial. Diabetes Care 2005;28: 2939–41.

43. Cornier M-A, Donahoo WT, Pereira R, et al. Insulin sensitivity determines the effectiveness of dietary macronutrient composition on weight loss in obese women. Obes Res 2005;13:703–9.

44. Ebbeling CB, Leidig MM, Feldman HA, et al. Effects of a low-glycemic load vs low-fat diet in obese young adults: a randomized trial. JAMA 2007;297:2092–102.

45. Jenkins DJ, Wolever TM, Taylor RH, et al. Glycemic index of foods: a physiological basis for carbohydrate exchange. Am J Clin Nutr 1981;34(3):362–6.

46. Das SK, Gilhooly CH, Golden JK, et al. Long-term effects of 2 energy-restricted diets differing in glycemic load on dietary adherence, body composition, and metabolism in CALERIE: a 1-y randomized controlled trial. Am J Clin Nutr 2007;85(4):1023–30.

47. Zeevi D, Korem T, Zmora N, et al. Personalized nutrition by prediction of glycemic responses. Cell 2015;163(5):1079–94.

48. Gardner CD, Kiazand A, Alhassan S, et al. Comparison of the Atkins, Zone, Ornish, and LEARN diets for change in weight and related risk factors among overweight premenopausal women: the A TO Z Weight Loss Study: a randomized trial. JAMA 2007;297:969–77.

49. Yancy WS Jr, Foy M, Chalecki AM, et al. A low-carbohydrate, ketogenic diet to treat type 2 diabetes. Nutr Metab 2005;2:34.

50. Shai I, Schwarzfuchs D, Henkin Y, et al. Weight loss with a low-carbohydrate, Mediterranean, or low-fat diet. N Engl J Med 2008;359:229–41.

51. Johnston BC, Kanters S, Bandayrel K, et al. Comparison of weight loss among named diet programs in overweight and obese adults. JAMA 2014;312:923.

52. Dansinger ML, Gleason JA, Griffith JL, et al. Comparison of the Atkins, Ornish, Weight Watchers, and Zone diets for weight loss and heart disease risk reduction: a randomized trial. JAMA 2005;293:43–53.

53. Foster GD, Wyatt HR, Hill JO, et al. Weight and metabolic outcomes after 2 years on a low-carbohydrate versus low-fat diet: a randomized trial. Ann Intern Med 2010;153:147–57.

54. Phelan S, Kanaya AM, Subak LL, et al. Weight loss prevents urinary incontinence in women with type 2 diabetes: results from the Look AHEAD trial. J Urol 2012; 187(3):939–44.

55. Foster GD, Borradaile KE, Sanders MH, et al. A randomized study on the effect of weight loss on obstructive sleep apnea among obese patients with type 2 diabetes: the Sleep AHEAD study. Arch Intern Med 2009;169(17):1619–26.

56. Promrat K, Kleiner DE, Niemeier HM, et al. Randomized controlled trial testing the effects of weight loss on nonalcoholic steatohepatitis. Hepatology 2010;51(1): 121–9.

57. Hall KD, Sacks G, Chandramohan D, et al. Quantification of the effect of energy imbalance on bodyweight. Lancet 2011;378(9793):826–37.

58. Foster GD, Wadden TA, Vogt RA, et al. What is a reasonable weight loss? Patients' expectations and evaluations of obesity treatment outcomes. J Consult Clin Psychol 1997;65(1):79–85.

59. Bartfield JK, Stevens VJ, Jerome GJ, et al. Behavioral transitions and weight change patterns within the PREMIER trial. Obesity 2011;19(8):1609–15.

60. Burke LE, Wang J, Sevick MA. Self-monitoring in weight loss: a systematic review of the literature. J Am Diet Assoc 2011;111(1):92–102.

61. Weinsier RL, Hunter GR, Zuckerman PA, et al. Energy expenditure and free-living physical activity in black and white women: comparison before and after weight loss. Am J Clin Nutr 2000;71(5):1138–46.

62. Grande F, Anderson JT, Keys A. Changes of basal metabolic rate in man in semi-starvation and refeeding. J Appl Physiol 1958;12(2):230–8.

63. James WP, Shetty PS. Metabolic adaptation and energy requirements in developing countries. Hum Nutr Clin Nutr 1982;36(5):331–6.

64. Hill JO, Wyatt HR, Peters JC. Energy balance and obesity. Circulation 2012; 126(1):126–32.

65. Weinsier RL, Wilson LJ, Lee J. Medically safe rate of weight loss for the treatment of obesity: a guideline based on risk of gallstone formation. Am J Med 1995; 98(2):115–7.

66. Everhart JE. Contributions of obesity and weight loss to gallstone disease. Ann Intern Med 1993;119(10):1029–35.

67. Johansson K, Sundstrom J, Marcus C, et al. Risk of symptomatic gallstones and cholecystectomy after a very-low-calorie diet or low-calorie diet in a commercial weight loss program: 1-year matched cohort study. Int J Obes 2014;38(2): 279–84.

68. Festi D, Colecchia A, Larocca A, et al. Review: low caloric intake and gall-bladder motor function. Aliment Pharmacol Ther 2000;14(Suppl 2):51–3.

69. Malkud S. Telogen effluvium: a review. J Clin Diagn Res 2015;9(9):WE01–3.

70. Thomas DM, Martin CK, Redman LM, et al. Effect of dietary adherence on the body weight plateau: a mathematical model incorporating intermittent compliance with energy intake prescription. Am J Clin Nutr 2014;100:787–95.

71. Jakicic JM, Marcus BH, Lang W, et al. Effect of exercise on 24-month weight loss maintenance in overweight women. Arch Intern Med 2008;168:1550–9 [discussion: 1559–60].

72. Ross R, Hudson R, Stotz PJ, et al. Effects of exercise amount and intensity on abdominal obesity and glucose tolerance in obese adults: a randomized trial. Ann Intern Med 2015;162:325–34.

73. Feinman RD, Fine EJ. Thermodynamics and metabolic advantage of weight loss diets. Metab Syndr Relat Disord 2003;1:209–19.

74. Ebbeling CB, Swain JF, Feldman HA, et al. Effects of dietary composition on energy expenditure during weight-loss maintenance. JAMA 2012;307:2627–34.

75. Aller EE, Larsen TM, Claus H, et al. Weight loss maintenance in overweight subjects on ad libitum diets with high or low protein content and glycemic index: the DIOGENES trial 12-month results. Int J Obes 2014;38(12):1511–7.
76. Blanck HM, Serdula MK, Gillespie C, et al. Use of nonprescription dietary supplements for weight loss is common among Americans. J Am Diet Assoc 2007; 107(3):441–7.
77. Blanck HM, Khan LK, Serdula MK. Use of nonprescription weight loss products: results from a multistate survey. JAMA 2001;286(8):930–5.
78. Pillitteri JL, Shiffman S, Rohay JM, et al. Use of dietary supplements for weight loss in the United States: results of a national survey. Obesity (Silver Spring) 2008;16(4):790–6.
79. Pittler MH, Ernst E. Dietary supplements for body-weight reduction: a systematic review. Am J Clin Nutr 2004;79(4):529–36.
80. Onakpoya IJ, Wider B, Pittler MH, et al. Food supplements for body weight reduction: a systematic review of systematic reviews. Obesity (Silver Spring) 2011; 19(2):239–44.
81. Torgerson JS, Hauptman J, Boldrin MN, et al. XENical in the prevention of diabetes in obese subjects (XENDOS) study: a randomized study of orlistat as an adjunct to lifestyle changes for the prevention of type 2 diabetes in obese patients. Diabetes Care 2004;27(1):155–61.
82. Poddar K, Kolge S, Bezman L, et al. Nutraceutical supplements for weight loss: a systematic review. Nutr Clin Pract 2011;26(5):539–52.

Index

Note: Page numbers of article titles are in **boldface** type.

Med Clin N Am 100 (2016) 1357–1370
http://dx.doi.org/10.1016/S0025-7125(16)37349-7
0025-7125/16/$ – see front matter

medical.theclinics.com

UNITED STATES POSTAL SERVICE® Statement of Ownership, Management, and Circulation
(All Periodicals Publications Except Requester Publications)

1. Publication Title	2. Publication Number	3. Filing Date
MEDICAL CLINICS IN NORTH AMERICA	337 – 340	9/18/2016

4. Issue Frequency	5. Number of Issues Published Annually	6. Annual Subscription Price
JAN, MAR, MAY, JUL, SEP, NOV	6	$255

7. Complete Mailing Address of Known Office of Publication (Not printer) (Street, city, county, state, and ZIP+4®)

ELSEVIER INC.
360 PARK AVENUE SOUTH
NEW YORK, NY 10010-1710

Contact Person
STEPHEN R. BUSHING

Telephone (Include area code)
215-239-3688

8. Complete Mailing Address of Headquarters or General Business Office of Publisher (Not printer)

ELSEVIER INC.
360 PARK AVENUE SOUTH
NEW YORK, NY 10010-1710

9. Full Names and Complete Mailing Addresses of Publisher, Editor, and Managing Editor (Do not leave blank)

Publisher (Name and complete mailing address)

ADRIANNE BRIGIDO, ELSEVIER INC.
1600 JOHN F KENNEDY BLVD. SUITE 1800
PHILADELPHIA, PA 19103-2899

Editor (Name and complete mailing address)

JESSICA MCCOOL, ELSEVIER INC.
1600 JOHN F KENNEDY BLVD. SUITE 1800
PHILADELPHIA, PA 19103-2899

Managing Editor (Name and complete mailing address)

PATRICK MANLEY, ELSEVIER INC.
1600 JOHN F KENNEDY BLVD. SUITE 1800
PHILADELPHIA, PA 19103-2899

10. Owner (Do not leave blank. If the publication is owned by a corporation, give the name and address of the corporation immediately followed by the names and addresses of all stockholders owning or holding 1 percent or more of the total amount of stock. If not owned by a corporation, give the names and addresses of the individual owners. If owned by a partnership or other unincorporated firm, give its name and address as well as those of each individual owner. If the publication is published by a nonprofit organization, give its name and address.)

Full Name	Complete Mailing Address
WHOLLY OWNED SUBSIDIARY OF REED/ELSEVIER, US HOLDINGS	1600 JOHN F KENNEDY BLVD. SUITE 1800 PHILADELPHIA, PA 19103-2899

11. Known Bondholders, Mortgagees, and Other Security Holders Owning or Holding 1 Percent or More of Total Amount of Bonds, Mortgages, or Other Securities. If none, check box. ▶ ☐ None

Full Name	Complete Mailing Address
N/A	

12. Tax Status (For completion by nonprofit organizations authorized to mail at nonprofit rates) (Check one)
The purpose, function, and nonprofit status of this organization and the exempt status for federal income tax purposes:
☐ Has Not Changed During Preceding 12 Months
☐ Has Changed During Preceding 12 Months (Publisher must submit explanation of change with this statement)

13. Publication Title	14. Issue Date for Circulation Data Below
MEDICAL CLINICS IN NORTH AMERICA	JULY 2016

15. Extent and Nature of Circulation			Average No. Copies Each Issue During Preceding 12 Months	No. Copies of Single Issue Published Nearest to Filing Date
a. Total Number of Copies (Net press run)			999	1017
b. Paid Circulation (By Mail and Outside the Mail)	(1)	Mailed Outside-County Paid Subscriptions Stated on PS Form 3541 (include paid distribution above nominal rate, advertiser's proof copies, and exchange copies)	401	473
	(2)	Mailed In-County Paid Subscriptions Stated on PS Form 3541 (include paid distribution above nominal rate, advertiser's proof copies, and exchange copies)	0	0
	(3)	Paid Distribution Outside the Mails Including Sales Through Dealers and Carriers, Street Vendors, Counter Sales, and Other Paid Distribution Outside USPS®	194	247
	(4)	Paid Distribution by Other Classes of Mail Through the USPS (e.g. First-Class Mail®)	0	0
c. Total Paid Distribution [Sum of 15b (1), (2), (3), and (4)]		▶	595	720
d. Free or Nominal Rate Distribution (By Mail and Outside the Mail)	(1)	Free or Nominal Rate Outside-County Copies included on PS Form 3541	82	97
	(2)	Free or Nominal Rate In-County Copies Included on PS Form 3541	0	0
	(3)	Free or Nominal Rate Copies Mailed at Other Classes Through the USPS (e.g. First-Class Mail)	0	0
	(4)	Free or Nominal Rate Distribution Outside the Mail (Carriers or other means)	0	0
e. Total Free or Nominal Rate Distribution (Sum of 15d (1), (2), (3) and (4))		▶	82	97
f. Total Distribution (Sum of 15c and 15e)		▶	677	817
g. Copies not Distributed (See Instructions to Publishers #4 (page #3))		▶	322	200
h. Total (Sum of 15f and g)		▶	999	1017
i. Percent Paid (15c divided by 15f times 100)			88%	88%

* If you are claiming electronic copies, go to line 16 on page 3. If you are not claiming electronic copies, skip to line 17 on page 3.

16. Electronic Copy Circulation	Average No. Copies Each Issue During Preceding 12 Months	No. Copies of Single Issue Published Nearest to Filing Date
a. Paid Electronic Copies ▶	0	0
b. Total Paid Print Copies (Line 15c) + Paid Electronic Copies (Line 16a) ▶	595	720
c. Total Print Distribution (Line 15f) + Paid Electronic Copies (Line 16a) ▶	677	817
d. Percent Paid (Both Print & Electronic Copies) (16b divided by 16c × 100) ▶	88%	88%

☒ I certify that 50% of all my distributed copies (electronic and print) are paid above a nominal price.

17. Publication of Statement of Ownership
☒ If the publication is a general publication, publication of this statement is required. Will be printed ☐ Publication not required.
in the NOVEMBER 2016 issue of this publication.

18. Signature and Title of Editor, Publisher, Business Manager, or Owner

STEPHEN R. BUSHING - INVENTORY DISTRIBUTION CONTROL MANAGER
Date 9/18/2016

I certify that all information furnished on this form is true and complete. I understand that anyone who furnishes false or misleading information on this form or who omits material or information requested on the form may be subject to criminal sanctions (including fines and imprisonment) and/or civil sanctions (including civil penalties).

PS Form 3526, July 2014 (Page 1 of 4 (see instructions page 4)) PSN: 7530-01-000-9931 PRIVACY NOTICE: See our privacy policy on www.usps.com.

PS Form 3526, July 2014 (Page 3 of 4)   PRIVACY NOTICE: See our privacy policy on www.usps.com.

Moving?

Make sure your subscription moves with you!

To notify us of your new address, find your **Clinics Account Number** (located on your mailing label above your name), and contact customer service at:

Email: journalscustomerservice-usa@elsevier.com

800-654-2452 (subscribers in the U.S. & Canada)
314-447-8871 (subscribers outside of the U.S. & Canada)

Fax number: 314-447-8029

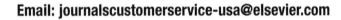

Elsevier Health Sciences Division
Subscription Customer Service
3251 Riverport Lane
Maryland Heights, MO 63043

*To ensure uninterrupted delivery of your subscription, please notify us at least 4 weeks in advance of move.

Printed and bound by CPI Group (UK) Ltd, Croydon, CR0 4YY

03/10/2024

01040390-0003